Landmark Papers
in Nephrology

Landmark Papers in ... series

Landmark Papers in Nephrology

Edited by

John Feehally

Christopher McIntyre

J. Stewart Cameron

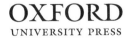

OXFORD
UNIVERSITY PRESS

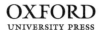

Great Clarendon Street, Oxford, OX2 6DP,
United Kingdom

Oxford University Press is a department of the University of Oxford.
It furthers the University's objective of excellence in research, scholarship,
and education by publishing worldwide. Oxford is a registered trade mark of
Oxford University Press in the UK and in certain other countries

First Edition published in 2013

Impression: 1

British Library Cataloging in Publication Data
Data available

ISBN 978–0–19–969925–4

Printed and bound by
CPI Group (UK) Ltd, Croydon, CR0 4YY

Preface

It has been our pleasure to edit this contribution to OUP's 'Landmarks' series. *Landmark Papers in Nephrology* has been designed to remind us all of the seminal observations and major steps forward that have led to the practice of nephrology as we know it today.

Inevitably, we cannot expect that the final product will meet with every reader's approval. How could it be that choosing a mere 200 papers from the whole oeuvre will satisfy every discerning student of the history of nephrology?

We have chosen first of all to divide nephrology into 20 chapters, itself an arbitrary selection. As perhaps would be expected, we start with chapters on the anatomy and physiology of the glomerulus and tubule, and the investigation of renal disease, and then follow with the achievements of recent years in unravelling the genetic basis for a range of inherited and congenital disorders of the kidney and urinary tract.

We have then committed three chapters to the remarkable story of the emergence of our current understanding of glomerular disease. The 1827 observations of Richard Bright remain the single most important clinico-pathological insight ever made into kidney disease, and one chapter covers the century either side of Bright's report during which were made some of the most fundamental pathological and clinical insights in the whole of renal disease (not just glomerular disease). We give over two further chapters to the explosion of new clinico-pathological observations that followed the introduction of renal biopsy in the 1950s, and which have led us to our modern understanding of the diagnosis, classification, and treatment of glomerular disease.

The next two chapters reflect the double jeopardy of the modern world: infection, or communicable disease, which remains a major cause and aggravating factor of renal disease, and the most potent of the nephropathic non-communicable diseases, diabetes.

There follow two chapters covering the broad clinical syndromes described in contemporary semantics as acute kidney injury and chronic kidney disease, and then four chapters covering the two great technological advances of the second half of the last century, dialysis and transplantation, which were the stimulus for the development of nephrology as the clinical speciality we know today. Further chapters reflect the consequences for the growing population whose lives are prolonged despite advanced or end-stage renal disease—which includes a unique pattern of high-risk cardiovascular disease, multifaceted bone and mineral disorders, and chronic anaemia. We end with two chapters on newer aspects of renal science, which are changing the framework in which nephrology is placed: a chapter that shows how epidemiology has provided important insights from databases mostly focused on those receiving renal replacement therapy, and finally, and perhaps surprisingly to some, we end with a chapter on the relatively new science of measuring and improving the quality of life for people with advanced kidney disease—a conceptual framework unconsidered by most physicians 50 years ago but now seen as a key element in offering the best possible care for people with chronic kidney disease.

The selection of the 20 chapter titles proved to be just the beginning of a lively debate with our contributors, each given the task of selecting only ten landmark papers for their chapter. An impossible task? Yes, of course, and we anticipate that every reader will have their own favourites, and will be mystified that in some cases we could have failed to include them. Therein lies the pleasure of this volume. There are no right answers; all we can say is that these 200 papers are among the great landmarks of our specialty, reflecting varying coincidences of brilliance, persistence, and good fortune; as always in medical science it is useful to be in the right place at the right time. Among them are a great variety of styles: ranging from observational experimental and clinical studies published more than a century ago through to recent randomized controlled clinical trials. However, such trials are in a minority, reflecting the disappointing lack of this sort of evidence to guide clinical care in nephrology, and emphasizing how, until very recently, seminal observations at the bench or in the clinic were needed to form a basis for our understanding.

We make no apology that two papers each appear twice—as landmarks in different chapters. The first, perhaps unsurprisingly, is Richard Bright's magisterial *Reports of Medical Cases* from 1827, chosen in Chapter 3 to exemplify the critical role played by morbid anatomy in the early investigation of renal disease, and again in Chapter 5 as the seminal work linking once and for all albuminuria, dropsy, and kidney disease. Perhaps less known to many readers will be Pierre Rayer's *Traité des Maladies des Reins* of 1839–1841, selected in Chapter 3 as the landmark paper introducing urine microscopy as an investigative tool, and again in Chapter 5 because it was in effect the first textbook of nephrology.

With a few exceptions, the papers in each chapter are presented chronologically, giving a sense of how progress unfolded, although not always in the systematic way we might imagine. For most papers, the abstract from the original publication is reproduced intact (although slightly truncated where required); for publications with no such abstract, a summary has been prepared. We then asked our contributors to provide commentaries that were succinct yet informative enough about the paper and its position in the history of nephrology to whet the reader's appetite. They have succeeded.

We hope you have the same sense of excitement as you read these chapters as we have had during their preparation. To see the breadth, range, and depth of the intellectual journey that precedes us is very properly to be reminded, as Sir Isaac Newton wrote to his fellow genius, Robert Hooke, in 1675: 'If I have seen further it is by standing on the shoulders of giants.'

John Feehally
Chris McIntyre
J. Stewart Cameron

Contents

Contributors

J. Stewart Cameron
Emeritus Professor of Renal Medicine, Guy's
Campus, King's College London, UK

Aisling Courteney
Regional Nephrology Unit, Belfast City
Hospital, Lisburn Road, Belfast, UK

John Cunningham
Centre for Nephrology, UCL Medical School,
Royal Free Campus, London, UK

Thomas A. Depner
Division of Nephrology, University of
California Davis, Sacramento, CA, USA

John Feehally
Consultant Nephrologist, University
Hospitals of Leicester, UK
Professor of Renal Medicine, University of
Leicester, UK

Fredric O. Finkelstein
Hospital of St Raphael, New Haven, CT, USA

Susan H. Finkelstein
Department of Psychiatry, Yale University,
New Haven, CT, USA

Robert N. Foley
United States Renal System, Minneapolis,
MN, USA

Richard J. Glassock
Department of Medicine, The David Geffen
School of Medicine at UCLA, Los Angeles,
CA, USA

Trevor Gerntholtz
Dumisani Mzamane African Institute
for Kidney Disease, Chris Hani
Baragwanath Hospital, Soweto,
Gauteng, South Africa

Kate A. Hillman
University of Manchester, Oxford Road,
Manchester, UK; and Central Manchester
University Hospitals, Manchester, UK

Dharmvir Jaswal
Division of Nephrology, University of British
Columbia Vancouver, British Columbia,
Canada

Sarah Jenkins
Sheffield Kidney Institute, Sheffield Teaching
Hospitals NHS Foundation Trust,
Sheffield, UK

Adeera Levin
Division of Nephrology, University of British
Columbia Vancouver, British Columbia,
Canada

Nathan W. Levin
Renal Research Institute, New York, NY, USA

Christopher W. McIntyre
Department of Renal Medicine, Royal Derby
Hospital, Uttoxeter Road, Derby, UK

Guy H. Neild
University College London Centre for
Nephrology, Royal Free Campus, London, UK

Eberhard Ritz
Sektion Nephrologie, Klinikum der Universitat
Heidelberg, Im Neuenheimer Feld 162,
Heidelberg, Germany

Andrew Salmon
Southmead Hospital, Southmead Road,
Westbury-on-Trym, Bristol, UK

Maarten Taal
Royal Derby Hospital, Uttoxeter Road,
Derby, UK

Jan H. M. Tordoir
Department of Surgery, Maastricht University Medical Center, P Debijelaan 25, Maastricht, the Netherlands

Robert J. Unwin
UCL Centre for Nephrology, University College London, Royal Free Campus, London, UK

Stephen B. Walsh
UCL Centre for Nephrology, University College London, Royal Free Campus, London, UK

Martin Wilkie
Sheffield Kidney Institute, Sheffield Teaching Hospitals NHS Foundation Trust, Sheffield, UK

Christopher G. Winearls
Oxford Kidney Unit, The Churchill, Oxford Radcliffe Hospitals NHS Trust, Old Road, Headington, Oxford, UK

Adrian S. Woolf
University of Manchester, Oxford Road, Manchester, UK; and Central Manchester University Hospitals, UK

Abbreviations

ABOi	ABO-incompatible
ACE	angiotensin-converting enzyme
ACEI	angiotensin-converting enzyme inhibitors
ACR	urine albumin-to-creatinine ratio
ACTH	adrenocorticotropic hormone
ADEMEX	Adequacy of Peritoneal Dialysis in Mexico
ADPKD	autosomal dominant polycystic kidney disease
AIDS	acquired immunodeficiency syndrome
AKI	acute kidney injury
AKIN	Acute Kidney Injury Network
APD	ambulatory peritoneal dialysis
AQP	aquaporin
ARB	angiotensin receptor blockers
ARPKD	autosomal recessive polycystic kidney disease
ATN	Acute Renal Failure Trial Network
ATN	acute tubular necrosis
AVP	arginine vasopressin
B2M	2-microglobulin
BDI	Beck Depression Inventory
BMI	body mass index
BP	blood pressure
BUN	blood urea nitrogen concentration
CAC	coronary artery calcification
CAD	coronary artery disease
CANUSA	Canada and USA study
CAPD	continuous ambulatory peritoneal dialysis
CaSR	calcium-sensing receptor
CBT	cognitive behavioural therapy
CES-D	Center for Epidemiologic Studies Depression
CHOICE	Choices for Healthy Outcomes in Caring for End-stage Renal Disease
CHOIR	Correction of Hemoglobin in Outcomes and Renal Insufficiency
CI	confidence interval
CIN	contrast-induced nephropathy
CKD	chronic kidney disease
CMV	cytomegalovirus
CREATE	Cardiovascular risk Reduction by Early Anemia Treatment with Epoetin Beta
CRI	catheter-related infection
CRRT	continuous renal replacement therapy
CyA	cyclosporin A
CYC	cyclophosphamide
DMSA	dimercaptosuccinic acid
DOPPS	Dialysis Outcomes and Practice Patterns Study
EARLI	Early Renal Service Involvement
EBCT	electron-beam computerized tomography
eGFR	estimated glomerular filtration rate
EPS	encapsulating peritoneal sclerosis
ESA	erythropoiesis-stimulating agent
ESRD	end-stage renal disease
FGF23	fibroblast growth factor 23
FSGS	focal segmental glomerulosclerosis
GAPDH	glyceraldehyde 3-phosphate dehydrogenase
GBM	glomerular basement membrane
GFR	glomerular filtration rate
HAART	highly active antiretroviral therapy
HBeAg	hepatitis B virus e antigen
HBsAg	hepatitis B virus surface antigen
HBV	hepatitis B virus
HCV	hepatitis C virus
HIV	human immunodeficiency virus
HIVAN	human immunodeficiency virus-associated nephropathy
HIVICK	human immunodeficiency virus immune complex kidney
HLA	human leukocyte antigen
HLAi	HLA-incompatible
HRQOL	health-related quality of life
ICD	International Classification of Diseases
ICU	intensive care unit

IDNT	Irbesartan Diabetic Nephropathy Trial		PD	peritoneal dialysis
IFN-α	alpha interferon		PET	peritoneal equilibration test
IVU	intravenous urography		PET	positron emission tomography
JGA	juxtaglomerular apparatus		PKD	polycystic kidney disease
KDOQI	Kidney Disease Outcomes Quality Initiative		PTFE	polytetrafluoroethylene
			PTH	parathyroid hormone
KDQOL-SF	Kidney Disease Quality of Life Short Form		PRCA	pure red-cell aplasia
			RAS	renin–angiotensin
LBW	low birth weight		RBF	renal blood flow
LDL	low-density lipoprotein		RCT	randomized controlled trial
LVM	left ventricular mass		REIN	Ramipril in Non-diabetic Renal Failure
MAG3	mercapto-acetyl-triglycine		rHuEPO	recombinant human erythropoietin
MAP	mean arterial pressure		RIFLE	Risk, Injury, Failure, Loss, and End-stage kidney disease
MBF	myocardial blood flow			
MCS	mental component scores		SCID	Structured Clinical Interview for Depression
MDRD	Modification of Diet in Renal Disease			
MMF	mycophenolate mofetil		SGLT	sodium-linked glucose transporters
MPGN	membranoproliferative glomerulonephritis		SNGFR	single-nephron glomerular filtration rate
			SPE B	streptococcal exotoxin B
NAC	N-Acetylcysteine		TREAT	Trial to Reduce Cardiovascular Events with Aranesp Therapy
NCDS	National Cooperative Dialysis Study			
NDI	nephrogenic diabetes insipidus		VHL	von Hippel–Lindau
pcr	protein catabolic rate		VUR	vesico-ureteric reflux
PCS	physical component score		WG	Wegener's granulomatosis

Chapter 1

Glomerular structure and function

Andrew Salmon

Introduction

In 1842, two reports dramatically redefined existing beliefs about glomerular structure and function, and provided the basic concepts for all modern investigations in the field. Carl Ludwig not only outlined the physical processes that result in the formation and subsequent modification of urine, but in so doing revolutionized scientific thinking and methodology with his mechanistic paradigm and hypothetico-deductive approaches. In the same year, William Bowman described the vascular system of the kidney, and demonstrated the intimate and functional relationship between the glomerulus and the proximal convoluted tubule.

Over the following 170 years, the structure of the glomerular capillary wall has been revealed in ever greater detail. The application of electron microscopy to glomerular investigations in the 1950s revealed the classic trilaminar structure of the glomerular capillary wall, and yet new structural insights continue to appear up to the present day, as a result of novel staining and imaging approaches in electron microscopy. The advent of the molecular era has further transformed our understanding of glomerular structure by allowing researchers to describe the composition of these anatomical structures at the molecular level.

Our understanding of glomerular function has also been dramatically advanced by insights obtained from micropuncture techniques, from studies of the clearance of macromolecular tracers, from manipulations of the molecular components of the glomerular capillary wall, and most recently from advances in fluorescence microscopy that allow the function of the glomerulus to be examined in real time *in vivo*, independent of tubular processes.

Throughout this time, a number of researchers have aimed to reconcile studies of glomerular structure and function, either through combining techniques (e.g. the use of electron-dense tracers to study functional pathways across the glomerular capillary wall) or by biophysical modelling approaches to ascribe resistances to the various layers of the glomerular capillary wall.

Nevertheless, despite these technical advances and many years of research, a comprehensive understanding of the process of glomerular filtration remains elusive, and even fundamental principles such as efficient retention of albumin by the glomerular capillary wall continue to be challenged by some. In the structural field, the notion that pores across the podocyte slit diaphragm have a regular size and arrangement has also been challenged, which may redefine the contribution that this structure makes to glomerular filtration. Moreover, in recent years, the glomerular capillary wall has been transformed in our thinking from a passive sieve with a fixed structure to a dynamic entity in which the cellular components of the wall move and paracrine interactions between the layers of the barrier allow the permeability of the barrier to be modified to meet physiological and pathophysiological demands.

1.1 De viribus physicis secretionem urinae adjuvantibus [On the physical forces that promote the secretion of urine]

Author

CFW Ludwig

Reference

Habilitation thesis, 1842, Marburg, Germany.

Summary

I have chosen to explain the physical laws governing renal secretion. A comparison of urine with the serum of the blood reveals great differences in the quality and quantity of solid and dissolved substances. All the substances present in urine are transferred into it from blood, and there is no substance found only in the kidneys and urine to which an attractive force can be attributed.

It is therefore necessary to examine an alternative force by which fluids are expressed from vessels, namely pressure. Blood flow in glomeruli is greatly impeded because the sum of the cross-sections of the individual vessels in the glomeruli is larger than that of the vas efferens. Therefore, the membranes of the vessels in the glomeruli are subjected to high pressure, resulting in a copious secretion from the delicate glomeruli. When kidneys were injected with wax, I detected discharge of the wax from the glomeruli.

The second physical process occurring in the kidney is an endosmotic action between the solution of salts secreted and the partly altered blood retained in the vessels. The first and best proof of endosmosis is the fact that, given the same composition of the blood, the concentration of urine depends on the urine flow rate.

It is clear that the process of expulsion of the urine is as follows: when the blood vascular system is filled with fluid, pressure is exerted against the walls of the glomeruli, and the water in the blood leaves the glomeruli and is taken up by the uriniferous ducts. It is here that endosmosis can occur as described above. The quantity of urine secretion is accelerated when the blood vascular system is filled with fluid, in which case the pressure against the walls of the glomeruli is increased.

Importance

Ludwig's description of urine formation is a landmark report in many respects (Davis *et al.*, 1994). At the time of Ludwig's habilitation thesis, much scientific reasoning was still based on the 'vitalist' view: that physicochemical processes alone could not explain life processes (such as urine formation) and that some non-physical 'vital force' was required. Ludwig assessed an alternative hypothesis that urine formation could be explained purely in terms of the laws of physics and chemistry. In so doing, Ludwig applied two new scientific approaches to human biology: the 'hypothetico-deductive' method, in which he used experimentation to test the validity of this hypothesis, and a 'mechanistic' paradigm' to evaluate whether human biological processes could be considered in purely mechanistic terms. These approaches to scientific enquiry form the basis for all modern scientific investigation.

Ludwig conducted a broad set of experiments to evaluate many of the individual components of urine formation and excretion. He examined the rate of fluid transfer across porous membranes in response to different hydrostatic pressures, and in combination with anatomical studies and hydraulic models to reconstruct the hydrostatic pressure profile across the renal circulation concluded that urine is formed by the movement of the fluid component of blood across pores in the membranes of the glomerular capillary wall under the influence of hydrostatic pressure. He also compared the chemical composition of serum and urine, and concluded not only that urine was derived from blood but also that the elevated concentration of various substances in urine relative to plasma (e.g. urea) were the result of reabsorption (or 'endosmosis') of filtered fluid from urinary tubules. Ludwig had thereby defined two of the major physiological processes involved in urine formation (it was not until 1906 that Metzner is reported to have recognized the additional contribution of tubular secretion in the formation of urine; Metzner, 1906). In broader terms, Ludwig had also defined the fundamental processes governing the exchange of fluids across capillary walls. This preceded Starling's classic descriptions of fluid exchange (Starling, 1896), based on essentially the same principles, by more than 50 years.

By deducing a number of the processes involved in urine formation, Ludwig's habilitation thesis is undoubtedly a landmark in nephrology. Moreover, the thesis can reasonably be considered a landmark in vascular physiology, and perhaps most importantly in scientific method. Ludwig's conclusion that 'Numerous problems are thus explained by purely physical laws' has far-reaching implications, and remains entirely justified.

References

Davis JM, Gottschalk CW, Haberle DA, Thurau K (1994). Carl Ludwig's revolutionary concept of renal function. *Kidney Int* **Suppl. 46**, 1–92.

Metzner K (1906). Die Absonderung und Herausbeforderung des Harnes. In: *Handbuch der Physiologie des Menschen*, pp. 207–335. Edited by Nagel W. Braunschweig: Vieweg.

Starling EH (1896). On the absorption of fluids from connective tissue spaces. *J Physiol* **19**, 312–326.

1.2 On the structure and use of the Malpighian bodies of the kidney, with observations on the circulation through that gland

Author

W Bowman

Reference

Philosophical Transactions of the Royal Society London 1842, **132**, 57–80.

Summary

This account has been drawn principally from my observations on the kidneys of mammalia, but it is intended to embrace the chief points in the anatomy of the Malpighian bodies in all the vertebrate tribes. In all these, I have ascertained the Malpighian body to consist of the dilated extremity of the uriniferous tube, with a small mass of blood vessels inserted into it. The tufts of vessels are a distinct system of capillaries inserted into the interior of the tube, surrounded by a capsule, formed by its membrane and closed everywhere except at the orifice of the tube. I injected some kidneys through the artery, and have since made numerous injections of the human kidney, and that of many of the lower animals, and in all, without exception, have met with the same disposition. The injected material had, in many instances, burst through the tuft, and, being extravasated into the capsule, had passed off along the tube.

The blood, leaving the Malpighian tufts, is conveyed by their efferent vessels to the capillary plexus surrounding the uriniferous tubes. Thus, there are two perfectly distinct systems of capillary vessels, and the efferent vessels may collectively be termed the portal system of the kidney.

Reflecting on this remarkable structure of the Malpighian bodies, and on their singular connection with the tubes, I was led to speculate on their use. It occurred to me that, as the tubes and their plexus of capillaries were probably the parts concerned with the secretion of that portion of the urine to which its characteristic properties are due (the urea etc.), the Malpighian bodies might be an apparatus designed to separate from the blood the watery portion.

Importance

As noted by Bowman in this report to the Royal Society in 1842, the relationship between the blood vessels and urinary tubules of the kidney had not until then been clear. A direct communication between the vasculature and urinary tubules ('arteries with open mouths') had been suggested, as had the possibility that there was no communication whatsoever between the two structures.

Bowman injected potassium dichromate and lead acetate solutions into the renal artery of kidneys from numerous species, and studied both the anatomy of the renal microcirculation and the nature of any communication between the microcirculation and the urinary tubules. Bowman noted that glomeruli were supplied by a single afferent arteriole and comprised a tuft of branching capillaries that reunited to form an efferent vessel, which forms a portal system by supplying a second, peritubular, capillary network. He remarked that the afferent and efferent arterioles on either side of the glomerulus act as a 'double valve' and result in a 'retardation of blood in the tuft'. He also noted that, when the injected material escapes from the vasculature (by bursting out), it forms a thin film enveloping the glomerulus and highlighting the inner surface of the capsule, before passing along the urinary tubule. Bowman thereby identified the glomerulus as the site for the separation of water from blood, and speculated that this process provided a diluent for secretion of salts and other products from the tubular epithelium—a view refined by Ludwig in the same year.

Whilst Bowman noted that previous researchers had used light microscopy and dye injections to examine the kidney (e.g. Ruysch), Bowman's findings were aided by improvements in light microscope design during the mid-nineteenth century. Some of Bowman's anatomical discoveries were refined over the following years, notably by Joseph von Gerlach, credited with demonstrating podocytes covering the outer surface of glomerular capillaries (Eknoyan, 1996), as well as parietal epithelial cells lining Bowman's capsule.

The next major step in defining glomerular structure resulted from electron microscopy images of the individual layers of the glomerulus in the mid-1950s. Structural insights from electron microscopy continue to appear with the use of new staining or reconstructive techniques, such as the ultrastructure of the podocyte slit diaphragm (Gagliardini *et al.*, 2010) and coverage of much of the glomerular capillary wall by the subpodocyte space (Neal *et al.*, 2005). Nevertheless, all subsequent studies accepted the basic structural relationship between the glomerulus and tubule identified by Bowman.

References

Eknoyan G (1996). Sir William Bowman: his contributions to physiology and nephrology. *Kidney Int* **50**, 2120–2128.

Gagliardini E, Conti S, Benigni A, Remuzzi G, Remuzzi A (2010). Imaging of the porous ultrastructure of the glomerular epithelial filtration slit. *J Am Soc Nephrol* **21**, 2081–2089.

Neal CR, Crook H, Bell E, Harper SJ, Bates DO (2005). Three-dimensional reconstruction of glomeruli by electron microscopy reveals a distinct restrictive urinary subpodocyte space. *J Am Soc Nephrol* **16**, 1223–1235.

1.3 Glomerular permeability. I. Ferritin transfer across the normal glomerular capillary wall

Authors
MG Farquhar, SL Wissig, GE Palade

Reference
Journal of Experimental Medicine 1961, **113**, 47–66.

Abstract

Ferritin was used as a tracer to investigate pathways and mechanisms for transfer across the layers of the glomerular capillary wall. Kidney tissue, fixed…following an intravenous injection of ferritin, was examined by electron microscopy.

The observations confirmed the existence of three distinct, successive layers in the glomerular capillary wall…In addition, they demonstrated a number of new structural features: namely (a) discrete fibrils in the subendothelial spaces; (b) a characteristic, highly elaborate, cytoplasmic organization in the visceral epithelium; and (c) special structures resembling "desmosomes" in the slits between foot processes.

In animals sacrificed at short time intervals (2 to 15 minutes) following ferritin administration, ferritin molecules were found at high concentration in the lumen and endothelial fenestrae, at low concentration in the basement membrane, and in very small numbers within the epithelium.

Later (1 to 2 hours), the tracer particles were still present in the lumen and within endothelial fenestrae, and, in addition, had accumulated on the luminal side of the basement membrane, especially in the axial regions of the vessels. Larger numbers of ferritin molecules were also found in the epithelium—in invaginations of the cell membrane at the base of the foot processes, and in various membrane-limited bodies…present within the cytoplasm.

These observations suggest that the endothelial fenestrae are patent and that the basement membrane is the main filtration barrier. Since the basement membrane has no demonstrable pores, it is probably not a simple sieve but presumably is a gel-like structure with two fine fibrillar components embedded in an amorphous matrix. Both the epithelium and endothelium may be concerned with building and maintaining this structure. Finally, the intracellular accumulation of particles in the epithelium suggests that the latter acts as a monitor that recovers, at least in part, the small amounts of protein which normally leak through the filter. [Extract.]

Importance

The ultrastructure of the glomerular capillary wall was redefined in the 1950s by electron microscopists (Hall, 1953; Haraldsson *et al.*, 2008) to reveal the now familiar multi-layered barrier comprising fenestrated endothelial cells and regularly arranged podocyte foot processes on either side of the glomerular basement membrane. However, insights into how this complex structure generated urine that was essentially protein-free remained largely theoretical until the novel approach described by Farquhar *et al.* to combine assessments of glomerular structure and function. The authors used ferritin as an electron dense tracer, such that they could visualize both the structure of the capillary wall and the pathways taken by the ferritin molecules across the wall.

Ferritin molecules were retained by the glomerular capillary wall, and specifically accumulated on the upstream side of the glomerular basement membrane. These findings were taken to indicate that the glomerular basement membrane is the principal filtration barrier. However, the authors also noted handling of ferritin by the cellular layers of the barrier, and speculated that 'each of the layers of the capillary wall appears to play a part in creating the functional characteristics observed'. Ever since, it has remained controversial which layer within the capillary wall dominates permselectivity, with the presumed 'dominant layer' changing as novel insights have emerged in each of the ensuing decades. It is noteworthy, however, that current views (e.g. Haraldsson *et al.*, 2008) tend to agree with the original interpretations of Farquhar and colleagues that the layers act together, and that filtration across the capillary wall 'could be affected by a change in the arrangement of any one of the components...singly or in combination'.

The authors also noted that the glomerular basement membrane acts as a filter, despite the fact that no clears 'tracks' were evident. Rather than being pierced by discrete and ultrastructurally visible pores in accordance with the initial descriptions of the 'pore theory' of capillary permeability (Pease and Baker, 1950), the glomerular basement membrane was therefore suggested to act as a gel-like matrix through which tortuous inter-fibre pathways have the functional capacity to retard the movement of molecules. Pore theory and fibre-matrix theories have both been employed to evaluate glomerular permeability, and current understanding remains far from complete (Pappenheimer *et al.*, 1951).

This report confirmed that the basement membrane of the glomerular capillary wall efficiently retards the passage of large macromolecules, but the questions addressed in this report remain challenging more than half a century later.

References

Hall B (1953). Studies of normal glomerular structure by electron microscopy. In: *5th Annual Conference on the Nephrotic Syndrome*, pp. 1–39. Philadelphia: National Nephrosis Foundation.

Haraldsson B, Nystrom J, Deen WM (2008). Properties of the glomerular barrier and mechanisms of proteinuria. *Physiol Rev* **88**, 451–487.

Pappenheimer JR, Renkin EM, Borrero LM (1951). Filtration, diffusion and molecular sieving through peripheral capillary membranes: a contribution to the pore theory of capillary permeability. *Am J Physiol* **167**, 13–46.

Pease DC, Baker RF (1950). Electron microscopy of the kidney. *Am J Anat* **87**, 349–389.

1.4 Composition of tubular fluid in the macula densa segment as a factor regulating the function of the juxtaglomerular apparatus

Authors

K Thurau, J Schnermann, W Nagel, M Horster, M Wahl

Reference

Circulation Research 1967, **21** (Suppl. 2), 79–90.

Abstract

Our recent micropuncture work with the rat kidney suggests that an intermediate functional connection between tubular and vascular structures operates through the juxtaglomerular apparatus and involves the renin-angiotensin system. In micropuncture experiments on the rat kidney, solutions of various electrolyte composition were injected toward the macula densa of single nephrons. In kidneys with a high renin content, the transient collapse of the proximal convolution of the same nephron occurred when sodium concentration was increased to 150 mM/L. This collapse indicated that glomerular filtration rate was interrupted. An increase in tubular fluid osmolality without a concomitant increase in sodium concentration had no effect on the filtration rate. This sodium-specific reaction was absent or markedly diminished in kidneys depleted of renin. These data demonstrate the operation of a sodium-sensitive feedback mechanism at the level of the juxtaglomerular apparatus in each single nephron unit. The physiological meaning of this mechanism may be to adjust glomerular filtration rate, and thereby tubular sodium load, to the reabsorptive capacity of the nephrons for sodium chloride; it may therefore be an intrarenal sodium conserving mechanism.

Importance

The specialization of the juxtaglomerular apparatus (JGA), and in particular its privileged anatomical location with connections to the early distal tubular lumen and terminal afferent arteriole of the same nephron, had led Goormaghtigh to speculate that this site acted as a functional connection between the tubular and glomerular components of the nephron (Goormaghtigh, 1937; Eknoyan *et al.*, 2009). In addition, preservation of both glomerular filtration rate and renal blood flow (Shipley and Study, 1951; Navar, 1978) in the face of haemodynamic and neural challenges indicated that adjustment of afferent arteriole tone was likely to mediate this renal autoregulation. Advances in renal micropuncture in the late 1950s and early 1960s had established that the sodium chloride concentration of tubular fluid in the vicinity of the JGA was considerably lower than that observed in plasma.

Thurau and colleagues postulated that sodium chloride sensing in the renal tubule was linked to changes in afferent arteriolar tone via renin release from the JGA. Increased sodium chloride concentration at the JGA (delivered by retrograde microperfusion of distal tubules) caused collapse of the proximal tubule of the same nephron (with no effect on adjacent nephrons), indicating complete cessation of glomerular filtration within that nephron. A graded relation between JGA, sodium chloride concentration, and proximal tubular diameter was noted. These effects were abolished by depleting renin from the JGA, indicating not only that the JGA was the locus for these effects (since the JGA-terminal afferent arteriole is a major source of intrarenal renin) but also that renin was involved in the effector mechanism.

The authors proposed a model in which an increase in sodium chloride concentration at the JGA led to a reduction in glomerular filtration and hence a reduction in tubular fluid flow rate, allowing the tubule to reabsorb a greater fraction of the filtered sodium load and therefore prevent excessive natriuresis. This demonstration of 'tubulo-glomerular feedback' therefore provided mechanistic insights into one of the fundamental homeostatic functions of the kidney—the ability to conserve salt and water. Adjusting filtered sodium load to match tubular reabsorptive capacity is essential to prevent excessive urinary sodium losses that would quickly result in cardiovascular collapse. Demonstration of this feedback loop between the tubular and glomerular portions of the same nephron provided a new dimension to understanding the nephron as a single, connected physiological unit.

References

Eknoyan G, Rubens R, Lameire N (2009). The juxtaglomerular apparatus of Norbert Goormaghtigh—a critical appraisal. *Nephrol Dial Transplant* **24**, 3876–81

Goormaghtigh N (1937). L'appareil neuro-myo-artériel juxtaglomérulaire du rein: ses réactions en pathologie et ses rapports avec le tube urinifère. *Compt Rend Soc Biol* **129**, 293–296.

Navar LG (1978). Renal autoregulation: perspectives from whole kidney and single nephron studies. *Am J Physiol* **234**, F357–F370.

Shipley RE, Study RS (1951). Changes in renal blood flow, extraction of inulin, glomerular filtration rate, tissue pressure and urine flow with acute alterations of renal artery blood pressure. *Am J Physiol* **167**, 676–688.

1.5 The dynamics of glomerular ultrafiltration in the rat

Authors

BM Brenner, JL Troy, TM Daugharty

Reference

Journal of Clinical Investigation 1971, **50**, 1776–1780.

Abstract

Using a unique strain of Wistar rats endowed with glomeruli situated directly on the renal cortical surface, we measured glomerular capillary pressures using servo-nulling micropipette transducer techniques. Pressures in 12 glomerular capillaries from 7 rats averaged 60 cm H_2O, or approximately 50% of mean systemic arterial values. Wave form characteristics for these glomerular capillaries were found to be remarkably similar to those of the central aorta. From similarly direct estimates of hydrostatic pressures in proximal tubules, and colloid osmotic pressures in systemic and efferent arteriolar plasmas, the net driving force for ultrafiltration was calculated. The average value of 14 cm H_2O is lower by some two-thirds than the majority of estimates reported previously based on indirect techniques. Single nephron GFR (glomerular filtration rate) was also measured in these rats, thereby permitting calculation of the glomerular capillary ultrafiltration coefficient. The average value of 0.044 nl sec^{-1} cm H_2O^{-1} $glomerulus^{-1}$ is at least fourfold greater than previous estimates derived from indirect observations.

Importance

As Ludwig had pointed out in 1842, glomerular capillary hydrostatic pressure is the dominant force driving the formation of primary ultrafiltrate across the glomerular capillary wall. Starling (1896) extended and quantified this relation by concluding that the balance of hydrostatic and osmotic forces regulates the movement of fluid across a capillary wall. Prior to 1971, many of these forces had been directly measured: for example, Wearn and Richards (1924) had micropunctured the frog nephron to demonstrate that primary ultrafiltrate is essentially protein-free, and Gottschalk and Mylle (1956) had measured the hydrostatic pressure within the lumen of the proximal convoluted tubule. However, mammalian glomeruli were too deep for direct micropuncture, and therefore glomerular capillary hydrostatic pressure had only been estimated indirectly in mammalian kidneys using the tubular stop-flow technique, and the cessation of tubular flow implicit in this technique will (according to Thurau and colleagues' theory of tubuloglomerular feedback) modify the value of the pressure being measured. Direct measurements of glomerular capillary hydrostatic pressure were therefore required.

Brenner and colleagues combined two relatively novel tools: a servo-null device for accurate measurement of capillary hydrostatic pressure (Wiederhielm *et al.*, 1964) and a strain of specially selected rats with superficially located glomeruli, i.e. with no overlying tubules. These two tools permitted direct measurement of the hydrostatic pressure within cannulated glomerular capillaries.

The authors found that glomerular capillary hydrostatic pressures were mostly within the range 55–65 cmH_2O, that glomerular capillary pressure was pulsatile, and that there was a significant pressure drop from the glomerular capillary to the efferent arteriole. These measurements were combined with assessments of tubular hydrostatic pressure and plasma oncotic pressure both to calculate the net force driving glomerular ultrafiltration and to estimate the hydraulic permeability of the glomerular capillary wall. These direct measurements were vastly different from previous estimates: the net force driving fluid movement across the glomerular capillary wall was approximately one-third of previous estimates and the hydraulic permeability was approximately four times greater than previous estimates.

These studies therefore radically redefined the process of glomerular filtration. Moreover, these techniques could subsequently be applied to understand the mechanisms by which a host of mediators, disease states, and therapies modified glomerular filtration, transforming our understanding of both the process and the regulation of glomerular filtration.

References

Gottschalk CW, Mylle M (1956). Micropuncture study of pressures in proximal tubules and peritubular capillaries of the rat kidney and their relation to ureteral and renal venous pressures. *Am J Physiol* **185**, 430–439.

Starling EH (1896). On the absorption of fluids from connective tissue spaces. *J Physiol* **19**, 312–326.

Wearn JT, Richards AN (1924). Observations on the composition of glomerular urine, with particular reference to the problem of reabsorption in the renal tubules. *Am J Physiol* **71**, 209–227.

Wiederhielm CA, Woodbury JW, Kirk S, Rushmer RF (1964). Pulsatile pressures in the microcirculation of frog's mesentery. *Am J Physiol* **207**, 173–176.

1.6 Porous substructure of the glomerular slit diaphragm in the rat and mouse

Authors

R Rodewald, MJ Karnovsky

Reference

Journal of Cell Biology 1974, **60**, 423–433.

Abstract

The highly ordered, isoporous substructure of the glomerular slit diaphragm was revealed in rat and mouse kidneys fixed by perfusion with tannic acid and gluteraldehyde. The slit diaphragm was similar in both animal species and appeared as a continuous junctional band, 300–450 Å wide, consistently present within all slits formed by the epithelial foot processes. The diaphragm exhibited a zipper-like substructure with alternating, periodic cross bridges extending from the podocyte plasma membranes to a central filament which ran parallel to and equidistant from cell membranes, the dimensions and spacings of the cross bridges defined a uniform population of rectangular pores approximately 40 by 140 Å in cross section and 70 Å in length. The total area of the pores was calculated to be about 2–3% of the total surface area of the glomerular capillaries. Physiological data indicate that the glomerular filter functions as if it were an isoporous membrane that excludes proteins larger than serum albumin. The similarity between the dimensions of the pores in the slit diaphragm and estimates for the size and shape of serum albumin supports the conclusion from tracer experiments that the slit diaphragm may serve as the principal filtration barrier to plasma proteins in the kidney.

Importance

A series of combined structure–function electron microscopy studies followed the initial report by Farquhar and colleagues, and employed electron-dense tracers that approximated the size of albumin (e.g. peroxidases; Deen, 2004). In contrast to Farquhar's demonstration that large molecules are excluded from the glomerular basement membrane, these studies showed that a structure traversing the filtration slit between adjacent foot processes appeared to act as the dominant sieve for molecules around the size of albumin.

Rodewald and Karnovsky applied a new staining procedure to their electron microscopy specimens to provide detailed images of this extracellular structure between adjacent podocyte foot processes, which they termed the 'slit diaphragm'. The classic electron micrographs, taken in a plane parallel to the glomerular basement membrane and at high resolution, show a central filament running along the length of the filtration slit and connected to the plasma membranes of the foot process on either side by bridges with a strikingly regular arrangement. The alternating arrangement of these bridges was described as a 'zipper-like appearance'. Moreover, the images were of sufficiently high quality to permit precise anatomical measurements: the 'pores' between the bridges of the diaphragm had cross-sectional dimensions of 40 × 140 Å. This structure was present in all filtration slits in which an appropriate section was obtained, and the pores of the diaphragm pores occupied 2–3% of the entire surface of the glomerular capillary wall.

The description of the podocyte slit diaphragm by Rodewald and Karnovsky has been the foundation for our understanding of this layer of the glomerular filtration barrier. Molecular studies have pieced together the individual components of the slit diaphragm (Gagliardini *et al.*, 2010), and biophysical models have used the anatomical measurements to develop detailed models of glomerular filtration (e.g. Wartiovaara *et al.*, 2004). These studies have enhanced our knowledge of the barrier enormously. However, whilst the dimensions of the pore are similar to those of an albumin molecule, the described pore is in fact too small to account for even the low quantities of albumin that do enter the urinary space (Graham and Karnovsky, 1966). Recent images of the slit diaphragm with scanning electron microscopy (Edwards *et al.*, 1999) have revealed considerably larger pores (of non-uniform dimensions), although in this study the pores were too large to account for the observed degrees of macromolecular sieving. Even the structure of the components of the glomerular filtration barrier therefore remains controversial to the present day.

References

Deen WM (2004). What determines glomerular capillary permeability? *J Clin Invest* **114**, 1412–1414.

Edwards A, Daniels BS, Deen WM (1999). Ultrastructural model for size selectivity in glomerular filtration. *Am J Physiol* **276**, F892–F902.

Gagliardini E, Conti S, Benigni A, Remuzzi G, Remuzzi A (2010). Imaging of the porous ultrastructure of the glomerular epithelial filtration slit. *J Am Soc Nephrol* **21**, 2081–2089.

Graham RC Jr, Karnovsky MJ (1966). Glomerular permeability. Ultrastructural cytochemical studies using peroxidases as protein tracers. *J Exp Med* **124**, 1123–1134.

Wartiovaara J, Ofverstedt LG, Khoshnoodi J, *et al.* (2004). Nephrin strands contribute to a porous slit diaphragm scaffold as revealed by electron tomography. *J Clin Invest* **114**, 1475–1483.

1.7 Control of glomerular hypertension limits glomerular injury in rats with reduced renal mass

Authors

S Anderson, TW Meyer, HG Rennke, BM Brenner

Reference

Journal of Clinical Investigation 1985, **76**, 612–619.

Abstract

Micropuncture and morphologic studies were performed in four groups of male Munich-Wistar rats after removal of the right kidney and segmental infarction of two-thirds of the left kidney. Groups 1 and 3 received no specific therapy. Groups 2 and 4 were treated with the angiotensin I converting enzyme inhibitor, enalapril, 50 mg/liter of which was put in their drinking water. All rats were fed standard chow. Groups 1 and 2 underwent micropuncture study 4 wk after renal ablation. Untreated group 1 rats exhibited systemic hypertension and elevation of the single nephron glomerular filtration rate (SNGFR) due to high average values for the mean glomerular transcapillary hydraulic pressure difference and glomerular plasma flow rate. In group 2 rats, treatment with enalapril prevented systemic hypertension and maintained the mean glomerular transcapillary hydraulic pressure gradient at near-normal levels without significantly compromising SNGFR and the glomerular capillary plasma flow rate, as compared with untreated group 1 rats. Groups 3 and 4 were studied 8 wk after renal ablation. Untreated group 3 rats demonstrated persistent systemic hypertension, progressive proteinuria, and glomerular structural lesions, including mesangial expansion and segmental sclerosis. In group 4 rats, treatment with enalapril maintained systemic blood pressure at normal levels over the 8-wk period and significantly limited the development of proteinuria and glomerular lesions. These studies suggest that control of glomerular hypertension effectively limits glomerular injury in rats with renal ablation, and further support the view that glomerular hemodynamic changes mediate progressive renal injury when nephron number is reduced.

Importance

Blockade of the renin–angiotensin system is one of the cornerstones of treatment in modern nephrology practice. Angiotensin-converting enzyme (ACE) inhibitors and angiotensin II receptor blockers slow the progression of proteinuric renal disease but are also widely used in a range of cardiovascular diseases. Hostetter *et al.* (1982) had proposed that progressive glomerular injury is, at least in part, due to sustained single nephron hyperfiltration, or to one of the haemodynamic determinants of this hyperfiltration (e.g. increased glomerular capillary pressure and/or flow rate). The study selected here therefore examined whether ACE inhibitors could modify glomerular haemodynamic changes *and* prevent progressive glomerular injury.

Five-sixths renal ablation in rats induced systemic hypertension, as well as increased glomerular capillary hydrostatic pressure, glomerular plasma flow rate and glomerular filtration rate. After 8 weeks, proteinuria and structural damage were also apparent. The ACE inhibitor enalapril not only reduced systemic blood pressure but also reduced the resistance of both afferent and efferent arterioles, and consequently reduced glomerular capillary hydrostatic pressure without compromising plasma flow rate, thereby maintaining the single-nephron glomerular filtration rate. Moreover, the progressive structural damage was also attenuated by enalapril. The authors subsequently reported that other combinations of antihypertensive therapy that selectively treated systemic hypertension without reducing glomerular capillary pressure did not protect animals from developing progressive structural renal damage (e.g. Anderson *et al.*, 1986), supporting their conclusion that it is the reduction in glomerular capillary hydrostatic pressure that protects the kidney from progressive injury.

This report is one in a series of reports from Brenner's laboratory that applied physiological investigations to understand the mechanisms driving progressive glomerular injury and to identify appropriate treatments to halt this progression. The direct clinical implications of these reports are that reducing intraglomerular capillary pressure can slow the progression of proteinuric nephropathy and that agents that block the renin–angiotensin system can achieve this benefit without compromising glomerular filtration rate, because of the pattern of changes in afferent and efferent arteriolar resistance. Maintaining glomerular filtration rate whilst slowing the progression of proteinuric disease is a frequently encountered challenge in renal disease management, and this study by Anderson and colleagues reveals the physiological processes by which these goals can be achieved.

References

Anderson S, Rennke HG, Brenner BM (1986). Therapeutic advantage of converting enzyme inhibitors in arresting progressive renal disease associated with systemic hypertension in the rat. *J Clin Invest* **77**, 1993–2000.

Hostetter TH, Rennke HG, Brenner BM (1982). The case for intrarenal hypertension in the initiation and progression of diabetic and other glomerulopathies. *Am J Med* **72**, 375–380.

1.8 The anionic matrix at the rat glomerular endothelial surface

Authors

PS Avasthi, V Koshy

Reference

Anatomical Records 1988, **220**, 258–266.

Abstract

The anionic macromolecules at the glomerular endothelial cell surface are visualized only when stained with cationic stains. We investigated the arrangement and composition of this anionic matrix at the luminal surface. Rat kidneys were perfused with anionic ferritin (PI 4.5), ferritin (PI 7.41), or cationized ferritin (CF, PI 8.3). Anionic ferritin (PI 4.5) did not bind to the capillary wall, ferritin (PI 7.4) bound discontinuously only to the laminae rarae of the basement membrane, but cationized ferritin (CF, PI 8.3) bound as a thick continuous layer to the cell plasmalemma and bound to the anionic matrix in the fenestral spaces. These observations show that an anionic matrix lines the entire capillary lumen surface, fills the fenestrae, and is interposed between the blood and the basement membrane at the fenestrae. The anionic constituents at the capillary luminal surface were identified by in vivo digestion with specific enzymes. Absence of CF binding following digestion with specific enzymes was taken to indicate the presence of the particular glycoprotein known to be susceptible to the enzyme used. Neuraminidase digestion revealed that anionic sites over the surface plasmalemma are mainly from sialoproteins. In contrast, the matrix in fenestral channels contains heparan sulfate, hyaluronic acid, and sialoproteins. Papain digestion showed no glycolipids at the luminal surface. The functions of this continuous anionic layer located at the luminal surface of glomerular capillaries have not yet been established.

Importance

Just as Rodewald and Karnovsky's careful electron microscopy study (see paper 1.6) revealed a novel and critical component of the glomerular capillary wall, so Avasthi and Koshy's study convincingly demonstrated that an extracellular matrix attached to the glomerular endothelial cell surface—the endothelial glycocalyx—is an integral structural component of the glomerular filtration barrier. Because the endothelial glycocalyx is only visible on electron micrographs when appropriate electron-dense labels are employed, it is frequently 'invisible' on routine electron microscopy. Whilst an endothelial glycocalyx layer had been previously demonstrated (Rennke *et al.*, 1975), Avasthi and Koshy reported that the endothelial glycocalyx was both present and specialized within the endothelial fenestrae: the fenestral glycocalyx comprised heparan sulfate, hyaluronan, and sialoprotein, whereas the glycocalyx covering the endothelial cell cytoplasm comprised predominantly sialoproteins. These findings underpin the concept that the endothelial glycocalyx of the glomerular capillary wall is a significant filtration barrier.

Avasthi and Koshy's findings supported the hypothesis, proposed at the beginning of the same decade, that the endothelial glycocalyx might act as a common macromolecular sieve in microvessels throughout the body (Curry and Michel, 1980). Subsequent studies have explored this functional importance of the glomerular endothelial glycocalyx. Enzymatic damage of the glomerular endothelial glycocalyx increases the passage of albumin across the glomerular capillary wall and affects both the size- and charge-selective aspects of the glomerular filtration (e.g. Jeansson and Haraldsson, 2006). In addition, loss of glomerular endothelial glycocalyx occurs in some proteinuric diseases (Jeansson *et al.*, 2009), and molecular correlates of these changes are now being identified. The decrease in albumin clearance that accompanies increased glomerular filtration rate (e.g. Lund *et al.*, 2003) provides indirect evidence that upstream layers of the barrier, including the endothelial glycocalyx, are likely to be an important functional barrier to albumin escape across the glomerular capillary wall.

References

Curry FE, Michel CC (1980). A fiber matrix model of capillary permeability. *Microvasc Res* **20**, 96–99.

Jeansson M, Haraldsson B (2006). Morphological and functional evidence for an important role of the endothelial cell glycocalyx in the glomerular barrier. *Am J Physiol—Renal Physiology* **290**, F111–F1116.

Jeansson M, Bjorck K, Tenstad O, Haraldsson B (2009). Adriamycin alters glomerular endothelium to induce proteinuria. *J Am Soc Nephrol* **20**, 114–122.

Lund U, Rippe A, Venturoli D, Tenstad O, Grubb A, Rippe B (2003). Glomerular filtration rate dependence of sieving of albumin and some neutral proteins in rat kidneys. *Am J Physiol—Renal Physiology* **284**, F1226–F1234.

Rennke HG, Cotran RS, Venkatachalam MA (1975). Role of molecular charge in glomerular permeability. Tracer studies with cationized ferritins. *J Cell Biol* **67**, 638–646.

1.9 Positionally cloned gene for a novel glomerular protein—nephrin—is mutated in congenital nephrotic syndrome

Authors

M Kestila, U Lenkkeri, M Mannikko, J Lamerdin, P McCready, H Putaala, V Ruotsalainen, T Morita, M Nissinen, R Herva, CE Kashtan, L Peltonen, C Holmberg, A Olsen, K Tryggvason

Reference

Molecular Cell 1998, **1**, 575–582.

Abstract

Congenital nephrotic syndrome of the Finnish type (NPHS1) is an autosomal-recessive disorder, characterized by massive proteinuria in utero and nephrosis at birth. In this study, the 150 kb critical region of NPHS1 was sequenced, revealing the presence of at least 11 genes, the structures of 5 of which were determined. Four different mutations segregating with the disease were found in one of the genes in NPHS1 patients. The *NPHS1* gene product, termed nephrin, is a 1241-residue putative transmembrane protein of the immunoglobulin family of cell adhesion molecules, which by Northern and in situ hybridization was shown to be specifically expressed in renal glomeruli. The results demonstrate a crucial role for this protein in the development or function of the kidney filtration barrier.

Importance

This report reconciled a molecular defect within the podocyte slit diaphragm with a devastating clinical condition and was at the forefront of a major research effort into understanding the importance of the podocyte in glomerular structure and function, both in health and disease. The authors identified four different coding defects within a single gene in patients with a distinct clinical syndrome: congenital nephrotic syndrome of the Finnish type. The gene product was named nephrin, and localized to the peripheral regions of glomeruli in embryonic human kidneys. Sequence analysis predicted that the molecule might span the plasma membrane and might serve as a signalling molecule.

Subsequent studies of nephrin have confirmed these predictions and revealed that nephrin is an integral component of the podocyte slit diaphragm. Nephrin molecules extend from the podocyte cell membrane and form the bridges of the slit diaphragm (Wartiovaara *et al.*, 2004). The intracellular portion of nephrin undergoes tyrosine phosphorylation, and interacts with podocin, CD2AP, and a host of other molecules to form a signalling complex (Huber *et al.*, 2001). In addition, nephrin interacts with the podocyte actin cytoskeleton (Jones *et al.*, 2006), and signalling through nephrin is therefore capable of modifying podocyte architecture. Knockout of nephrin in mice essentially reproduces the human phenotype of fatal congenital nephrotic syndrome (Putaala *et al.*, 2001). Whilst the individual layers of the barrier act in concert to retain albumin, these studies confirmed that nephrin is an essential component of the podocyte slit diaphram and, in turn, that an intact slit diaphragm is required for normal glomerular function.

In clinical terms, the report was also the first in a series of studies identifying mutations in genes encoding podocyte proteins in patients with hereditary forms of nephrotic syndrome. The role of genetic testing in appropriately selected paediatric patients, for instance to guide the use of cytotoxic therapies and transplantation, is being developed. Finally, the *NPHS1* gene has become an indispensable tool in glomerular research, as the relatively specific expression of the gene product in podocytes has enabled a raft of transgenic models to be developed in which podocyte-specific expression/removal of a desired target has been achieved under the control of the *NPHS1* promoter region.

This landmark report initiated wide-ranging advances in our understanding of the molecular basis of glomerular structure and function using novel research tools, and also led to changes in clinical practice for patients with hereditary nephropathy.

References

Huber TB, Kottgen M, Schilling B, Walz G, Benzing T (2001). Interaction with podocin facilitates nephrin signaling. *J Biol Chem* **276**, 41543–41546.

Jones N, Blasutig IM, Eremina V, *et al.* (2006). Nck adaptor proteins link nephrin to the actin cytoskeleton of kidney podocytes. *Nature* **440**, 818–823.

Putaala H, Soininen R, Kilpelainen P, Wartiovaara J, Tryggvason K (2001). The murine nephrin gene is specifically expressed in kidney, brain and pancreas: inactivation of the gene leads to massive proteinuria and neonatal death. *Hum Mol Genet* **10**, 1–8.

Wartiovaara J, Ofverstedt LG, Khoshnoodi J, *et al.* (2004). Nephrin strands contribute to a porous slit diaphragm scaffold as revealed by electron tomography. *J Clin Invest* **114**, 1475–1483.

1.10 A high-powered view of the filtration barrier

Authors

J Peti-Peterdi, A Sipos

Reference

Journal of the American Society of Nephrology 2010, **21**, 1835–1841.

Abstract

Multiphoton excitation fluorescence microscopy is a powerful noninvasive imaging technique for the deep optical sectioning of living tissues. Its application in several intact tissues is a significant advance in our understanding of organ function, including renal pathophysiological mechanisms. The glomerulus, the filtering unit in the kidney, is one good example of a relatively inaccessible and complex structure, with cell types that are otherwise difficult to study at high resolution in their native environment. In this article, we address the application, advantages, and limitations of this imaging technology for the study of the glomerular filtration barrier and the controversy it recently generated regarding the glomerular filtration of macromolecules. More advanced and accurate multiphoton determinations of the glomerular sieving coefficient that are presented here dismiss previous claims on the filtration of nephrotic levels of albumin. The sieving coefficient of 70-kD dextran was found to be around 0.001. Using a model of focal segmental glomerulosclerosis, increased filtration barrier permeability is restricted only to areas of podocyte damage, consistent with the generally accepted role of podocytes and the glomerular origin of albuminuria. Time-lapse imaging provides new details and important in vivo confirmation of the dynamics of podocyte movement, shedding, replacement, and the role of the parietal epithelial cells and Bowman's capsule in the pathology of glomerulosclerosis.

Importance

Multiphoton microscopy has given new insights into key aspects of glomerular physiology *in vivo* (e.g. Dunn *et al.*, 2002). Whilst a number of these processes are appraised in the article, revelationary new experimental evidence is also provided.

Firstly, functioning mouse glomeruli are visualized, opening the door to combining multiphoton microscopy with transgenic mouse models. These transgenic models have already transformed our understanding of the glomerular filtration barrier, for example by revealing a highly dynamic structure in which molecular crosstalk between individual layers of the barrier is required to maintain normal physiology (Eremina *et al.*, 2003): the combination of multiphoton microscopy and transgenic manipulation is likely to reveal a wealth of new insights.

Secondly, the report brings a new dimension to the dynamic nature of the glomerular filtration barrier, by showing what appear to be podocytes moving along the glomerular capillary wall. Our understanding of glomerular permeability is currently incomplete, but learning how the highly selective filtration of plasma is maintained when the components of the barrier move is likely to require a re-evaluation of current models. The importance of understanding how the glomerular capillary wall functions under these circumstances is highlighted by the authors' third observation that focal streams of macromolecular leak occur at sites where podocytes detach from the capillary wall (as a result of puromycin aminonucleoside-induced nephropathy). Whilst the tracer macromolecule employed (dextran) exhibits some important differences from albumin, these findings raise the possibility that macromolecular leak, apparent in renal disease as albuminuria, may arise not just from glomeruli, nor indeed just from some glomeruli, but rather may arise (at least in part) from a series of short-lived, dynamic leaks from small, focally damaged areas of the glomerular capillary wall.

Finally, the authors also report that these focally damaged areas were reconstituted by cells migrating onto the capillary wall from Bowman's capsule. These findings provide important evidence for the concept that progenitor cells can regenerate the glomerulus, and that parietal epithelial cells may serve as podocyte progenitors (Appel *et al.*, 2009; Ronconi *et al.*, 2009). Harnessing this process would clearly have important implications for the treatment of glomerular disease.

This report provides important new insights into the dynamic nature of the glomerular capillary wall, in both health and disease, and highlights a new strategy for investigating these processes by combining modern imaging and genetic manipulation technologies.

References

Appel D, Kershaw DB, Smeets B, *et al.* (2009). Recruitment of podocytes from glomerular parietal epithelial cells. *J Am Soc Nephrol* **20**, 333–343.

Dunn KW, Sandoval RM, Kelly KJ, *et al.* (2002). Functional studies of the kidney of living animals using multicolor two-photon microscopy. *Am J Physiol—Cell Physiology* **283**, C905–C916.

Eremina V, Sood M, Haigh J, *et al.* (2003). Glomerular-specific alterations of VEGF-A expression lead to distinct congenital and acquired renal diseases. *J Clin Invest* **111**, 707–716.

Ronconi E, Sagrinati C, Angelotti ML, *et al.* (2009). Regeneration of glomerular podocytes by human renal progenitors. *J Am Soc Nephrol* **20**, 322–332.

Chapter 2

Tubular structure and function

Robert J. Unwin and Stephen B. Walsh

Introduction

Whilst renal physiology began with, and depended critically on, anatomical descriptions of the kidney and the elegant depiction of the nephron by Bowman in 1842, it was the 'clearance concept' (although not a new idea), as formulated and applied to urea by Van Slyke, that really formed the basis for the rapid advances in renal physiology from the late 1920s onwards. Indeed, Homer Smith, one of the founders of modern renal physiology, is quoted as saying that the word 'clearance' has, in his own words, '… been more useful to renal physiology than all the equations ever written'. Using this concept, Homer Smith and others were able to find substances suitable for determining glomerular filtration rate (GFR) and renal blood flow.

However, the papers that we have chosen for this section illustrate several technical advances, such as tubule micropuncture *in vivo* and *in vitro*, which both still use this concept but have extended its application, and which also required the development of new analytical methods, and other key concepts around the transport of solutes and ions. It was the advances in these areas of thinking and experimentation that led to our current understanding and models of the axial properties and functions of the renal tubule, and the central role of the kidney in maintaining fluid and electrolyte homeostasis, including acid–base balance.

In our choice of 'landmark' papers, we have tried to reflect this important 'tubular' aspect of renal physiology, which continues to accelerate with the 'new genetics' and other technological advances, particularly in structural imaging and molecular analysis. The papers we have included begin with a description of the techniques of renal micropuncture and isolated tubule microperfusion, which were essential in mapping the transport properties along the nephron, integrating the later and more recent findings (and cell models) derived from cellular- and molecular-based studies *in vitro*.

Emphasizing the continuing place and virtues of integrative and observational studies in whole animals and in humans are papers on glucose reabsorption and the concept of a 'tubular maximum', and a specific rate-limited transport mechanism for glucose; the importance of potassium secretion in the distal nephron and its critical role in potassium balance; and acid handling by the kidney in various metabolic disorders, including 'renal tubular acidosis', which formed the basis for the ammonium chloride acidification test that is still used in patients.

Another key element and advance in renal physiology was a series of papers describing the hypothesis, testing, and validation of the countercurrent mechanism for concentrating (and diluting) the urine. Finally, one of the most insightful papers describes active transport of sodium across an epithelial cell layer (frog skin) and the 'sodium pump' (Na^+,K^+-ATPase) on which almost all other modes of transcellular transport depend.

2.1 Methods of collecting fluid from known regions of the renal tubule of amphibia and of perfusing the lumen of a single tubule

Authors

AN Richards, AM Walker

Reference

American Journal of Physiology 1936, **118**, 111–120.

Abstract

Procedures have been described by which fluid, in amounts sufficient for analysis, can be collected from various identified levels of the renal tubule of Necturi and frogs. Methods are also described for perfusing different parts of the lumen of a single tubule with artificial solutions.

Importance

This landmark paper by Richards and Walker is a technical account describing the essentials of renal tubule micropuncture *in vivo* under anaesthesia and reflected light illumination, later widely applied to the smaller mammalian tubules of the rat. It not only describes the apparatus they designed, including how to puncture tubules with glass micropipettes with a tip diameter of 20 μm, but also the use of ink to identify the tubule segments punctured (proximal versus distal) and oil blocks to prevent backflow and contamination of tubule fluid samples, as well as the technique of microperfusion *in vivo* using artificial solutions. It was the next step from whole-kidney clearance, which treated the kidney as something of a 'black box', and it was the beginning of studies that investigated individual nephron function and defined the axial and segmental model of transport along the nephron that we understand today.

One of the later technical advances that built on this approach, and which was necessary for study of those parts of the nephron inaccessible to direct micropuncture *in vivo*, was development of the isolated renal tubule technique *in vitro* described by Burg 30 years later. In a subsequent review of this technique, Burg (1982) puts its development in historical context, as well providing an entertaining personal account of why and how the technique was developed. His initial work with kidney slices showed how resilient kidney cells were, and studies at the time had already described tubules dissected from fish kidneys or chick embryos using dyes to show visual evidence of transport. He began by finding ways of separating and isolating tubules using collagenase and produced tubules in suspensions, but these were a mixture of different tubule segments, and he eventually obtained single tubules by dissection after perfusing a kidney with collagenase. He confirmed tubule viability and went on to develop the apparatus (concentric holding and perfusion glass pipettes) necessary to suspend, perfuse, and bathe single-tubule segments. This required a great deal of collaboration, and trial and error, until the apparatus still used today was designed and built. Rabbit tubules were chosen for most of the early studies because they were easy to microdissect, even without collagenase. Progress had to be coupled with a better understanding and knowledge of the different segments of the rabbit nephron, as well as the composition of perfusing and bathing solutions, measurement of transtubular (lumen versus bath) potential difference—an important driving force for any measured ion transport—and a variety of ultramicroanalytical techniques.

These two single-nephron techniques opened the way to defining fluid, electrolyte, and solute transport along the mammalian nephron and led to much of our current knowledge of renal function. The techniques are complementary in that renal micropuncture has the limitation of accessibility (surface tubule segments only), but it is *in vivo*, whereas isolated tubule microperfusion can examine almost all tubule segments, but it is *in vitro*. Moreover, the technique of isolating tubules by microdissection has had even wider applications in studies of tubule cell metabolism, enzymology, receptor binding, mRNA analysis, and transcriptomics.

Reference

Burg M (1982). Introduction: background and development of microperfusion technique. *Kidney Int* **22**, 417–424.

2.2 Active transport of sodium as the source of electric current in the short circuited isolated frog skin

Authors

HH Ussing, K Zerahn

Reference

Acta Physiologica Scandinavica 1951, **23**, 110–127.

Abstract

1. A technique is described by which it is possible to determine, simultaneously, the current that can be drawn from the totally short-circuited frog skin, and, using Na^{24} as a tracer, the influx or outflux of sodium.

2. Under normal conditions, with Ringer solution on both sides of the skin, the Na-influx is on an average 105 % of the current, whereas the outflux is some 5 % of the current. It follows that, within the accuracy of the methods used the current is equal to the net active transport of sodium.

3. Even when the current is increased to more than 150 % its normal value by the addition of neurohypophyseal extract, or decreased to zero by a raised CO_2 tension, the identity between current and net Na-transport still holds.

4. The question, whether the current-Na-transport identity holds exactly when current is increased by addition of adrenaline, cannot be answered from material at hand.

5. With increasing potential difference (the inside positive) the Na-influx decreases and the outflux increases, so that around 100 mV, the two quantities become equal. The extrapolated voltage represents the electromotive force (E_{Na}) of the Na-transporting mechanism.

6. A hypothesis is developed according to which it is possible to calculate E_{Na} as well as the resistance to the Na-current (R_{Na}) from the Na-outflux and the short-circuit current.

Importance

The importance of Hans Ussing to the field of epithelial transport physiology cannot be overstated. His 1958 paper with Koefoed-Johnsen established the concept of epithelial polarity, but his earlier 1951 paper chosen here is just as important because of the methodology he introduced in an elegant set of experiments demonstrating active sodium transport across the short-circuited frog skin; he used apparatus that became widely applied and known as the 'Ussing chamber', and 'short-circuit current' became synonymous with active sodium transport.

Ussing mounted frog skin epithelium between two fluid-filled chambers that allowed access to both sides of the membrane to administer pharmacological agents, and measured the transport of isotopic $^{24}Na^+$ across it. This system allowed a short circuit to abolish any potential difference across the epithelium and eliminate voltage-dependent ion transport; as the solutions on either side were also identical (high-NaCl Ringer's solution), there was no concentration-dependent ion flow. Thus, any current flow across this short-circuited skin had to be active transport. When compared with $^{24}Na^+$ flux, it was found to account for all of the current, demonstrating that active Na^+ transport is the driving force for the potential difference across frog skin and that Na^+ transport across this epithelium is active. Furthermore, Ussing hypothesized that the electromotive force of the Na^+ transporter, as well as the epithelial resistance to Na^+, could be calculated from just the Na^+ efflux and the short-circuit current.

This work led directly to Ussing's 1958 paper with Koefoed-Johnsen, which not only established polarity of the epithelial membrane but also correctly deduced that the apical membrane had highly selective passive Na^+ transport, whilst the basolateral membrane exchanged Na^+ for K^+ against the Na^+ concentration gradient. These observations foreshadowed the discovery of the apical epithelial Na^+ channel and the basolateral Na^+/K^+-ATPase by over 30 years. Moreover, the Ussing chamber has become a standard experimental tool in the field of epithelial physiology—at the time of writing, the term 'Ussing chamber' is in the title of over 8000 publications.

2.3 The renal tubular reabsorption of glucose in the dog

Authors

JA Shannon, S Fisher

Reference

American Journal of Physiology 1938, **122**, 765–774.

Abstract

1. The transtubular reabsorption of glucose has been examined by the simultaneous determination of glucose and creatinine clearances at various arterial plasma glucose concentrations in the normal dog.

2. The essential limitation in the reabsorptive process lies in the circumstance that the tubules are able to transfer only a certain maximal quantity of glucose from the tubular urine to the blood per unit time. When the rate of glomerular filtration of glucose is such that glucose is delivered to the tubules at less than maximal rate, reabsorption is essentially complete.

3. This relationship has been discussed in relation to an hypothesis suggested to describe a similar limitation in the tubular secretion of certain substances.

Importance

The importance of glycosuria had been appreciated at least as early as medieval times, but the physiology of glucose transport in the nephron was only understood in rudimentary terms in the 1930s, when Walker and Reisinger (1933) showed that glucose was freely filtered at the glomerulus. Walker and Hudson (1938) then showed that this filtered glucose was reabsorbed in the proximal tubule in amphibians. Ni and Rehberg (1930) had demonstrated that the glycosuria occurring in hyperglycaemia was not due to cessation of glucose reabsorption but to more glucose being filtered than can be reabsorbed; however, in their studies venous blood samples were used to estimate the filtered load of glucose and there was marked variation in both GFR and plasma glucose concentration.

Shannon and Fisher wanted to provide a more accurate and quantitative description of glucose reabsorption; so they made observations on urinary glucose filtration, reabsorption and excretion in dogs (two trained animals and four decerebrate animals) during steady-state infusions of intravenous glucose to achieve varying plasma glucose concentrations over a tenfold range, and using creatinine clearance as their measure of GFR. They found that the maximum rate of transport (transport maximum or T_m) of glucose was stable in individual dogs and that the T_m was reproducible under different experimental conditions. These experiments showed elegantly that, as plasma glucose concentration rises, tubular reabsorption of glucose also rises linearly until the T_m is reached, when absorption no longer increases (reaches a plateau) and glycosuria occurs. Shannon concluded, '…in the process of reabsorption glucose enters into a reversible combination with some element in the tubule cells, present in constant but limited amount, and that the subsequent decomposition of this complex limits the rate of glucose transfer from tubular urine to the blood'.

The saturability of glucose reabsorption (and to some extent its specificity for glucose) led to the concept of an enzyme-like reaction determining glucose transport, underlining the widely used kinetic approach (see paper 2.6) to define coupled transport mechanisms in renal and intestinal epithelial cells. Subsequent studies showed that glucose (using galactose) was taken up against its concentration gradient, and that this process was not due to glucose metabolism inside the cell (using a non-metabolizable glucose analogue) but to an 'active' process, later shown to couple Na^+ with glucose. It was another 20 years before sodium-linked glucose transporters (SGLTs) were characterized and identified at the molecular level. One of these, SGLT2, is now a therapeutic target in the treatment of type 2 diabetes mellitus.

References

Ni TG, Rehberg PB (1930). On the mechanism of sugar excretion: glucose. *Biochemical Journal* **24**, 1039–1046.

Walker AM, Hudson C (1938). The reabsorption of glucose from the renal tubule in amphibia and the action of phlorhizin upon it. *Am J Physiol* **118**, 130–143.

Walker AM, Reisinger JA (1933). Quantitative studies of the composition of glomerular urine. IX. Concentration of reducing substances in glomerular urine from frogs and necturi determined by an ultramicroadaptation of the method of Sumner. Observations on the action of phlorhizin. *J Biol Chem* **101**, 23–37.

2.4 Renal tubular secretion of potassium in the normal dog

Authors

R Berliner, T Kennedy

Reference

Proceedings of the Society of Experimental Biology 1948, **67**, 542–545.

Abstract

A constant rate of potassium excretion, dissociated from filtered load, occurring after salygran [a mercurial diuretic] administration suggested a tubular secretory mechanism located, presumably, in the distal tubule. The presence of such a mechanism has been demonstrated by the administration of hypertonic KCl solutions which yielded rates of potassium excretion considerably above rates of filtration of potassium at the glomerulus.

Importance

This elegant and, on the face of it, simple study in dogs by Berliner and Kennedy in 1948 provided evidence for renal tubular secretion of potassium. Using the mercurial diuretic salyrgan to cause a natriuresis and diuresis, they showed that, following an initial rise in potassium excretion, the rate of potassium excretion remained pretty constant, despite a fall in the filtered load of potassium calculated from its plasma concentration and GFR estimated by creatinine clearance. Moreover, in some experiments, it was possible to show that the amount of potassium excreted exceeded that filtered, again supporting the notion of tubular secretion of potassium. It was also pointed out that correction of the estimates of filtered potassium for the Donnan equilibrium across the filtration barrier (charged protein on one side and not on the other) would lower the filtered load and make the relative increase in excreted potassium even greater.

Following up on these observations, and with some guidance from Berliner, Giebisch and co-workers published a series of ground-breaking renal micropuncture studies from 1964 to 1971 that defined potassium transport along the rat nephron and confirmed the interpretation by Berliner of his earlier dog experiments (Stanton, 2010). These studies showed that the proximal tubule and loop of Henle reabsorb a constant fraction of the filtered load of potassium and that it is in the distal tubule that potassium secretion is regulated. They also showed that, while there is an inverse relationship between H^+ and K^+ secretion, these ions are not tightly coupled, and that in the case of Na^+ reabsorption and K^+ secretion along the distal tubule, K^+ secretion does not depend directly on Na^+ reabsorption (i.e. K^+ and Na^+ transport are also not directly linked or coupled) but on the electrical potential difference across the distal tubule, which does depend on Na^+ reabsorption. They also provided indirect evidence for potassium reabsorption by the collecting duct, which was later shown to be mediated by a K^+/H^+-ATPase, similar to the one present in the stomach.

Thus, Berliner and Giebisch were the leading figures whose work established beyond doubt the process of K^+ secretion by the distal renal tubule, which determines the final urinary excretion of potassium. From these studies has come the identification and characterization of renal

K$^+$ channels—the renal outer medullary K$^+$ (ROMK) and calcium- and voltage-activated large conductance K$^+$ (BK) channels among others—and their role in tubular cell function, as well as potassium excretion by the kidney, and in disease [e.g. ROMK in Bartter type 2 syndrome, and KCNJ10 in EAST (epilepsy, ataxia, sensorineural deafness, and tubulopathy) syndrome].

Reference

Stanton B (2010). Renal potassium transport: the pioneering studies of Gerhard Giebisch. *Am J Physiol* **98**, F233–F234.

2.5 The excretion of acid in renal disease

Authors

OM Wrong, HEF Davies

Reference

Quarterly Journal of Medicine 1959, **28**, 259–313.

Abstract

A short test using ammonium chloride has been employed to assess the ability of the kidney to excrete ammonium and an acid urine. Ten normal subjects, and over 50 patients with different forms of renal disease, have been studied.

Patients with the classical syndrome of renal tubular acidosis were unable to excrete urine of normal minimum pH. The same impairment was found in severely potassium-depleted subjects, in some patients with persistent hypercalcaemia, and in one patient recovering from acute anuria. Most patients with severe general renal failure excreted urine as acid as those with normal renal function.

The rate of ammonium excretion after ammonium chloride was proportional to the glomerular filtration rate, and was invariably depressed in renal failure. Reduced ammonium excretion was found in eight out of nine patients with renal tubular acidosis, but did not appear to be a specific abnormality of this syndrome, as glomerular filtration rate was correspondingly reduced.

We have studied three patients who have what appears to be an incomplete form of the syndrome of renal tubular acidosis. These patients had generalised nephrocalcinosis, and were unable to excrete urine of normal minimum pH, but they had no extracellular acidosis. All three had relatively normal glomerular filtration rates and high levels of ammonium excretion, which appeared to prevent them from developing acidosis.

The findings in two patients with the Fanconi syndrome suggest that the acidosis frequently reported in this condition has multiple causes. One of our patients was severely depleted of potassium, and the other had advanced renal failure; their responses to ammonium chloride were characteristic of these two abnormalities.

Importance

The renal regulation of acid–base balance was recognized and well described by the early twentieth century, but the effect of kidney disease on this physiological process had been explored in only a limited way until Wrong's seminal case-based clinical study was published in 1959. It is a large paper (over 50 pages in length) and its scope is broad; it is primarily a study designed to examine the efficacy and reliability of using oral ammonium chloride to determine the kidney's ability to excrete acid. However, not only did Wrong and Davies observe important differences in urinary acidification in what they classified as glomerular and tubular disease, they also documented for the first time the existence of the syndrome of 'incomplete distal renal tubular acidosis', in which there is an inability to acidify the urine in response to an acid challenge, but no systemic acidosis (normal or preserved blood bicarbonate concentration). Another important finding was that patients with chronic renal failure could acidify their urine but could not increase net acid excretion, the sum of phosphate (titratable acid) and ammonium excretion. The acute or short ammonium chloride challenge that Wrong and Davies used became the 'gold standard' test for the diagnosis of 'classical' (also known as hypokalemic) distal renal tubular acidosis (RTA), especially the incomplete form.

In distal RTA, the main defect in acidification was a failure to increase urine pH with reduced titratable acid excretion and a modest reduction in ammonium excretion, in contrast to patients with renal failure and reduced GFR, who had significant reductions in both titratable acid and ammonium excretion. In distal RTA, titratable acid excretion could be increased by intravenous phosphate infusion, but was normally limited by the impaired H^+ secretion and elevated urine pH. Patients with incomplete distal RTA had normal or raised ammonium excretion, which is probably why they did not develop a systemic acidosis.

This paper properly characterized disorders of acid excretion in renal disease and was a comprehensive study of the clinical pathophysiology of proximal and distal RTA. It described the syndrome of incomplete distal RTA, as well reporting then novel observations on patients with impaired GFR, hypercalcaemia, nephrocalcinosis, and renal Fanconi syndrome. It even anticipated genetic defects in renal acidification, describing several pedigrees. It was not only pioneering, it also became a citation classic, establishing the short ammonium chloride test as *the* reference clinical test of renal acidification, which it remains to this day.

2.6 Properties of the Na$^+$-H$^+$ exchanger in renal microvillus membrane vesicles

Authors

J Kinsella, P Aronson

Reference

American Journal of Physiology 1980, **238**, F461–F469.

Abstract

Transport of Na$^+$ and H$^+$ was evaluated in brush border membrane vesicles isolated from the rabbit renal cortex. Na$^+$ transport was assayed by a rapid filtration technique; H$^+$ transport was monitored with 5,5-dimethoxazolidine-2,4-dione by flow analysis. Uphill Na$^+$ uptake was induced by imposition of an in > out H$^+$ gradient, and uphill H$^+$ efflux by imposition of an out > in Na$^+$ gradient, consistent with the action of a Na$^+$-H$^+$ exchanger. The uptake of Na$^+$ was electroneutral either in the presence or absence of a H$^+$ gradient, indicating a fixed 1:1 stoichiometry for the exchange process. Na$^+$ transport was saturable and inhibited by Li$^+$ and NH$_4^+$ but not by K$^+$, Rb$^+$, Cs$^+$, or choline. Uphill H$^+$ efflux was induced by imposition of an out > in Li$^+$ gradient. Neither the uptake of Na$^+$ nor H$^+$ efflux were influenced by out > in gradients of Cl$^-$ compared to gradients of SCN$^-$ or SO$_4^{2-}$. If transport systems mediating Na$^+$-Cl$^-$ co-transport and/or Cl$^-$-OH$^-$ exchange are present in the microvillus membrane, their respective rates must be slow compared to the rate of Na$^+$-H$^+$ exchange. Transport of Na$^+$ was inhibited by harmaline and amiloride, but not by acetazolamide, furosemide, or 4-acetamido-4'-isothiocyanostilbene-2,2'-disulfonate. We conclude that isolated renal microvillus membranes contain a tightly coupled Na$^+$-H$^+$ exchanger that may play an important role in proximal tubular acidification.

Importance

Peter Aronson had been working on Na$^+$–glucose transport and intended to use renal brush border membrane vesicles to study sodium-coupled glucose transport in more detail. However, his influential study with Kinsella on Na$^+$–H$^+$ transport was prompted not only by the earlier suggestion by Berliner that bicarbonate reabsorption along the proximal tubule was mediated by an exchange of Na$^+$ for H$^+$ (although it was not known if this was directly coupled) but also by a more recent report from the group of Heini Murer showing that Na$^+$–H$^+$ exchange was present in both intestinal and renal brush border membrane vesicles, although this was still controversial.

What the vesicle membrane preparation technique could achieve, which studies of the intact renal tubule cannot, was to define the transport mechanisms at the cell membrane level, apical or basolateral. Renal brush border membranes are derived from proximal tubules; by a complex and comprehensive series of manipulations of their membrane vesicle preparation, Kinsella and Aronson defined an electroneutral Na$^+$–H$^+$ exchanger that was independent of Cl$^-$. They also cleverly showed not only that an outward H$^+$ gradient would drive the uptake of Na$^+$ into vesicles but that an inward Na$^+$ gradient would generate an inside alkaline pH (from H$^+$ extrusion), an effect also produced by Li.

Amiloride was originally used to block Na$^+$ channels, but, surprisingly at the time, it caused inhibition and it was only later realized to be an inhibitor of Na$^+$–H$^+$ exchange. NH$_4^+$ was also shown to be transported by the exchanger. They concluded that '... isolated renal microvillus membranes contain a tightly coupled Na$^+$-H$^+$ exchanger that may play an important role in proximal tubular acidification'.

This work led to the recognition that Na$^+$–H$^+$ exchange is the major (although not the only) mechanism for bicarbonate reabsorption along the proximal tubule, and the characterization of the renal brush border membrane Na$^+$–H$^+$ exchanger as NHE3, the renal isoform of the NHE family of Na$^+$–H$^+$ exchangers found in almost all cells, as well as its regulation by a complex of intracellular signalling and scaffolding molecules (such as NHERF and PDZ proteins) now known to be shared with other renal transporters, channels, and receptors or signalling molecules. Moreover, the vesicle membrane technique has continued to identify novel organic ion exchange mechanisms in the proximal tubule, and it remains a valuable functional tool for studying coupled ion and solute transport along the proximal tubule and intestine.

2.7 The mechanism of bicarbonate reabsorption in the proximal and distal tubules of the kidney

Authors

FC Rector, N Carter, Seldin D

Reference

Journal of Clinical Investigation 1965, **44**, 278–290.

Abstract

The mechanism of HCO_3^- reabsorption in proximal and distal tubules was examined in rats undergoing $NaHCO_3$ diuresis. The steady-state intratubular pH was measured with pH-sensitive glass microelectrodes and compared with the equilibrium pH calculated from the HCO_3^- concentration of the tubular fluid (measured with quinhydrone electrodes) and plasma PCO_2.

In the proximal tubule the intratubular pH and the equilibrium pH were identical, indicating no accumulation of excess H_2CO_3. After inhibition of carbonic anhydrase, however, intratubular pH was significantly lower (0.85 pH U) than the equilibrium pH. It was concluded that HCO_3^- reabsorption in the proximal tubule was mediated by H^+ secretion, but that carbonic anhydrase located in the luminal membrane of the cell prevented H_2CO_3 from accumulating in the tubular fluid.

In the distal tubule the intratubular pH was 0.85 U lower than the equilibrium pH. This difference could be obliterated by an intravenous injection of carbonic anhydrase. It was concluded that HCO_3^- reabsorption in this segment was also accomplished by H^+ secretion. The accumulation of excess H_2CO_3 in the tubular fluid indicated that, in contrast to the proximal tubule, carbonic anhydrase was not located in the luminal membrane of distal tubular cells.

Importance

Berliner had proposed in the early 1950s that bicarbonate reabsorption occurred predominantly in the proximal tubule and that it depended on H^+ secretion and required the enzyme carbonic anhydrase. In the tubule lumen, secreted H^+ titrates filtered bicarbonate to form carbonic acid (H_2CO_3), which dissociates to form CO_2 and H_2O. However, for this mechanism to work in the steady state, the rate at which H_2CO_3 is formed and dissociates must equal the rate of bicarbonate reabsorption. A later calculation by Walser and Mudge based on the uncatalysed rate of H_2CO_3 breakdown to CO_2 and H_2O indicated that, for the H_2CO_3 breakdown rate to equal the rate of bicarbonate reabsorption, the concentration of H_2CO_3 would have to be ten times higher than the value existing were H_2CO_3 in equilibrium with the CO_2 tension of tubule fluid and plasma. This predicted an intraluminal pH one pH unit lower than would be expected from the luminal concentration of HCO_3^- and the CO_2 tension of plasma, assuming equilibration of luminal H_2CO_3 with plasma CO_2, a so-called disequilibrium pH.

Using the *in vivo* renal tubule micropuncture technique (see paper 2.1) and the recently developed pH-sensitive glass microelectrodes, Rector and colleagues decided to characterize the mechanism of bicarbonate reabsorption in the proximal tubules of rats infused with $NaHCO_3$ and to test the hypothesis of a disequilibrium pH. They compared the directly measured steady-state intraluminal pH with the calculated equilibrium pH estimated from the luminal concentration of HCO_3^- and plasma CO_2 tension.

In the proximal tubule, no disequilibrium pH was found, but when carbonic anhydrase was inhibited, and although bicarbonate reabsorption itself was partially inhibited, tubule fluid pH became 0.8 pH units more acid than the predicted equilibrium pH, thus revealing a disequilibrium pH. However, in the distal tubule, a disequilibrium pH was already present (no luminal carbonic anhydrase). These findings clearly indicated that in both the proximal and distal tubules HCO_3^- reabsorption depends on H^+ secretion, but that in the proximal tubule carbonic anhydrase prevents H_2CO_3 from accumulating in the tubule fluid and limiting reabsorption.

By 1965, the evidence for H^+ secretion in the proximal and distal parts of the nephron was convincing. Over the next 35 years, the cellular and molecular basis of this H^+ secretion has been characterized and defined with the identification of the apically located Na^+–H^+ exchanger in the proximal tubule (see paper 2.6) and the electrogenic H^+-ATPase in the distal tubule and collecting duct, the latter recently shown to be a cause of inherited (recessive) distal renal tubular acidosis (see paper 2.5).

2.8 Das Multipikationsprinzip als Grundlage der Harnkonzentrierung in der Niere [The multiplication principle as the basis for concentrating urine in the kidney]

Authors

B Hargitay, W Kuhn

Reference

Zeitschrift für Elektrochemie und Angewandte Physikalische 1951, **55,** 539–558. [Translated from German by Thomas R, Rossi T, Hargitay B. *Journal of the American Society of Nephrology* 2001, **12,** 1566–1586.]

Summary

The system formed in the kidney from Henle's loops and the collecting ducts represents a device which, by multiplication of a small concentration effect, makes possible the production of the relatively concentrated solutions excreted, as we know, by the kidney. The feasibility of elaborating concentrated solutions using such a 'Hairpin-Countercurrent-System' is confirmed by studies using an experimental model and is dealt with quantitatively in a theoretical treatment.

Importance

The senior author of this landmark paper, Werner Kuhn, was a physical chemist who had been a research fellow with the eminent theoretical physicist Niels Bohr in Copenhagen and later with Lord Rutherford in Cambridge, one of many examples of a well-trained chemist or physicist turning his attention and expertise to important questions of biology. As early as 1936, Kuhn had begun to think about a countercurrent system in the kidney, which had been prompted by his earlier experience of how to enrich an isotope (using repeated separation and concentration) and his awareness of the hairpin structure of the loop of Henle. Indeed, he had been able to enrich sugar in water using a countercurrent system with two semipermeable membranes and phenol, and no other driving force. However, although he had published his concept of countercurrent multiplication some 10 years earlier, it was not until this paper with Hargitay in 1951, which also included a working model, that the idea became widely known. Moreover, the fact that these publications were originally in German, and in non-biological journals, may also have delayed an even wider appreciation of this pivotal concept.

Hargitay, then a new young fellow in Kuhn's laboratory, was given the task of proving the countercurrent principle by achieving solute concentration using not more than one semipermeable membrane and any chosen driving force; he chose hydrostatic pressure. The model depended on this pressure to produce a single effect across a semipermeable membrane separating two compartments, which would then be multiplied by countercurrent flow. The inflowing fluid corresponded to the descending limb of the loop of Henle (compartment 1) and the outflowing fluid corresponded to the ascending limb of the loop of Henle (compartment 2). Hydrostatic pressure applied to the inflow fluid or solvent (water) containing an impermeable solute (salt) would (by forcing water across the semipermeable membrane) cause a small increase in concentration in compartment 1 and dilution in compartment 2, an osmotic difference that will eventually slow and stop the passage of water; this is the single effect. As this process is repeated many times during continuous flow, fluid near the tip, connecting inflow to outflow, will become progressively more concentrated. However, knowing that the hydrostatic pressure to the loop of Henle would probably not be sufficient, the authors proposed that their model would also work with active salt transport in the opposite direction, that is, from ascending to descending limbs of the loop of Henle.

Later work (see paper 2.10) established active salt transport from the medullary thick ascending limb as the 'single-effect' driving force in the outer medulla, but we still do not really know what the driving force is in the inner medulla. Passive transport of urea from the terminal collecting ducts into the papillary interstitium does not quite fit with what we now know of the measured tubule permeabilities for urea.

2.9 Micropuncture study of the mammalian urinary concentrating mechanism: evidence for the countercurrent hypothesis

Authors

C Gottschalk, M Mylle

Reference

American Journal of Physiology 1959, **196**, 927–936.

Abstract

The osmolality was determined of fluid collected by micropuncture from proximal and distal convolutions, loops of Henle, collecting ducts and vasa recta of kidneys of various rodents with and without osmotic diuresis. Proximal tubular fluid was isosmotic; in the presence of antidiuretic hormone, early distal fluid was hypo-osmotic due to the prior reabsorption of sodium chloride, and late distal fluid again isosmotic. The hyperosmotic concentration of the urine is established in the collecting ducts, apparently as a consequence, in part at least, of the hyperosmotic reabsorption of sodium chloride in the loops of Henle. Fluid from the bends of loops of Henle, and from collecting ducts and vasa recta at the same level were equally hyperosmotic, consistent with the hypothesis that the mammalian nephron functions as a countercurrent multiplier system. The vasa recta are believed to play an important role in the concentration of the urine by functioning as countercurrent diffusion exchangers.

Importance

Hargitay and Kuhn had proposed a theory and model of urine concentration based on the idea that the U-shaped loop of Henle acted as a countercurrent multiplier (see paper 2. 8). Wirz had also reported that the osmolality of distal tubule fluid taken from water-deprived rats with concentrated urine was hypo-osmolar. Using kidney slices and freezing point depression to measure osmolality, Wirz and his colleagues also demonstrated an increasing osmotic gradient from cortex to medulla.

Against this backdrop, Gottschalk and Mylle reinvestigated and extended these observations using *in vivo* renal tubule micropuncture in Wistar rats with mainly short-looped cortical nephrons, and in hamsters and kangaroo rats with more accessible papillae containing long-looped juxtamedullary nephrons, as well as fat sand (desert) rats with only long-loop nephrons. During a range of manipulations from hydropenia to saline and osmotic (mannitol or glucose) diuresis, they found that proximal tubule fluid was always isosmotic with plasma and that distal tubule fluid was always hypo-osmotic; indeed, distal tubule fluid osmolality decreased further during saline diuresis, leading to the conclusion that distal tubule fluid hypotonicity is generated by NaCl reabsorption in the loop of Henle, rather than by secretion of water into the tubule lumen. Moreover, late distal tubule fluid had become isosmotic, meaning that its later hyperosmotic concentration (as evident from a concentrated urine) occurred in the collecting duct and was dependent in part on the '… hyperosmotic reabsorption of sodium chloride in the loops of Henle'.

A final and key observation was that fluid taken from the tips (bends) of loops of Henle had the same *increased* osmolality as collecting ducts and vasa recta at the same level, in keeping with the countercurrent multiplier hypothesis and with the vasa recta behaving as countercurrent (by diffusion) exchangers. Gottschalk and Mylle also speculated that, in addition to its effect on water permeability in the late distal tubule and collecting duct, vasopressin (antidiuretic hormone) might directly increase sodium transport in the loop of Henle. This has since been shown to be correct, although they dismissed the thick ascending limb, where vasopressin acts, in favour of the thin ascending limb.

This important and technically difficult study *in vivo* confirmed all the elements of the proposed urinary concentrating mechanism, ensuring that the countercurrent hypothesis would be widely acknowledged and accepted.

2.10 Sodium chloride and water transport in the medullary thick ascending limb of the loop of Henle

Authors

A Rocha, JJ Kokko

Reference

Journal of Clinical Investigation 1973, **52**, 612–623.

Abstract

Transport of NaCl and water was examined in isolated rabbit medullary thick ascending limb of Henle (ALH) segments in vitro. Net transport of fluid was zero when segments were perfused with isotonic ultrafiltrate in a bath of rabbit serum with an osmolality increased by addition of either 239±8 mos-mol/liter of raffinose or 232±17 mosmol of NaCl, indicating that the thick ALH is impermeant to osmotic flow of water. When tubules were perfused at slow rates with an isosmolal ultrafiltrate of rabbit serum, effluent osmolality was consistently less than perfusate and bath. The decrease in collected fluid osmolality represented salt transport, since sodium and chloride concentrations were decreased when compared with perfusate. The simultaneously determined transtubular potential difference (PD) was lumen positive and depended on perfusion rate. At flow rates above 2 nl.min^{-1} mean transtubular PD was equal to 6.7±0.34 mV. During stop-flow PD became more positive. Ouabain and cooling reversibly decreased the PD. The PD remained positive when choline was substituted for Na in both perfusion fluid and bathing media. These results suggest that the active transport process is primarily an electrogenic chloride mechanism. The isotopic permeability coefficient for Na was $6.27 \pm 0.38 \times 10^{-5}$ cm.s^{-1} and so the thick ALH is as permeable to Na as the proximal convoluted tubule. The chloride permeability coefficient for the thick ALH was $1.06 \pm 0.12 \times 10^{-5}$ cm.s^{-1}, significantly less than the chloride permeability of the proximal tubule.

Thus, the medullary thick ALH is water impermeable and actively transports solute outward as a consequence of an electrogenic chloride pump. These characteristics allow this segment to generate a dilute tubular fluid and make it the energy source for operation of the countercurrent multiplication system. [Adapted.]

Importance

Although the mechanism of the countercurrent multiplication system of the loop of Henle was already well described (see papers 2.8 and 2.9), and the concept of active transport of sodium from the lumen of the ascending limb of the loop of Henle was supported by micropuncture work showing that the fluid in the early distal tubule was hypo-osmolar when compared with plasma (see paper 2.9), this had not been demonstrated directly, nor had the mechanism been described. In this excellent and thorough set of experiments, Rocha and Kokko used isolated perfused segments of the rabbit nephron *in vitro* and measured the osmotic permeability, transtubular electrical potential difference (p.d.), isotopic fluxes of Na$^+$ and Cl$^-$, and NaCl transport rates against concentration gradients.

They showed that the thick ascending limb of the loop of Henle was completely impermeable to water, even when an osmotic or NaCl gradient was applied across it. They also showed that the thick ascending limb could transport NaCl without water, thus generating hypo-osmolar tubular fluid. Furthermore, they measured the transtubular potential difference arising from NaCl transport and found it to be an active process inhibited by cooling or the addition of the Na^+/K^+-ATPase inhibitor ouabain. They also suggested that the main transported ion was Cl^-, because the positive transtubular potential difference persisted after removal of Na^+ from both the perfusion and bath solutions. With some foresight, they rejected the idea that Na^+ transport was driven passively by the electrical gradient generated by active Cl^- transport, because they observed that the isotopic flux ratio for Na^+ was greater than that predicted the Ussing equation (see paper 2.2).

Rocha and Kokko set the scene for the discovery of the bumetanide-sensitive co-transporter (BSC), now known as the Na–K–Cl co-transporter (NKCC), discovered over a decade later, which was the first candidate gene for Bartter syndrome type 1. It also provided the molecular basis for the role of countercurrent multiplication and the part played by the medullary thick ascending limb in establishing the cortico-medullary osmotic gradient without which vasopressin cannot act.

Chapter 3

Investigation of renal disease

Guy H. Neild

Introduction

In the late eighteenth century, investigation of dropsy or gross dependent oedema led to the recognition that some forms were associated with massive proteinuria ('serum in urine'). It was Bright who, by systematically performing autopsies on his patients who had died, correlated the morbid anatomy (gross macroscopic appearance) with clinical signs and symptoms in life. He was the first to connect dropsy and proteinuria with the universal finding of abnormal renal pathology. With these new insights, uroscopy, which had been the first clinical 'investigation' in medicine, and widely used for 4000 years was consigned to oblivion.

Advances in microscopy in the mid-nineteenth century led to the examination of renal autopsy tissue (histology) and the examination of urine (cells and casts). Studies of blood chemistry had begun in the late eighteenth century and thereafter urea was described, found in large quantities in urine, and was found to be reduced in urine of chronic renal disease, raised in the blood of animals following nephrectomy and then in patients with chronic renal disease, although blood urea measurement was not in clinical practice until 1920. The period between the two World Wars saw the concepts of clearance develop and the advantages of creatinine emerge as an endogenous marker of renal disease. The analysis of blood presented huge problems. Protein-free filtrates had to be produced, and large volumes were required to measure the small quantities of chemicals to be found. All methods involved multiple manual steps that took days to complete.

In the 1960s, modern nephrology took off with the flame photometer, the development of automated clinical chemistry by Leonard Skeggs, renal biopsy, and the modern classifications of glomerular disease. Then came the advances in immunology that led to diagnostic blood tests (such as the antinuclear antibody test) and immunofluorescence for renal biopsies. By the 1980s, ultrasound began to replace the intravenous urogram as a simple tool to establish renal anatomy. More recently, with worldwide interest in the pandemic of renal disease and diabetes, screening using urine dipsticks for blood and protein, estimated glomerular filtration rate (eGFR) and urine protein:creatinine ratio have made global epidemiology possible.

The choice of landmark papers in this chapter is based on a clinical approach to investigating renal disease: if any patient has significant damage to their kidneys then: (i) there may be blood or protein in the urine; (ii) if the damage is severe enough to cause renal impairment, then urea and creatinine levels are raised; and (iii) patients often have hypertension. All renal disease can be categorised by the three Us: ultrasound, urine analysis (dipstick), and urine microscopy. Specific diagnosis is then made with renal imaging, renal biopsy, and immunological tests. This approach gives a series of topics for each of which I have identified landmark papers.

In choosing the most important landmark papers, I have generally sided with Sir William Osler: 'In science the credit goes to the man who convinces the world, not to the man to whom the idea first occurs.'

3.1 Reports of medical cases, vol. 1

Author

R Bright

Reference

Published by Longman Green, London, UK (1827).

Summary

There are other appearances to which I think too little attention has hitherto been paid. They are those evidences of organic change that occasionally present themselves in the structure of the kidney, and which, whether they are to be considered as the cause of the dropsical effusion or as the consequence of some other disease, cannot be unimportant. Where those conditions of the kidney to which I allude have occurred, I have often found the dropsy connected with secretion of albuminous urine more or less coaguable on the application of heat.

Importance

Apart from the knowledge of renal failure that we now get from measuring the serum urea and creatinine, nothing is more synonymous with kidney disease than the finding of protein in the urine.

It was towards the end of the eighteenth century that clinical investigation of dropsy showed that some cases were associated with protein in the urine. Dropsy is a syndrome in which there is gross dependent oedema, and we now appreciate the difference between the salt and water retention of heart failure or of renal failure, and the hypoalbuminaemic state of nephrotic syndrome.

It was in 1765 that Domenico Cotungo first demonstrated in a patient with acute dropsy that the urine, when heated, appeared to coagulate to produce a material like egg white (albumen) (see paper 5.1). There are several claimants to be the first clinical chemist, but for the scientific investigation of the chemistry of urine, William Cruickshank in London is foremost and he showed in 1797 that protein in urine could be demonstrated by adding concentrated nitric acid. The nitric acid test and heating of urine remained the standard methods for 150 years. In England, Cruickshank, Wells (in 1811) (see paper 5.2), and Blackall (in 1813) independently described 'serum' in urine of patients with dropsy.

However, it was Richard Bright's work in 1827 on the morbid anatomy of his deceased patients, combined with their clinical histories and the observation of protein in the urine, that first made clear the connection between kidney disease and proteinuria. He made detailed post-mortem inspection of the viscera (hence 'morbid anatomy'). This was not normal practice, and what Bright pointed out was the obvious abnormalities of the kidneys, when attention had previously focused on the liver and heart. He was able to link these observations back to his records of protein found in the urine. The advent of histology was not for another 30 years.

Although history has awarded Bright all the prizes, it is important to note that his books were extremely expensive and Volume I (on the kidney) sold only 243 copies. It was never translated into French or German, and much of Bright's work was reproduced on the continent, principally by Rayer, without knowledge of this publication.

From his dissections, Bright described many other novel pathologies from almost every organ, and his second volume, which sold 171 copies, concerned other viscera and the brain. He also described fatty stools and glycosuria in pancreatic disease.

3.2 Über den Niederschlag welchen Pikrinsäure in normalem Harn erzeugt und über eine neue Reaction des Kreatinins [Concerning both the precipitation caused in normal urine by picric acid and a new reaction with creatinine]

Author

M Jaffe

Reference

Zeitschrift für Physikalische Chemie 1886, **10**, 391–400.

Summary

If one mixes a solution of creatinine together with a little aqueous solution of picric acid and adds a few drops of potassium or sodium hydroxide, then immediately an intense red colour develops even in the cold. Depending on the concentration of the creatinine solution the intensity of the colour varies from red-orange to dark blood-red, intensifies greatly over a few minutes and remains unchanged for hours; only when an excess of alkali is added, does the solution, when exposed to light, turn yellow after a time. Acidification with acetic acid or hydrochloric acid changes the red colour yellow in a few minutes. [Extract translated from the paper.]

Importance

Creatinine was first isolated and named Kreatinin in 1847 by the German chemist Justus von Liebig. Jaffe's great contribution was to report that creatinine in a solution of alkaline picrate produced an intense red colour. Jaffe was an eminent physician and chemical pathologist but did not exploit this observation further (Delanghe and Speeckaert, 2011). Its first clinical application was from the laboratory of Folin, the Swedish-born pioneer of all twentieth-century analytical chemistry, who worked in Boston, USA. In 1904, he introduced the colorimeter into analytical practice to compare the colours generated by what he named the Jaffe reaction.

In 1910, creatinine was reported in blood, but this was disputed for another 20 years. It was Folin who developed practical methods that by 1914 had become commonplace. It became clear that blood contained other Jaffe-positive material ('chromogens'), but it was not until 1934 that Zacherl and Lieb were able to show definitely that chromogens in blood are mainly creatinine. In 1945, Bosnes and Taussky described for the first time standard optimal conditions for a rapid colorimetric Jaffe reaction.

The whole of clinical chemistry underwent a series of revolutions during the 1940s and 1950s. The introduction of the flame photometer had made the measurement of electrolytes simple, cheap, and easy. But what took clinical chemistry methods out of the research laboratories and into the public hospitals as a daily routine was the automated auto-analyser method developed in 1957 by Leonard Skeggs (Skeggs, 2000). He used serum and on-line dialysis to remove protein, although this method did introduce a further pseudo-chromogen effect.

In the meantime, in 1971 more specific definitive measurements of 'true' blood creatinine were developed using an enzymatic, kinetic-rate reaction, which utilized different rates of formation of colour for creatinine versus other chromogen substrates. This method produced results 20% lower than standard Jaffe methods. In addition, high-pressure liquid chromatography was developed in

1977, liquid chromatography/mass spectrometry in 2003, and isotope dilution mass spectrometry in 2007, which has become the new standard.

Whilst urea is the *fons et origo* of renal chemistry and had a 100-year start on creatinine, creatinine is today *primus inter pares* in the investigation of renal disease. Although Folin takes credit for the method, he honoured Jaffe by naming the reaction after him. One hundred and twenty-five years later, so do we.

References

Delanghe JR, Speeckaert MM (2011). Creatinine determination according to Jaffe—what does it stand for? *NDT Plus* **4**, 83–86.

Skeggs LT Jr (2000). Persistence … and prayer: from the artificial kidney to the AutoAnalyzer. *Clin Chem* **46**, 1425–1436.

3.3 Albumin excretion as a measure of glomerular dysfunction in children

Authors

TM Barratt, PN McLaine, JF Soothill

Reference

Archives of Disease in Childhood 1970, **45**, 496–501.

Abstract

The urine albumin/creatinine concentration ratio (U_A/U_C) and the albumin excretion rate per unit weight ($U_A V/Wt$) have been compared with the theoretically ideal parameter for measuring glomerular damage, clearance of albumin/clearance of creatinine (C_A/C_C), using a simple sensitive immunochemical technique for albumin. It is shown that U_A/U_C on random urine specimens can be as satisfactorily used to predict C_A/C_C as $U_A V/Wt$. Normal data over a wide range of body size of this simple parameter are presented; higher values in the newborn reflect increased permeability of the neonatal glomerulus.

Importance

For 200 years, proteinuria has been a test for kidney disease. For 150 years, physicians had detected proteinuria qualitatively by either heating and acidifying urine, or by adding concentrated nitric acid and observing the white precipitate. This became a little safer in 1923 when sulphosalicylic acid could be added instead.

Quantitative tests were time-consuming and prone to interference; they involved precipitating and washing the protein and then measuring it either with a biuret reaction (violet colour with alkaline copper sulphate, developed in 1847) or the Kjeldahl method (digestion of protein with concentrated sulphuric acid, developed in 1883), followed by measuring the ammonium liberated by a Nessler reaction (yellow colour with mercury iodide salt, developed in 1856). Folin in Boston, USA (who had also worked on the Jaffe reaction for measurement of creatinine), collaborating with Hsien Wu from China, discovered that the reagent phosphotungstic-phosphomolybdic acid could precipitate all the protein in blood without absorbing non-protein constituents (known as the Folin–Wu method). This was developed for the analysis of blood samples, but the same methodology was used for quantitative measurements of proteinuria. In 1951, Lowry modified this reaction by adding alkaline copper solution and produced the most cited paper ever (over 200,000 citations; Lowry *et al.*, 1951). Immunoassays developed in 1963 offered a more specific answer, and other protein-binding colour reactions such as Coomassie blue also came into use in the same year.

With the development of nephrology as a speciality, quantification of proteinuria became important: nephrotic-range proteinuria was defined as >3 g/day, and the trajectory of proteinuria became important in the management of glomerulonephritis and later the treatment of progressive renal failure with angiotensin-converting enzyme (ACE) inhibitors. However, 24 h collections of urine were difficult for both patient and clinician.

In 1983, Ginsberg and colleagues published a paper on the 'Use of single voided urine samples to estimate quantitative proteinuria' (Ginsberg *et al.*, 1983). It was a huge advance to show that one could measure proteinuria easily and accurately at every clinic visit and follow the trajectory of proteinuria, although it took more than 20 years for this method to render the 24 h protein collection obsolete. But, in fact, the methodology had been designed, investigated, and reported 13 years earlier by paediatricians at The Hospital for Sick Children, Great Ormond Street, London, so on this occasion I have ignored Osler's adage and selected the paper of Barratt, McLaine, and Soothill.

References

Ginsberg JM, Chang BS, Matarese RA, Garella S (1983). Use of single voided urine samples to estimate quantitative proteinuria. *N Engl J Med* **309**, 1543–1536.

Lowry OH, Rosebrough NJ, Farr AL, Randall RJ (1951). Protein measurement with the Folin phenol reagent. *J Biol Chem* **193**, 265–275.

3.4 Measurement of glomerular filtration rate in man using a ^{51}Cr-edetic-acid complex

Authors

ES Garnett, V Parsons, N Veall

Reference

Lancet 1967 **i**, 818–819.

Abstract

^{51}Cr complexed with edetic acid (^{51}Cr-E.D.T.A.) can be prepared in a form which is stable when auto-claved and in vivo. It does not bind to protein or enter red blood-cells and excretion via the gut is insignificant. The renal clearance, as measured by the continuous-infusion technique, is the same as that of inulin. Equilibration with interstitial fluid in non-oedematous patients takes less than 2 hours and there is no detectable extrarenal uptake so that the "slope" method based on 2–4-hour plasma-activity measurements can be used as a simple routine procedure. Results obtained in this way accord well with 24-hour endogenous creatinine clearance data, but the technique is not applicable to oedematous patients where equilibration is delayed. ^{51}Cr-E.D.T.A. seems to be eminently suitable for clinical use.

Importance

The concept of renal (urea) clearance had been described in France by Ambard and Weil in 1912 by comparing urea concentration in blood and urine. This was developed by Van Slyke in New York, who produced the standard method for blood urea clearance (volume of blood that excretion by kidneys clears of urea per minute). In 1921, they reported its clinical validity when performed during water diuresis, and then standardized it to the surface area (1.73 m^2) of the average American person aged 25 years (McIntosh *et al.*, 1928). Until this time, opinions had been divided between urine as a pure secretion and a process that involved filtration and reabsorption.

In 1926, Rehberg, in Copenhagen, noted that creatinine was the substance with the highest concentration ratio according to the values given for blood and urine. The amount of creatinine in blood was, however, so small, and its estimation so uncertain, that he used exogenous (ingested) creatinine and proposed that its clearance was equivalent to the GFR. In 1937, Popper and Mandel described endogenous 'chromogen' clearance as a measure of GFR (see paper 3.2).

In 1935, Shannon and Smith compared the renal excretion of (exogenous) creatinine in man with inulin and showed that tubular secretion of creatinine could be blocked by phlorizin. In the same paper, they also reported that the sugar inulin was an ideal substance to examine pure glomerular filtration, and this method remains the gold standard for measuring GFR (Shannon and Smith, 1935).

The problem with all clearances methods was that they depended on accurate, timed urine collections (sometimes with catheterization) and often the constant infusion of molecules like inulin. In the 1940s, many groups investigated single injection techniques using inulin and mannitol, but the methods for measuring blood concentrations were not appropriate for routine clinical use. The advance came with radionuclides conjugated to tracer molecules that could be injected safely either as a constant infusion or as a single shot. ^{51}Cr-EDTA and ^{125}I-iothalamate have been most widely used.

In 1967, Garnett and colleagues first described the use of ^{51}Cr-EDTA in man. Their paper in the *Lancet* principally compared inulin clearance with ^{51}Cr-EDTA using the same continuous infusion technique and timed urine collection. The techniques showed excellent correlation (r . 0.995). They went on to examine the correlation between a 'single-shot' technique and 24 h creatinine clearance and found a good correlation. Further studies soon confirmed that the single-shot technique correlated well with inulin clearance (Chantler *et al.*, 1969).

References

Chantler C, Garnett ES, Parsons V, Veall N (1969). Glomerular filtration rate measurement in man by the single injection methods using 51Cr-EDTA. *Clin Sci* **37**, 169–180.

McIntosh JF, Möller E, van Slyke DD (1928). Studies of urea excretion. III: the influence of body size on urea output. *J Clin Invest* **6**, 467–843.

Shannon JA, Smith HW (1935). The excretion of inulin, xylose and urea by normal and phlorizinized man. *J Clin Invest* **14**, 393–401.

3.5 Using standardized serum creatinine values in the Modification of Diet in Renal Disease study equation for estimating glomerular filtration rate

Authors

AS Levey, J Coresh, T Greene, LA Stevens, YL Zhang, S Hendriksen, JW Kusek, F Van Lente

Reference

Annals of Internal Medicine 2006, **145**, 247–254.

Abstract

Background: Glomerular filtration rate (GFR) estimates facilitate detection of chronic kidney disease but require calibration of the serum creatinine assay to the laboratory that developed the equation. The 4-variable equation from the Modification of Diet in Renal Disease (MDRD) Study has been re-expressed for use with a standardized assay.

Objective: To describe the performance of the revised 4-variable MDRD Study equation and compare it with the performance of the 6-variable MDRD Study and Cockcroft-Gault equations.

Patients: 1628 patients with chronic kidney disease participating in the MDRD Study.

Measurements: Serum creatinine levels were calibrated to an assay traceable to isotope-dilution mass spectrometry. GFR was measured as urinary clearance of ^{125}I-iothalamate.

Results: Mean measured GFR was 39.8 mL/min per 1.73 m^2 (SD, 21.2). Accuracy and precision of the revised 4-variable equation were similar to those of the original 6-variable equation and better than in the Cockcroft-Gault equation, even when the latter was corrected for bias, with 90%, 91%, 60%, and 83% of estimates within 30% of measured GFR, respectively. Differences between measured and estimated GFR were greater for all equations when the estimated GFR was 60 mL/min per 1.73 m^2 or greater.

Conclusions: The 4-variable MDRD Study equation provides reasonably accurate GFR estimates in patients with chronic kidney disease and a measured GFR of less than 90 mL/min per 1.73 m^2. By using the re-expressed ff Study equation with the standardized serum creatinine assay, clinical laboratories can report more accurate GFR estimates.

Importance

Although by 1935 inulin clearance had been established as the gold standard for measuring GFR in research, for routine clinical purposes a 24 h creatinine clearance was the best available test until the mid-1960s. Apart from its inconvenience for doctor and patient alike, it had a large error of around ±20%.

In 1957, Effersoe, in Copenhagen, found a close arithmetic correlation between log-transformed serum creatinine and log creatinine clearance. From this relationship, he derived nomograms that predicted the clearance from the serum creatinine.

It seems to have been Edwards and Whyte (1959), in Sydney, Australia, who first recognised that GFR correlated closely with the reciprocal creatinine and derived a simple equation for estimating GFR [(96.8/serum creatinine) – 4, for males]. In 1971, Jellife modified these equations and added a factor for age, but nobody seems to have taken much notice until Cockcroft and Gault published their equation in 1976. Although their formula ruled for 30 years, it was derived from data on hospitalized men with more or less normal renal function, whose mean weight was 72 kg, with a guestimate correction for women (15% less). If it were to be used today, the creatinine value should be increased by 30% to correlate with the contemporary methods of 1976. Also in 1976, Schwartz, Haycock and colleagues published a method for eGFR in children that is still in use:

eGFR = k (constant) × height/creatinine.

During the 1990s, a series of papers was published with data from the Modification of Diet in Renal Disease (MDRD) Study. Over 1600 patients were enrolled, and part of their evaluation was serial clearance tests using the renal clearance of ^{125}I-iothalamate. From these data, new formulae were derived in 1999 that were more suitable for estimating GFR of <60 ml/min and required creatinine, age, urea, and albumin with correction for gender and race. In this landmark paper (2006), a simplified version was published that did not require urea and albumin and this 'four-variable' method (for eGFR) has been widely adopted in the routine reporting of urea and creatinine results:

eGFR = $175 \times$ standardized $S_{cr}^{-1.154} \times$ age$^{-0.203} \times 1.212$ (if black) $\times 0.742$ (if female).

The simplicity, and therefore wide applicability, of this equation has been pivotal in generating a swathe of novel data about the epidemiology of chronic kidney disease. Although not without controversy, these data have transformed the way that chronic kidney disease is studied on a population basis.

3.6 Aspiration biopsy of the kidney

Authors

P Iversen, C Brun

Reference

American Journal of Medicine 1951, **11**, 324–330.

Abstract

The authors describe a technic [sic] for aspiration biopsy of renal tissue in man. Biopsies from two normal individuals and from five patients with various renal disorders are reported in preliminary form. At the same time determinations of discrete kidney functions were made in these patients. The authors consider that continued studies of material removed by aspiration biopsy of the kidney may contribute materially to solution of the pathophysiologic problems of the heterogeneous group of renal diseases generally termed 'lower nephron nephrosis.'

Importance

'Biopsy' (first defined by Besnier in 1895) became useful towards the end of the nineteenth century with the development of good histology and microbiology. Surgical biopsy of the kidney at incidental operations, particularly the then-fashionable renal decapsulation, was performed from 1900 to 1930.

Needle biopsy of the liver, although first performed in 1895, was adopted after the report by Iversen and Roholm in 1939. Percutaneous needle renal biopsy followed after successful liver biopsy, and also after demonstration of the value of aspiration needle biopsy in tumours of the kidney. In addition, a number of physicians obtained renal tissue by accident and without problems during intended biopsies of the liver. Nils Alwall of Sweden performed the first systematic aspiration needle biopsies of the kidney in 1944, but did not publish his results because of an early death of one of his patients, which led him to abandon the technique. However, when Iversen and Brun in Copenhagen, using the same technique that they described for liver biopsy, published their results in 1951, a number of physicians around the world immediately began to attempt renal biopsy, using cutting as well as aspiration techniques. Success was inconsistent and operator dependent: the refinements of technique and needles were introduced by the group in Chicago led by Robert Kark, and their advocacy of the technique and their training of many physicians in its performance rapidly led to widespread acceptance (Cameron and Hicks, 1997).

New techniques of immunofluorescence (in 1956) and electron microscopy (in 1957) arrived at the same time, so that the technique could be fully exploited. The performance and interpretation of renal biopsies became, along with classical whole-organ and nephron physiology and the introduction of dialysis and transplantation, powerful agents determining the emergence of nephrology as a specialty around 1960 (Cameron and Hicks, 1997). In 1961, the CIBA Foundation organized a meeting on 'Renal biopsy: clinical and pathological significance' to which all the key international groups were invited. Together, the participants already had experience of over 5000 renal biopsies.

Reference

Cameron JS, Hicks J (1997). The introduction of renal biopsy into nephrology from 1901 to 1961: a paradigm of the forming of nephrology by technology. *Am J Nephrol* **17**, 347–358.

3.7 Ultrasonics in renal biopsy: an aid to determination of kidney position

Author

GM Berlyne

Reference

Lancet 1961, **ii**, 750–751.

Abstract

The use of a simple ultrasonic flaw-detector is described to determine depth and position of kidney as an aid to renal biopsy. This method may make biopsy in uraemic patients more practicable.

Importance

Until the late 1970s, kidneys were imaged radiologically either by plain abdominal X-ray (1896), retrograde pyelogram (1906), or intravenous urogram (1929). Before that, there was only cystoscopy (1885). This was fine for urological investigation as the excretion of radiocontrast by the kidneys gave good definition of the calyces and collecting system and information about the parenchyma as well. Unfortunately, as renal function deteriorates, nephrological information decreases so that in acute renal failure little more than a vague nephrogram might be seen. If obstruction was suspected, delayed films (up to 24 h later) were taken or a cystoscopy and retrograde examination might be necessary.

With the development of ultrasound, all this changed. Ultrasound had originally been developed as a clinical tool in obstetrics, allowing imaging of the fetus without exposure to radiation (Woo, 2006), and was soon applied in nephrology. In a few seconds, the difference between chronic renal failure, obstruction or normal-sized kidneys suggesting an acute problem could readily be obtained. The impact of ultrasound was so clear and overwhelming that it seems it did not require people to write papers to convince others. As a result, there is almost no literature. Berlyne's seminal paper is the first identified report of renal ultrasound and focuses mainly on the value of ultrasound in aiding renal biopsy, rather than its broad applicability in the investigation of renal disease. This was published, as a letter to the *Lancet*, in 1961; yet it was another 20 years before ultrasound was adopted widely into clinical practice and its diagnostic value was properly appreciated. Why did it take 20 years to reach the ward? The early machines were expensive, but, more importantly, the poor resolution of these early images meant that few were at first convinced of the full potential of the technique.

Reference

Woo J (2006). A short history of the development of ultrasound in obstetrics and gynecology. http://www.ob-ultrasound.net/history1.html

3.8 Urography versus DMSA scan in children with vesicoureteric reflux

Authors

NP Goldraich, OL Ramos, IH Goldraich

Reference

Pediatric Nephrology 1989, **3**, 1–5.

Abstract

Following the diagnosis of primary vesicoureteric reflux, identified as part of the investigation of urinary tract infection, 299 refluxing kidneys in 202 children (aged 0–14 years) were prospectively evaluated using intravenous urography (IVU) and the DMSA renal scan at least 4 weeks after urine infection. There was 88% concordance between IVU and the DMSA scan, but in 12% there were discrepancies manifested in 37 kidneys from 31 children. Thirty-four kidneys were normal on IVU but showed scars of reflux nephropathy (RN) on the technetium 99m-dimercaptosuccinic acid (DMSA) renal scan; 4 of these (2 infants and 2 pre-school children) had severe generalized changes on scanning. Three kidneys were normal on DMSA scan and, although abnormal on initial IVU, were considered to be normal when this was repeated. During a follow up period of 5 years an annual DMSA was undertaken in 194 patients and the renal scars remained unchanged in all except 1 child. The IVU was repeated 1–3 years after the initial study in 31 children in which the results of the first imaging did not agree. In 28 patients (34 kidneys) in which the initial IVU was normal but the DMSA abnormal, IVU evidence of scarring emerged in 30 of 34 kidneys, including the 4 patients with severe generalized damage on the DMSA. We conclude that abnormalities detected by the DMSA scan may precede the radiological findings, especially in young children. Even severe RN can be established in kidneys that appear normal on the IVU.

Importance

The use of radioisotopes to image body organs has a short history. Most commonly used today is technetium-99m (^{99m}Tc), which was only discovered in 1937. The first isotope renograms provided qualitative information on dynamic renal function (renal blood flow, ureteric obstruction). In 1956, Taplin, in Los Angeles, used radio contrast (diodrast) labelled with ^{131}I. This was soon followed by ^{125}I-hippuran, which was rapidly eliminated by tubular secretion, and between 1960 and 1964, its role in acute renal failure, obstruction and renal transplant became established. Hippuran was eventually replaced in 1970 by ^{99m}Tc-diethylene triamine pentaactate (^{99m}Tc-DTPA), which was excreted by glomerular filtration, and in 1986 by ^{99m}Tc- mercapto-acetyl-triglycine (^{99m}Tc-MAG3), which was excreted by tubular secretion.

Renal imaging (scintigraphy) required a compound that was taken up and retained by the kidneys. This was first achieved with mercurial salts in 1960: with ^{203}Hg- chlormerodrin and then ^{197}Hg-chlormerodrin. ^{99m}Tc-dimercaptosuccinic acid (^{99m}Tc-DMSA) was introduced in 1974 as a cortical marker that was extracted by tubular cells (by a different mechanism to hippuran and MAG3). It provided both morphological information and quantitative measurement of individual renal function. It avoided some of the problems of intravenous urography (IVU): it did not require preparation of the patient, was not affected by bowel gas, and avoided exposure to contrast medium; it also gave better visualization of the renal parenchyma than IVU due to the combination of posterior and oblique views, and the radiation dose was significantly less than with IVU.

From the start, it was promoted as providing superior imaging of the renal cortex, but it was this paper by Goldraich and her colleagues from Porto Alegre, Brazil, that established DMSA as the 'gold standard' in renal imaging for the detection of scarring and asymmetry in children with vesico-ureteric reflux. Their study provided powerful evidence that DMSA scanning was more sensitive than IVU in identifying renal parenchymal scars in infants and children.

3.9 Studies with a new colorimetric test for proteinuria

Authors

AH Free, CO Rupe, I Metzler

Reference

Clinical Chemistry 1957, **3**, 716–727.

Abstract

A color reaction of protein has been formulated into two simple colorimetric tests for protein in urine; one is a tablet test, consisting of a salicylate buffer and bromphenol blue, and the other is a strip test, consisting of a paper strip impregnated with a citrate buffer and tetrabromphenol blue. The basic principle in both tests is that of 'protein error of indicators.' Experiments with approximately 5000 urines, taken from both hospital patients and normal subjects, reveal that these tests are simple, rapid, accurate, sensitive, specific, and capable of being used with turbid urines.

Importance

Given the primacy of detecting proteinuria for the diagnosis of renal disease, dipstick testing for proteinuria has had a huge impact (Voswinckel, 1994).

In the mid-nineteenth century, testing urine for protein or blood used 'wet chemical' methods that were time-consuming and impractical. Reagents had to be made up freshly (copper sulfate and alkali solutions for sugar) or were dangerous (concentrated nitric acid for protein). In 1850, Maumené, in Paris, used wool strips impregnated with stannous chloride that, when dipped in urine containing sugar, turned black when heated. Developing the theme of dry chemistry, in 1880, Pavy at Guy's Hospital in London, developed pellets containing copper sulfate and caustic potash (potassium hydroxide) that could be dropped into urine to detect sugar. Even more successful was George Oliver, who practised in Harrogate, Yorkshire, in the UK, when he was not doing physiology research at University College London and discovering adrenaline (in 1883). His urinary test papers were strips of filter paper impregnated with different reagents required to test for sugar and protein. In his *Lancet* article (Oliver, 1883, and then best-selling book) 'On bedside urine testing', he reported that potassio-mercuric-iodide (white precipitate) or potassium ferrocyanide were equally effective in acidified urine (using citric acid). This technology then seems to have moved to Germany and the methods are not found in British textbooks.

Unrelated to this entrepreneurial science, Sørensen in 1902 described a colour reaction that occurs on adding protein to a solution containing a colour indicator, independent of any change in pH, that was called the 'protein error of indicators' (Sørensen, 1909). But the hero of spot-testing analysis (Tüpfelreaktion) is Fritz Feigl (1891–1971), Professor of Chemistry in Vienna until he had to leave in 1938. His career eventually continued in Brazil. His method was first published in 1921 and was followed by over 300 more papers. In 1937, he described the detection of protein using tetrabromophenolphthalein, which produced a deep blue colour independent of any change in urinary pH.

Subsequently, dipstick technology was developed by the pharmaceutical industry. In 1941, the Ames' 'Clinitest' for sugar was, despite all the patents taken out, a recapitulation of Pavy's tablets.

On dipsticks for protein, there have been very few publications. In fact, there is probably only one of significance, selected here, written by Free and his colleagues working at the Ames Corporation. Their new test for protein was colorimetric and could be performed on turbid urines without filtration. The first strip test or stick (Albustix) was yellow and turned green in the presence of protein—as it still does. Their paper cites none of the preceding history except for Sørensen's paper.

The emphasis in management of kidney disease is shifting to early detection and primary care intervention, and the dipstick test of urine to find protein and blood is a cornerstone of this approach.

References

Oliver G (1883). On bedside urinary tests. *Lancet* **i**, 139–140, 190–192.

Sørensen SP (1909). Über die Messung und die Bedeutung der Wasserstoff ionen Konzentration bei Enzymatischen Prozessen. *Biochem Z* **21**, 131–304.

Voswinckel P (1994). A marvel of colors and ingredients. The story of urine test strip. *Kidney Int* (Suppl.) **47**, S3–S7.

3.10 Traité des maladies des reins [Treatise on kidney diseases]

Author

P Rayer

Reference

Three volumes. Published by J. B. Baillière, Paris (1839–1841).

Summary

The microscopic examination (of urine) shall promptly determine the number and nature of the elements of deposits, particularly aided when the case requires, by the use of reactive chemicals. Without microscopic inspection, the search for organic materials, mucus, debris epithelium, small amounts of pus or blood, spermatic animalcules, offers insurmountable difficulties, and determination of amorphous or crystalline material in urine, uric acid, urates, phosphates, of cystine, may be made in the ordinary chemists, with the aid of several analysis long and complicated. So I cannot understand the reluctance of most doctors to use a microscope for the examination of urine.

Importance

The first description of microscopy applied to urinalysis was in 1630 by Nicolaus de Peiresc in Provence, who observed crystalluria (Cameron, 2010). Subsequent contributions often relied on novel advances in optics. In 1665, Robert Hooke, in London, using a compound microscope with three lenses, published in his book *Micrographia* a detailed description of crystalluria, whilst Hermann Boerhaave observed in 1744 that crystals could form from normal urine.

The introduction of achromatic lenses in 1820 reduced distortion from 19 to 3%, and Paris, led by the work of Alfred Donné in 1831, became the centre of the new science of urine microscopy. Vigla and Rayer, in 1837 at the Hôpital de la Charité, used microscopy routinely to examine urine and described its cellular components in health and disease. These findings were first reported by Vigla in 1837 and then extended and illustrated in Rayer's three-volume text selected here. Becquerel, in 1841 in Paris, described dysmorphic red cells in Bright's disease, whilst Simon, in Berlin in 1842, described tubular casts in urine.

In 1890s, the introduction of apochromatic lenses, which reduced chromatic aberration and improved magnification, brought further advances. In 1897, Rieder showed the benefits of staining the centrifuged urine (with Sudan black), whilst in 1925, the new technique of polarized light led to the description by Fritz Munk of birefringent bodies in the (vague) shape of a Maltese cross that were caused by lipid droplets in tubular cells.

Some of the most important work ever performed on the make-up of urine was by Thomas Addis, the Scottish born physician, who settled in San Francisco and, *inter alia*, produced in 1926 detailed quantitation of normal ranges of cellular components in healthy students that are still used as reference values today.

In 1966, the new science of immunofluorescent-labelled antibodies was used by McQueen to described Tamm–Horsfall protein (uromodulin) as the main constituent of a tubular cast.

What finally liberated the subject from the specialist laboratory to a routine bedside investigation was the availability of phase-contrast microscopy described in 1968 by Brody, Webster, and Kark. Using this technique, Fairley and Birch, in Melbourne in 1982, rediscovered dysmorphic red cells as a feature of glomerular bleeding.

However, it is Pierre François Olive Rayer who should be recognized as the father of renal microscopy (Androutsos, 2001). He became a good friend of Richard Bright, but at the outset of his studies was probably unaware of Bright's findings and reproduced many of them. It was probably Rayer who first used the term Bright's disease (*maladie de Bright*).

References

Androutsos G (2001). Pierre-François-Olive Rayer (1793–1867): one of the founders of modern uro-nephrology. *Prog Urol* **11**, 562–567.

Cameron JS (2010). Historical introduction. In: *The Urinary Sediment: an Integrated Review*, 3rd edn, pp. 1–16. Edited by G Fogazzi. Milano: Elsevier-Masson.

Chapter 4

Inherited renal disease

Katherine A. Hillman and Adrian S. Woolf

Introduction

It is evident that most children with end-stage renal disease (ESRD) have congenital structural kidney malformations, which may have a genetic basis, or have epithelial diseases such as congenital nephrotic syndrome or the nephronophthises, which are clearly heritable. Other children have inherited kidney disorders, such as salt- or water-losing tubulopathies, which, although not usually causing ESRD, can nevertheless cause much morbidity. In adult nephrology, genetic disease may sometimes be less well appreciated, but it can certainly be present, most obviously in kindreds with cystic kidney disease and Alport syndromes. Major discoveries about the genetic bases of well-known kidney and renal tract diseases have been made over the past few decades, and several of the highlights are discussed in this chapter. In addition, 'new' renal genetic and familial disorders continue to be described, and more will surely follow.

The best reference tool for nephrologists wanting to learn about clinical and genetic aspects of inherited kidney and renal tract diseases is certainly the web-based, constantly updated resource Online Mendelian Inheritance in Man (OMIM; http://www.ncbi.nlm.nih.gov/omim). In clinical practice, it is feasible to seek mutations in an increasing selection of genes associated kidney disease, for example through the UK Genetic Testing Network (http://www.ukgtn.nhs.uk/gtn/Home). Nephrologists are not currently trained in genetic counselling, so such testing should be undertaken in close consultation with experts trained in clinical genetics, ideally in joint clinics (Adalat *et al.*, 2010). As well as helping physicians and patients understand why a disease has occurred, finding mutations opens up the possibility of earlier diagnosis, which is useful if there are prospects for therapeutic interventions. The better understanding of renal cell biology and pathogenesis that follow genetic insights are now generating knowledge that can lead to the design of novel therapies.

The landmark papers selected for this chapter cover genetic aspects of renal development, cystic disease, and glomerular and tubular disorders. We have chosen to present them chronologically, as this highlights the importance of early studies based on careful and thorough clinical and laboratory observations. Such studies have laid the phenotypic groundwork that facilitated the explosion of knowledge about single-gene disorders from the mid-1980s onwards. In particular, in papers 4.6 and 4.10, we see how investigating aberrant biological pathways controlled by mutated genes opens the potential for therapeutic intervention.

Reference

Adalat S, Bockenhauer D, Ledermann SE, Hennekam RC, Woolf AS (2010). Renal malformations associated with mutations of developmental genes: messages from the clinic. *Pediatr Nephrol* **11**, 2242–2255.

4.1 Hereditary familial congenital haemorrhagic nephritis

Author

AC Alport

Reference

British Medical Journal 1927, **i**, 504–506.

Abstract

Hereditary familial or congenital nephritis is a definite entity, and the kidneys in these patients are more susceptible to damage by the toxin of an unknown organism than is the case in the normal person. The organism probably belongs to the streptococcal group…Deafness is a marked feature in nearly all these cases. The male members of a family tend to develop nephritis and deafness and do not as a rule survive. The females have deafness and haematuria and live to an old age. [Extract.]

Importance

Cecil Alport wrote this landmark paper when based at St Mary's Hospital in London. It is the 'classical' clinical description of what we now call Alport syndrome, although several of his, and similar, cases had been reported previously in the medical literature. Alport detailed the clinical features of a four-generation kindred, with women passing on the disorder to their sons. He noted that males were severely affected with 'nephritis' (haematuria, proteinuria, and renal failure), together with deafness, whereas the affected females had a milder clinical course. Looking back, we can see this explained by the transmission of a mutated gene located on the X chromosome, and over 60 years later it was reported that X-linked Alport syndrome is caused by mutations of the *COL4A5* gene (Barker *et al.*, 1990), coding for a collagen chain normally found in the mature glomerular basement membrane (GBM), as well as in the ear. We now realize that 'Alport syndrome' is heterogeneous, with rarer, autosomal recessive forms associated with mutations of genes coding for α3(IV) and α4(IV) collagen chains (Mochizuki *et al.*, 1994) also present in mature GBM; hence, heterozygous carriers also have haematuria, although they only rarely get renal failure, having only thinning of the GBM rather than the major structural disruptions found in the full-blown Alport syndrome present in homozygotes. More recently, another hereditary proteinuric nephropathy, called Pierson syndrome, has been found to be caused by mutations of *LAMB2* encoding a laminin chain also found in the mature GBM (Zenker *et al.*, 2004). Interestingly, Alport himself considered that the inherited renal disease he described might be triggered, or even caused, by the kidney being attacked by external agents. Although there is no evidence to support his specific hypothesis in Alport syndrome itself, we do now know that certain genetic glomerular diseases, as for example in some forms of atypical haemolytic uraemic syndrome, are indeed caused by external attack. In some such cases, the glomerular architecture is damaged by a cascade of events, including microangiopathic haemolytic anaemia, associated with genetic deficiency or malfunction of complement factor H (Warwicker *et al.*, 1998; Ying *et al.*, 1999).

References

Barker DF, Hostikka SL, Zhou J, *et al.* (1990). Identification of mutations in the COL4A5 collagen gene in Alport syndrome. *Science* **248**, 1224–1227.

Mochizuki T, Lemmink HH, Mariyama M, *et al.* (1994). Identification of mutations in the α3(IV) and α4(IV) collagen genes in autosomal recessive Alport syndrome. *Nat Genet* **8**, 77–81.

Warwicker P, Goodship TH, Donne RL, *et al.* (1998). Genetic studies into inherited and sporadic hemolytic uremic syndrome. *Kidney Int* **53**, 836–844.

Ying L, Katz Y, Schlesinger M, *et al.* (1999). Complement factor H gene mutation associated with autosomal recessive atypical hemolytic uremic syndrome. *Am J Hum Genet|* **65**, 1538–1546.

Zenker M, Aigner T, Wendler O, *et al.* (2004). Human laminin β2 deficiency causes congenital nephrosis with mesangial sclerosis and distinct eye abnormalities. *Hum Mol Genet* **13**, 2625–2632.

4.2 Hyperplasia of the juxtaglomerular complex with hyperaldosteronism and hypokalemic alkalosis. A new syndrome

Authors

FC Bartter, P Pronove, JR Gill Jr, RC MacCardle

Reference

American Journal of Medicine 1962, **33**, 811–828.

Abstract

A new syndrome, characterized by hypertrophy and hyperplasia of the juxtaglomerular apparatus of the kidneys, aldosteronism resulting from adrenal cortical hyperplasia, and persistently normal blood pressure is described in two patients. Overproduction of aldosterone could not be prevented by sodium loading or by administration of albumin intravenously; it was associated with hypokalemic alkalosis and pitressin-resistant impairment of urinary concentrating ability. In both subjects, increased amounts of circulating angiotensin were demonstrated; infusion of angiotensin II produced rises of blood pressure in both subjects considerably less than the rises induced by comparable doses in normal subjects. The sequence of events, (1) primary resistance to the pressor action of angiotensin, (2) compensatory overproduction of renin and thus of angiotensin, and (3) stimulation of adrenal cortex by angiotensin is consistent with all the information available about the syndrome.

Importance

This landmark paper constitutes the first description of what would become known as 'Bartter syndrome', which ultimately would lead the way to the clinical and then genetic definition of several varieties of this disorder and better understanding of the physiology of the distal tubular epithelia of the nephron. It is now evident that 'Bartter syndrome' is not one disease (Seyberth *et al.*, 2011), and includes the Gitelman-like syndrome variants as well as the recently described EAST (epilepsy, ataxia, sensorineural deafness, tubulopathy) syndome (Bockenhauer *et al.*, 2009). All, however, are characterized by a salt-losing tendency, with the particular additional features (e.g. urinary magnesium wasting and hypo/hypercalciuria) dependent on whether the mutated gene is normally expressed and active in the thick ascending limb of Henle, the distal convoluted tubule, or the cortical collecting duct. So far, all defined genetic varieties of Bartter syndrome are autosomal recessive. In 1996, it was reported that the Gitelman variant of the syndrome is caused by mutation of the gene encoding the thiazide-sensitive Na-Cl co-transporter (Simon *et al.*, 1996a), and in the same year, a classic form of Bartter syndrome was reported to be caused by mutation of the gene encoding the Na-K-2Cl co-transporter (Simon *et al.*, 1996b) normally expressed in the loop of Henle. These genetic studies have also given insights about the function of diuretics, because the various biochemical derangements can be mimicked by actions of specific diuretics—furosemide, thiazide, and amiloride—each targeting different parts of the tubule implicated in Bartter syndromes (Seyberth *et al.*, 2011).

References

Bockenhauer D, Feather S, Stanescu HC, *et al.* (2009). Epilepsy, ataxia, sensorineural deafness, tubulopathy, and KCNJ10 mutations. *N Engl J Med* **360**, 1960–1970.

Seyberth HW, Schlingmann KP (2011). Bartter- and Gitelman-like syndromes: salt-losing tubulopathies with loop or DCT defects. *Pediatr Nephrol* **26**, 1789–1802.

Simon DB, Nelson-Williams C, Bia MJ, *et al.* (1996a). Gitelman's variant of Bartter's syndrome, inherited hypokalaemic alkalosis, is caused by mutations in the thiazide-sensitive Na-Cl cotransporter. *Nat Genet* **12**, 24–30.

Simon DB, Karet FE, Hamdan JM, DiPietro A, Sanjad SA, Lifton RP (1996b). Bartter's syndrome, hypokalaemic alkalosis with hypercalciuria, is caused by mutations in the Na-K-2Cl cotransporter NKCC2. *Nat Genet* **13**, 183–188.

4.3 Normal and abnormal development of the kidney

Author

EL Potter

Reference

Published by Year Book Medical Publishers, Chicago, USA (1972).

Abstract

The more complicated an organ in its development the more subject it is to maldevelopment, and in this respect the kidney outranks most other organs. For a kidney to develop properly, a normal ureteral bud must come in contact with normal metanephric blastema and the two must interact in a normal manner. To understand the structure and function of the mature kidney, it is necessary to understand all aspects of development. The type I (cystic) kidney is an inherited abnormality, usually fatal in the newborn period, which results from a secondary disturbance in newly formed collecting tubules. The intrahepatic bile ducts are increased in size and number. Type II (cystic) kidney is a non-inherited abnormality, fatal in the newborn period if bilateral but ordinarily producing no symptoms in early life if unilateral or segmental. The kidneys are of extremely variable appearance and range from those that grossly seem to be small nubbins of solid tissue to those composed almost entirely of large cysts. The condition appears to result from severe inhibition of function of the ampulla of the ureteral bud. It is characterised by complete abnormality of all collecting tubules and nephrons within affected areas. The type III cystic kidney is most commonly recognised as an inherited abnormality occurring in adult life. It is characterised by the presence of a great number of variably sized cysts in collecting tubules and all portions of nephrons in both kidneys. The most characteristic feature of the type II kidney is the intimate intermixture of normal and abnormal structures. The type IV (cystic) kidney is a non-inherited abnormality characterised by the presence of one or more layers of thin walled supcapsular cysts caused by urinary back pressure exerted during intrauterine life on nephrons in the S stage of development. [Adapted.]

Importance

From the 1930s, Edith Potter worked as a perinatal pathologist in the Chicago Lying-in Hospital where she undertook microdissection and histology studies on human fetuses. She showed how the mechanisms of kidney development and maldevelopment can begin to be deduced from such descriptive data. She documented normal developmental stages, from the kidney's origin at 5 weeks' gestation, to the formation of the first glomeruli at 8 weeks, through to late gestation when nephron formation finishes. She emphasized that new nephrons formed next to ureteric bud branch tips and that the distal of the forming nephron fused with the adjacent collecting duct, which formed from the bud. Potter for the first time clearly distinguished four varieties of cystic kidney. Type I is what we now call autosomal recessive polycystic kidney disease (ARPKD), and type III is predominantly autosomal dominant polycystic kidney disease (ADPKD) but with similar appearances in certain syndromes including tuberous sclerosis. She put to rest the idea that such cysts resulted from nephrons developing in separation from the collecting system. In type I and III kidneys, cysts arose after the main stages of kidney development had been completed. By contrast, cystogenesis in type II and IV kidneys represented aberrant development. The former, exemplified by the multicystic dysplastic kidney, represented a primary failure of nephron induction, while the latter, typically associated with bladder outflow obstruction and urethral valves, was caused by impairment of fetal urine flow with secondary nephron dilatation. As Potter was making her observations, two fundamental scientific breakthroughs were occurring. Firstly, mechanisms of DNA replication (Watson and Crick, 1953) and the genetic code were being unravelled. Secondly, it was demonstrated that the collecting ducts and nephrons arose from mutual induction between epithelial and mesenchymal tissues in embryonic kidneys (Grobstein, 1953). We now know that these tissues signal to each other, for example by secreting growth factors and matrix molecules, and that that when this cross-talk goes wrong, kidney malformations occur (Kerecuk *et al.*, 2008). In retrospect, Potter was not correct about everything—for example, she did not appreciate the familial nature of some type II cystic malformations (e.g. Bingham *et al.*, 2000)—nevertheless, most of her observations and incisive conclusions have stood the test of time.

Her name has been given to 'Potter syndrome', more properly termed 'Potter sequence', where external deformations occur in fetuses, which, because they have severe bilateral kidney malformations, fail to generate urine, which normally constitutes amniotic fluid in the second half of gestation.

References

Bingham C, Ellard S, Allen L, *et al.* (2000). Abnormal nephron development associated with a frameshift mutation in the transcription factor hepatocyte nuclear factor-1β. *Kidney Int* **57**, 898–907.

Grobstein C (1953). Inductive epitheliomesenchymal interaction in cultured organ rudiments of the mouse. *Science*, **118**, 52–55.

Kerecuk L, Schreuder MF, Woolf AS (2008). Human renal tract malformations: perspectives for nephrologists. *Nat Clin Pract Nephrol* **4**, 312–325.

Watson JD, Crick FH (1953). Molecular structure of nucleic acids; a structure for deoxyribose nucleic acid. *Nature* **17**, 737–738.

4.4 A highly polymorphic DNA marker linked to adult polycystic kidney disease on chromosome 16

Authors

ST Reeders, MH Breuning, KE Davies, RD Nicholls, AP Jarman, DR Higgs, PL Pearson, DJ Weatherall

Reference

Nature 1985, **317**, 542–544.

Abstract

Adult polycystic kidney disease (APCKD) is a common and often lethal multi-organ disease with an autosomal dominant pattern of inheritance; approximately 1 in 1,000 people carry the mutant gene. The major pathological abnormality is the development and progressive enlargement of cysts in several organs including the liver, pancreas and spleen as well as the kidneys. The basic biochemical defect which leads to the formation of cysts remains unknown. Cyst development, which is not retarded by any known therapy, leads to irreversible renal failure and death at a mean age of 51 unless dialysis or transplantation are used. Patients with the disease account for 9% of chronic dialysis requirement. The first symptoms tend to occur in the fourth decade, after most patients have reproduced. Presymptomatic diagnosis depends on the ultrasonographic detection of cysts, but exclusion cannot be achieved by this means; 34% of at-risk patients in the second decade and 14% in the third will go on to develop cysts after negative diagnosis. The low sensitivity of diagnostic techniques in this critical age-range imposes severe limitations on genetic counselling and the condition cannot be identified prenatally. Hence we have searched for a linkage marker for APCKD; we show here that the APCKD locus is closely linked to the α-globin locus on the short arm of chromosome 16 ($\zeta = 25.85$, $\theta = 0.05$).

Importance

Previous work had clarified that ADPKD was familial and transmitted in a dominant manner (Dalgaard *et al.*, 1957). This landmark paper is the original description of the genetic linkage of ADPKD to chromosome 16. It focused on several large families from the UK and the Netherlands and employed, fortuitously, DNA probes produced using fragments of the highly polymorphic region of the α-globin gene on chromosome 16, which had just been cloned and partially sequenced in Oxford, UK. The probes hybridized to two allelic fragments of genomic DNA digests from affected families, which segregated with linkage to disease phenotype according to Mendelian laws. This was an early application of this newly designed technology to nephrology research, and led to the possibility of genetic screening for ADPKD. About a decade later, the exact location of the gene, now known as *PKD1*, was pinpointed, again rather fortuitously, in a family in which the gene was bisected by a translocation (16p 13.3), with polycystic kidney disease (PKD) manifesting in individuals with a balanced exchange (Harris *et al.*, 1995). The subsequent identification of the *PKD1* gene and *PKD2*, encoded by the second ADPKD locus, enabled a deeper understanding of the pathogenesis of cyst formation, eventually implicating aberrant function of primary cilia (Nauli *et al.*, 2003) as a key mechanism in ADPKD. Abnormalities of the primary cilia are also now known to be critical in the pathogenesis of other diseases that can feature renal cysts, including ARPKD, oral-facial-digital syndrome type 1, and Meckel–Gruber, Joubert, and Bardet–Biedl syndromes, as well as the nephronophthises (Hildebrandt, 2010). Furthermore, a particularly severe form of PKD is now known to be caused by a 'contiguous' deletion of *PKD1* and the adjacent gene *TSC2* (Brook-Carter *et al.*, 1994), itself implicated in causing tuberous sclerosis.

References

Brook-Carter PT, Peral B, Ward CJ, *et al.* (1994). Deletion of the *TSC2* and *PKD1* genes associated with severe infantile polycystic kidney disease—a contiguous gene syndrome. *Nat Genet* **8**, 328–332.

Dalgaard OZ (1957). Bilateral polycystic disease of the kidneys; a follow-up of 284 patients and their families. *Dan Med Bull* **4**, 128–133.

Harris PC, Ward CJ, Peral B, Hughes J (1995). Polycystic kidney disease. 1: Identification and analysis of the primary defect. *J Am Soc Nephrol* **6**, 1125–1133.

Hildebrandt F (2010). Genetic kidney diseases. *Lancet* **375**, 1287–1295.

Nauli SM, Alenghat FJ, Luo Y, *et al.* (2003). Polycystins 1 and 2 mediate mechanosensation in the primary cilium of kidney cells. *Nat Genet* **33**, 129–137.

4.5 Germline mutations in the Wilms' tumor suppressor gene are associated with abnormal urogenital development in Denys-Drash syndrome

Authors

J Pelletier, W Bruening, CE Kashtan, SM Mauer, JC Manivel, JE Striegel, DC Houghton, C Junien, R Habib, L Fouser, RN Fine, BL Silverman, DA Haber, D Housman

Reference

Cell 1991, **67**, 437–447.

Abstract

Denys-Drash syndrome is a rare human condition in which severe urogenital aberrations result in renal failure, pseudohermaphroditism, and Wilms' tumor (nephroblastoma). To investigate its possible role, we have analyzed the coding exons of the Wilms' tumor suppressor gene (*WT1*) for germline mutations. In ten independent cases of Denys-Drash syndrome, point mutations in the zinc finger domains of one *WT1* gene copy were found. Nine of these mutations are found within exon 9 (zinc finger III); the remaining mutation is in exon 8 (zinc finger II). These mutations directly affect DNA sequence recognition. In two families analyzed, the mutations were shown to arise de novo. Wilms' tumors from three individuals and one juvenile granulosa cell tumor demonstrate reduction to homozygosity for the mutated *WT1* allele. Our results provide evidence of a direct role for WT1 in Denys-Drash syndrome and thus urogenital system development.

Importance

In 1990, it was reported that mutations of the Wilms' tumour gene (*WT1*) on chromosome 11p13 were associated with the commonest type of childhood kidney cancer, known as Wilms' tumour (Call *et al.*, 1990; Gessler *et al.*, 1990). *WT1* encodes a transcription factor that is normally expressed in mammalian kidneys in cells destined to form nephrons (Pritchard-Jones *et al.*, 1990). Indeed, studies in mutant mice that lacked functional WT1 showed that their embryonic kidneys regressed soon after they began to form. The gene is active in developing podocytes, which normally maintain WT1 expression through adult life. When WT1 is mutated, by mechanisms still poorly understood, kidney precursor cell growth and differentiation are reregulated, one result being cancer. WT1 is also normally expressed in fetal gonads (Pritchard-Jones *et al.*, 1990). In the current landmark paper, researchers based in North America defined point mutations of *WT1* in Denys–Drash syndrome, a rare but clinically striking syndrome comprising external sex reversal in males, gonadal tumours, Wilms' tumour, and renal failure associated with mesangial sclerosis and progressive glomerulopathy. Subsequently, *WT1* mutations were also demonstrated in Frasier syndrome, also characterized by male pseudo-hermaphroditism and childhood proteinuria, and nephrotic syndrome, with focal and segmental glomerular sclerosis on renal biopsy, progressing to ESRD in adolescence or early adulthood (Barbaux *et al.*, 1997). Collectively, these studies point to a remarkable multifaceted role for WT1 functioning at multiple levels in the kidney; it is essential first for normal renal development, then acts as a tumour suppressor gene, and finally is required to maintain the healthy biology of the glomerulus.

References

Barbaux S, Niaudet P, Gubler MC, *et al*. (1997). Donor splice-site mutations in WT1 are responsible for Frasier syndrome. *Nat Genet* **17**, 467–470.

Call KM, Glaser T, Ito CY, *et al*. (1990). Isolation and characterization of a zinc finger polypeptide gene at the human chromosome 11 Wilms' tumor locus. *Cell* **60**, 509–520.

Gessler M, Poustka A, Cavenee W, Neve RL, Orkin SH, Bruns GA (1990). Homozygous deletion in Wilms tumours of a zinc-finger gene identified by chromosome jumping. *Nature* **343**, 774–778.

Pritchard-Jones K, Fleming S, Davidson D, *et al*. (1990). The candidate Wilms' tumour gene is involved in genitourinary development. *Nature* **346**, 194–197.

4.6 Molecular identification of the gene responsible for congenital nephrogenic diabetes insipidus

Authors

W Rosenthal, A Seibold, A Antaramian, M Lonergan, MF Arthus, GN Hendy, M Birnbaumer, DG Bichet

Reference

Nature 1992, **359**, 233–235.

Abstract

Antidiuretic hormone (arginine vasopressin) binds to and activates V2 receptors in renal collecting tubule cells. Subsequent stimulation of the Gs/adenylyl cyclase system promotes insertion of water pores into the luminal membrane and thereby reabsorption of fluid. In congenital nephrogenic diabetes insipidus (CNDI), an X-linked recessive disorder, the kidney fails to respond to arginine vasopressin. Here we report that an affected male of a family with CNDI has a deletion in the open reading frame of the V2 receptor gene, causing a frame shift and premature termination of translation in the third intracellular loop of the receptor protein. A normal receptor gene was found in the patient's brother. Both the normal and the mutant allele were detected in his mother. A different mutation, causing a codon change in the third transmembrane domain of the V2 receptor, was found in the open reading frame of an affected male but not in the unaffected brother belonging to another family suffering from CNDI.

Importance

In paper 4.10, we discuss the cell biological effects of arginine vasopressin (AVP) signalling through its type 2 receptor (AVPR2), which induces deregulated growth of collecting duct epithelia in the context of PKD. Long before that insight, nephrologists were aware of nephrogenic diabetes insipidus (NDI), where polyuria and polydipsia were associated with failure of the kidney to concentrate urine when challenged with AVP. In this landmark paper, the gene for a form of congenital X-linked NDI was discovered—it encoded *AVPR2*, normally expressed on the plasma membrane of collecting ducts. Other reports of mutations in different families soon followed. One very large North American kindred of great interest was affected by congenital NDI and shared an Ulster Scot ancestor who arrived in Halifax, Nova Scotia, in 1761 on a ship called *Hopewell* (Bode and Crawford, 1696); the entire kindred share the same stop mutation in *AVPR2* (Bichet *et al.*, 1993). This is a striking example of the 'founder effect', whereby an ancestral mutation is passed on over many generations, becoming pervasive in that population. After AVP binds to its type 2 receptor, water channels are upregulated and inserted into the apical epithelial membrane, allowing passage of water from the lumen, a critical step in urine concentration. Rarer forms of congenital NDI are caused by autosomal recessive or dominant mutations of this aquaporin-2 channel (Deen *et al.*, 1994). Unravelling these pathways gives the exciting prospect of designing drugs that ameliorate some of the severe clinical effects of NDI. For example, some *AVPR2* mutations do not disrupt the gene completely but instead generate an altered protein retained in the endoplasmic reticulum.

Certain cell-permeable antagonists or 'pharmacological chaperones' can stabilize such mutant proteins, allowing them to reach, and function within, the plasma membrane (Los *et al.*, 2010).

References

Bichet DG, Arthus MF, Lonergan M, *et al.* (1993). X-linked nephrogenic diabetes insipidus mutations in North America and the Hopewell hypothesis. *J Clin Invest* **92**, 1262–1268.

Bode HH, Crawford JD (1969). Nephrogenic diabetes insipidus in North America. The Hopewell hypothesis. *N Engl J Med* **280**, 750–754.

Deen PM, Verdijk MA, Knoers NV, *et al.* (1994). Requirement of human renal water channel aquaporin-2 for vasopressin-dependent concentration of urine. *Science* **264**, 92–95.

Los EL, Deen PM, Robben JH (2010). Potential of nonpeptide (ant)agonists to rescue vasopressin V2 receptor mutants for the treatment of X-linked nephrogenic diabetes insipidus. *J Neuroendocrinol* **22**, 393–399.

4.7 Identification of the von Hippel-Lindau disease tumor suppressor gene

Authors

F Latif, K Tory, J Gnarra, M Yao, FM Duh, ML Orcutt, T Stackhouse, I Kuzmin, W Modi, L Geil, L Schmidt, F Zhou, H Li, MH Wei, F Chen, G Glenn, P Choyke, MM Walther, Y Weng, DDR Duan, M Dean, D Glava, FM Richards, PA Crossey, MA Ferguson-Smith, D Le Paslier, I Chumakov, D Cohen, AC Chinault, ER Maher, WM Linehan, B Zbar, MI Lerman

Reference

Science 1993, **260**, 1317–1320.

Abstract

A gene discovered by positional cloning has been identified as the von Hippel-Lindau (VHL) disease tumor suppressor gene. A restriction fragment encompassing the gene showed rearrangements in 28 of 221 VHL kindreds. Eighteen of these rearrangements were due to deletions in the candidate gene, including three large nonoverlapping deletions. Intragenic mutations were detected in cell lines derived from VHL patients and from sporadic renal cell carcinomas. The VHL gene is evolutionarily conserved and encodes two widely expressed transcripts of approximately 6 and 6.5 kilobases. The partial sequence of the inferred gene product shows no homology to other proteins, except for an acidic repeat domain found in the procyclic surface membrane glycoprotein of Trypanosoma brucei.

From Latif F, Tory K, Gnarra J, Yao M, Duh FM, Orcutt ML, Stackhouse T, *et al* (1993) Identification of the von Hippel-Lindau disease tumor suppressor gene. *Science*, **260**, 1317–1320. Reproduced with permission from AAAS.

Importance

Von Hippel–Lindau (VHL) disease confers a dominantly inherited predisposition to tumours including renal cell carcinoma, phaeochromocytoma, and haemoangioblastomas of the central nervous system and retina (Arjumand and Sultana, 2012). The potential to treat effectively or at least ameliorate some of these conditions if detected early, along with almost complete penetrance by the age of 65 years, makes a reliable genetic test invaluable to detect carriers. Previous studies had implicated chromosome 3p25–p26 in VHL, and this landmark paper used positional cloning to investigate over 200 VHL families. It was the discovery of constitutional genetic deletions in several unrelated individuals that led the investigators to look at a more specific region where the VHL gene resides.

The discovery of the gene for this rare cancer syndrome has implications far beyond the scope of VHL disease itself. Individuals with VHL disease are born with all their somatic cells containing a single aberrant allele. During life, a minority of cells lose the second—normal—VHL allele, and these cells are then prone to give rise to tumours. A similar 'two-hit' mechanism may operate in determining whether a kidney tubule will become cystic in ADPKD (Qian *et al.*, 1996). Mutations in VHL are now known to be present in the majority of sporadic renal-cell carcinomas. Functional studies of the VHL protein revealed that it has a central role in modulating the cellular response to hypoxia (Maxwell *et al.*, 1999; Schofield and Ratcliffe, 2004). VHL protein binds to and speeds the degradation of hypoxia-inducible factors, which are transcription factor proteins normally only stabile in the presence of hypoxia. When VHL is mutated and non-functional, the cell is 'fooled' into thinking it is hypoxic and upregulates expression of, for example, erythropoietin and vascular endothelial growth factor, the latter stimulating angiogenesis, allowing tumour growth. A better understanding of these complex intracellular pathways may lead to potential therapies for VHL and other cancers (Arjumand and Sultana, 2012).

References

Arjumand W, Sultana S (2012). Role of VHL gene mutation in human renal cell carcinoma. *Tumour Biol* **33**, 9–16.

Maxwell PH, Wiesener MS, Chang GW, *et al.* (1999). The tumour suppressor protein VHL targets hypoxia-inducible factors for oxygen-dependent proteolysis. *Nature* **399**, 271–275.

Qian F, Watnick TJ, Onuchic LF, Germino GG (1996). The molecular basis of focal cyst formation in human autosomal dominant polycystic kidney disease type I. *Cell* **87**, 979–987.

Schofield CJ, Ratcliffe PJ (2004). Oxygen sensing by HIF hydroxylases. *Nat Rev Mol Cell Biol* **5**, 343–354.

4.8 Dent's disease; a familial proximal renal tubular syndrome with low-molecular-weight proteinuria, hypercalciuria, nephrocalcinosis, metabolic bone disease, progressive renal failure and a marked male predominance

Authors

OM Wrong, AG Norden, TG Feest

Reference

Quarterly Journal of Medicine 1994, **87**, 473–493.

Abstract

We describe a familial form of renal Fanconi syndrome characterized by hypercalciuria, low-molecular-weight proteinuria, nephrocalcinosis and slowly progressive renal failure. Males are much more severely affected than females. The patients studied included 15 males and 10 females, and five families with up to three generations involved. Studies of the two largest families described here have already shown that their disease is inherited on the X-chromosome. The series contains the two unrelated patients originally described by Dent and Friedman in 1964 as 'hypercalcuric rickets'.

Importance

In this paper, Oliver Wrong and colleagues, based in London and Bristol, UK, described several families with members affected by a kidney disorder characterized by nephrocalcinosis, hyper-calciuria, and chronic renal failure. The finding of low-molecular-weight proteinuria further pointed to a primary defect in the proximal tubule of the nephron. Although the condition had originally been described by Charles Dent, a London physician, in 1964, it was Wrong's detailed approach that allowed the phenotype to be defined with sufficient precision to facilitate the sub-sequent genetic studies. Although the other landmark papers in this chapter that are phenotypic descriptions are from earlier generations, this paper demonstrates the enduring value of such an approach. A wonderful feature of this paper is the wealth of clinical blood and urinary biochemi-cal data presented for each patient. A few years later, the genetic basis of this form of familial Fanconi syndrome was revealed as a mutation of the X chromosome gene called *CLCN5*, coding for a chloride channel (Lloyd *et al.*, 1996). A similar condition, comprising vitamin D-resistant rickets and aminoaciduria, is found as part of Lowe's oculocerebrorenal syndrome, caused by mutation of another X-linked gene, *OCRL1*, which encodes an intracellular protein, inositol polyphosphate-5-phosphatase (Attree *et al.*, 1992). Oliver Wrong turned a similar, detailed clini-cal eye to familial renal tubular acidosis (Richards and Wrong, 1972), opening a pathway for eventual discoveries regarding the genetic bases of distal renal tubular acidosis (e.g. Bruce *et al.*, 1997).

References

Attree O, Olivos IM, Okabe I, *et al.* (1992). The Lowe's oculocerebrorenal syndrome gene encodes a protein highly homologous to inositol polyphosphate-5-phosphatase. *Nature* **358**, 239–242.

Bruce LJ, Cope DL, Jones GK, *et al.* (1997). Familial distal renal tubular acidosis is associated with mutations in the red cell exchanger (band 3, AE1) gene. *J Clin Invest* **100**, 1693–1707.

Lloyd SE, Pearce SH, Fisher SE, *et al.* (1996). A common molecular basis for three inherited kidney stone diseases. *Nature* **379**, 445–449.

Richards P, OM Wrong (1972). Dominant inheritance in a family with familial renal tubular acidosis. *Lancet* **ii**, 998–999.

4.9 Mutation of the *PAX2* gene in a family with optic nerve colobomas, renal anomalies and vesicoureteral reflux

Authors

P Sanyanusin, LA Schimmenti, LA McNoe, TA Ward, ME Pierpont, MJ Sullivan, WB Dobyns, MR Eccles

Reference

Nature Genetics 1995, **9**, 358–364.

Abstract

Paired box (*PAX*) genes play a critical role in human development and disease. The *PAX2* gene is expressed in primitive cells of the kidney, ureter, eye, ear and central nervous system. We have conducted a mutational analysis of *PAX2* in a family with optic nerve colobomas, renal hypoplasia, mild proteinuria and vesicoureteral reflux. We report a single nucleotide deletion in exon five, causing a frame-shift of the *PAX2* coding region in the octapeptide domain. The phenotype resulting from the *PAX2* mutation in this family was very similar to abnormalities that have been reported in *Krd* mutant mice. These data suggest that *PAX2* is required for normal kidney and eye development.

Importance

The renal coloboma syndrome had been described several decades earlier, and in this paper, a group from New Zealand were the first to define associated mutations that were inherited in an autosomal dominant manner, tracking with clinical disease. The syndrome includes renal hypoplasia with congenital small kidneys, which can cause ESRD. The mutated gene is called paired-box 2 (*PAX2*) and is a member of a family that is highly conserved from flies to humans. The gene is active, or 'expressed', in early kidney development, where it encodes a transcription factor protein that prevents apoptotic death of kidney progenitor cells. Thus, when the gene is non-functional, fewer nephrons than normal are generated. *PAX2* is also expressed in the developing eye, explaining why affected individuals are sometimes blind; on ophthalmoscopy, optic discs are characteristically very pale. This landmark paper was 'proof of principle' that, in humans, when a nephrogenic gene is mutated, kidney tract malformations can arise. Since publication of this paper in the mid-1990s, the genetic bases of many other human syndromes featuring kidney malformations have been defined. It is currently thought that dominant mutations of hepatocyte growth factor 1β and PAX2 together account for around 10% of children with hypoplastic or dysplastic renal malformations (Weber *et al.*, 2006; Adalat *et al.*, 2009). Rarer genetically defined diseases featuring renal malformations include autosomal dominant branchio-oto-renal syndrome (Abdelhak *et al.*, 1997) and autosomal recessive Fraser syndrome (McGregor *et al.*, 2003). As renal coloboma syndrome can feature vesico-ureteric reflux (VUR), it was hoped that *PAX2* mutations might prove critical in the development of primary (non-syndromic) VUR. However, no PAX mutations have been found in primary VUR, and the genetic basis of this common familial condition, which affects at least 1% of babies, remains elusive.

References

Abdelhak S, Kalatzis V, Heilig R, *et al.* (1997). A human homologue of the *Drosophila eyes* absent gene underlies branchio-oto-renal (BOR) syndrome and identifies a novel gene family. *Nat Genet* **15**, 157–264.

Adalat S, Woolf AS, Johnstone KA, *et al.* (2009). *HNF1B* mutations associate with hypomagnesemia and renal magnesium wasting. *J Am Soc Nephrol* **20**, 1123–1131.

McGregor L, Makela V, Darling SM, *et al.* (2003). Fraser syndrome and mouse blebbed phenotype caused by mutations in *FRAS1/Fras1* encoding a putative extracellular matrix protein. *Nat Genet* **34**, 203–208.

Weber S, Moriniere V, Knüppel T, *et al.* (2006). Prevalence of mutations in renal developmental genes in children with renal hypodysplasia: results of the ESCAPE study. *J Am Soc Nephrol* **17**, 2864–2870.

4.10 Vasopressin directly regulates cyst growth in polycystic kidney disease

Authors

X Wang, Y Wu, CJ Ward, PC Harris, VE Torres

Reference

Journal of the American Society of Nephrology 2008, **19**, 102–108.

Abstract

The polycystic kidney diseases (PKD) are a group of genetic disorders causing renal failure and death from infancy to adulthood. Arginine vasopressin (AVP) V2 receptor antagonists inhibit cystogenesis in animal models of cystic kidney diseases, presumably by downregulating cAMP signaling, cell proliferation, and chloride-driven fluid secretion. For confirmation that the protective effect of these drugs is due to antagonism of AVP, PCK (*Pkhd1*$^{-/-}$) and Brattleboro (*AVP*$^{-/-}$) rats were crossed to generate rats with PKD and varying amounts of AVP. At 10 and 20 weeks of age, PCK *AVP*$^{-/-}$ rats had lower renal cAMP and almost complete inhibition of cystogenesis compared with PCK *AVP*$^{+/+}$ and PCK *AVP*$^{+/-}$ rats. The V2 receptor agonist 1-deamino-8-D-arginine vasopressin increased renal cAMP and recovered the full cystic phenotype of PCK *AVP*$^{-/-}$ rats and aggravated the cystic disease of PCK *AVP*$^{+/+}$ rats but did not induce cystic changes in wild-type rats. These observations indicate that AVP is a powerful modulator of cystogenesis and provide further support for clinical trials of V2 receptor antagonists in PKD.

Importance

This elegant study provided direct evidence of the importance of AVP as a modulator of renal cytogenesis. Cyclic AMP, which is upregulated in collecting duct epithelia when AVP binds to AVPR2, had been identified as a modulator of cystic epithelial growth *in vitro* (Mangoo-Karim *et al.*, 1989). Strikingly, pharmacological blockade of this receptor ameliorates PKD in several animal models (e.g. Gattone *et al.*, 2003), as does reduction of endogenous circulating AVP levels mediated simply by increased water intake (Nagao *et al.*, 2006). This landmark study crossed a genetic PKD rat with the AVP-deficient Brattleboro rat, which suffers from central diabetes insipidus, and found that progression of kidney cysts was remarkably delayed. The cystic phenotype could then be re-induced by treating these double-mutant rats with synthetic AVP. Not only does this provide direct evidence of the role of AVP in cystogenesis and add support to the use of therapeutic blockade of AVPR2 *in vivo*, but the findings raise the possibility of modifying PKD disease progression by manipulating water intake and lowering circulating AVP levels. Indeed, therapeutic studies in humans with ADPKD are now underway, based on the rationale developed from these observations.

References

Gattone VH II, Wang X, Harris PC, Torres VE (2003). Inhibition of renal cystic disease development and progression by a vasopressin V2 receptor antagonist. *Nat Med* **9**, 1323–1326.

Mangoo-Karim R, Uchic ME, Grant M, *et al.* (1989). Renal epithelial fluid secretion and cyst growth: the role of cyclic AMP. *FASEB Jl* **3**, 2629–2632.

Nagao S, Nishii K, Katsuyama M, *et al.* (2006). Increased water intake decreases progression of polycystic kidney disease in the PCK rat. *J Am Soc Nephrol* **17**, 2220–2227.

Chapter 5

Glomerular disease—before 1950

J. Stewart Cameron

Introduction

Nephrology as we know it today was a twentieth-century development. Both dialysis and trans-plantation had their intellectual birth around 1900, and evolved into foci of organized activity around 1950. In contrast, both knowledge of the intimate anatomy and the physiology of the kidney, and the story of the understanding of nephritis and the destruction of the renal parenchyma, both began a century earlier, around 1800 (see Chapters 1 and 2). Thus, it is valuable to glance back at some of the landmark publications before 1950 in clinical aspects of nephritis, the nephrotic syndrome, and renal sclerosis or 'granular kidney', before renal biopsy and new microscopic techniques redefined the field.

This was another era, in which knowledge was disseminated in ways very different from today. Firstly, the number of clinicians and scientists publishing papers and books was tiny. Until 1850, there were only a handful of medical journals, and many authors wrote books or pamphlets, often quite small by today's standards, to publicize their work. Secondly, the epicentre of medical progress was decidedly in Europe during this period, with London, Paris, and a number of German universities from Strasburg in the west to Dorpat in the east contributing new ideas. The USA was relatively barren of major advances in nephrology until almost 1900, except perhaps Tyson and Delafield in the 1880s, and then the effects of the Flexner revolution in US medical education burst out.

Science and academic medicine are today overwhelmingly Anglophone, but this is a recent development. Until 1900 and in some disciplines even 1950, English-speaking physicians usually had to have some command of at least written German or French, in which from 1850 to 1920 many of the major advances were reported.

Publishing was also very different in the nineteenth century. Papers were in general longer, to our ears and eyes often verbose, and subjected to very little editing and, one suspects, little or no review by outside sources; sometimes the author and editor of the journal were the same person! Books were also published more or less as the authors submitted them. The origins of outside peer review (i.e. other than the editor's scrutiny) are obscure, and penetrated slowly and variably during the first half of the twentieth century into medical publishing. The late example of *The Lancet*, which even in the 1960s rarely used outside reviewers, is well known. However, despite many valid criticisms, no superior system than some form of peer review as we know it today has yet been identified.

As elsewhere in this book, selection of papers or books for inclusion in this chapter was arbitrary and personal, and one might change several of the choices without losing much. For example, Cruickshank could be included rather than Wells, George Johnson could be replaced by Samuel Wilks, and Theodor Frerichs or Jacob Loehlein added. German authors of the second half of the nineteenth century suffer from the masterly summary of their work in the book of Volhard and Fahr.

5.1 De ischiade nervosa: commentarius [A commentary on the sciatic nerve]

Author

D Cotugno

Reference

Published by Graeffer, Vienna (1770), pp. 28–29.

Narrative from the text

A soldier, twenty-eight years old, was stationed for many years at Baiae [which is] very mild and damp. About the end of August he was seized with an intermittent quotidian fever, which strangely broke out in dropsy in five days. At the beginning of September he was brought to my sanatorium. He was suffering at this time with immense watery swellings of his whole body, and overwhelmed by the hitherto daily attacks of fever. The dropsy seemed to increase daily, shortly before the paroxysms. The excreta were dry, there was but little urine and he was wholly cast down in mind…[he was treated with ipecac, squills, Peruvian bark and sassafras]…but the urine flowed much less and finally the dropsical swellings seemed to grow…In this case it seemed best to use cream of tartar…the output of urine was increased so that the sick man passed ten or twelve pints of concentrated urine in a night. However since…his drinking had been very slight, it was certain that the enormous quantities of urine were being drawn especially from the waters collected in the dropsy. Although this was shown by the decrease in the distension of the body, it seemed best to settle the argument by a definite experiment, heating the urine. For I had often conclusively shown that the fluid collected under the skin of such dropsical cadavers contained material capable of coagulation, and I hoped that if the sick man passed such fluid by the way of the urine, coagulation would be seen if the material which flowed out were heated; which, as I anticipated, was proved by experiment. For with two pints of this urine exposed to the fire, when scarcely half evaporated, the remainder made a white mass, like egg albumin…[Translated.]

Importance

This small book in Latin contains not only a commentary on the sciatic nerve but also a number of clinical observations on body fluids. The interest for nephrologists of this apparently obscure and irrelevant work is that here we find the first convincing description of urine coagulation under heat and, moreover, in a clinical setting, of the nephrotic syndrome following malaria, common in Italy well into the twentieth century. Cotugno was born in Ruvo, near Bari in Southern Italy in 1736 and died in 1822. He had a notable and productive career (Schena, 1994), married a duchess and became physician to the King of the Two Sicilies, publishing many influential works, particularly in anatomy, including one describing the cochlea.

Cotugno's is the first unequivocal description of coagulable urine, although claims have been made for earlier descriptions by Paracelsus (Eknoyan, 1996) and Frederick Dekkers (Dock, 1922) in the sixteenth and seventeenth centuries, whose observations were, however, muddled and inconclusive. Swelling (or 'dropsy'), described by a number of clinicians from Hippocrates onwards, was regarded as a disease entity in itself. The exception is Theodor Zwinger (1658–1724), a Swiss paediatrician, who, amazingly, described changes in the renal tubules ('*urinae parcae propter obstructus vel compressos tubulos renales*') in accurately described nephrotic children as early as 1722 (Cameron, 2003), a report that remained unknown until rediscovered in 1931. The idea of diseases arising in or from a particular organ awaited Giovanni Battista Morgagni's huge tome of 1761, *De Sedibus et Causis Morborum* [*On the Seats and Causes of Disease*].

Moreover, Cotugno's observation was made as part of a pre-planned 'experiment', characteristic of the new manner of the Enlightenment. The fact that Cotugno's interpretation of the benign significance of coagulable urine was totally wrong does not detract from the modernity of his approach to the problem. His results were widely quoted and discussed during the next half century, notably by Erasmus Darwin in his *Zoonomia,* which had wide readership, and contemporary French observers including Dupuytren. Cotugno's study also donated to us the words 'albuminous' and 'albuminuria', still used today. 'Proteinuria' is an upstart of more than a century later.

References

Cameron JS (2003). Milk or albumin: the history of proteinuria before Bright. *Nephrol Dial Transplant* **18**, 1281–1285.

Dock W (1922). Some early observers of proteinuria. *Ann Med Hist* **4**, 287–290.

Eknoyan G (1996). On the contributions of Paracelsus to nephrology. *Nephrol Dial Transplant* **11**, 1388–1394.

Schena P (1994). Domenico Cotugno and his interest in proteinuria. *Am J Nephrol*, **14**, 325–329.

5.2 On the presence of the red matter and serum of the blood in the urine of dropsy which has not originated in scarlatina

Author

WC Wells

Reference

Transaction of the Society for Improvement in Medical and Chirurgical Knowledge 1812, **3**, 194–240 (read 4 June 1811).

Summary

Wells had already described post-scarlatinal nephritis and its complications (Wells, 1812), and identified not only the 'red' but also the 'serous matter' of blood in the urine in such patients. In this second paper, Wells discusses at length a patient having swollen 'ancles' who suffered an episode of uraemia with reddish, turbid, coagulable urine and appeared likely to die, yet made a recovery; but nine years later still had coagulable urine. Wells had become aware of Cruickshank's work only 'several years' after its publication and used 'nitrous' (actually nitric) acid and heat in 130 dropsical patients, finding serum in the urine of 78. He estimated the quantity by allowing the coagulum to settle, and studied diluted serum to establish that a 1:640 dilution gave a just visible coagulum—a concentration of 120 mg/dl, which corresponds to the limit of 'normal' proteinuria used today, whilst 1:5 gave a solid mass. A large number of healthy people and patients with other disorders were clear, except in patients with venereal disease, three of four showing serum in their urine. All had been treated with mercury, so Wells examined the urine of six similar patients at St Thomas' before and after treatment with mercury: five showed coagulable urine: 'my suspicion…was now confirmed'. Wells ends with patients treated with cantharides, some with success, others without. The patient, Henry Norton, although adult (50 years old), appears to have gone into complete remission. Wells was, of course, aware of the origins of urine, and observed alterations in the kidneys in more than one patient: but he wrote '… the kidneys were much harder than they usually are. The cortical part was thickened and changes in its structure…I do not conclude, however, from these appearances…that the kidnies are always diseased when the urine in dropsy contains much serum'.

Importance

Wells (1757–1817) had an interesting although in many ways sad, lonely, and disappointing life (George, 1996). He was born in Charleston, South Carolina, but went twice to his ancestors' land of Scotland to study, graduating in medicine from Edinburgh in 1780 with an MD thesis. He returned to Charleston, now an independent loyalist state, but when it exchanged sides, he went to loyal Florida and then when the war finished back to now American Charleston, where he was promptly arrested but then rescued by the British Navy. Again he returned to Britain, eventually to St Thomas' Hospital in London where he practised from 1795, without much success, financially or socially, although he was elected a fellow of the Royal Society in 1793. A confirmed bachelor, he was 'a tall thin scraggy personage with long arms and legs he hardly knew what to do with and he wore a brown scratch wig which was never in place'. His papers, now seen as important, were little quoted, although it is clear that his work on renal disease was quietly influential on those who usually never cited him, including Richard Bright.

Wells was the first to study a substantial number of people with and without dropsy for coagulable urine, and, independently of William Cruickshanks's earlier description (Neild, 1996) to have discovered that the urine coagulability depended upon serum leaking into the urine. He narrowly—but decisively—missed the connection between proteinuria, dropsy, and diseased kidneys. The Scots ordnance chemist Cruickshank (died *c*.1811), working in the Woolwich arsenal, might well have been an alternative choice for this selection of landmark papers. Although mainly an able and versatile chemist, he was the first to make the distinction, later also emphasized by Brande in 1806 (Brande, 1812), between dropsy from liver disease (morbid viscera) in which the urine did not coagulate and the 'general' then supposed inflammatory dropsy, in which the urine coagulated with heat or threw a precipitate with several chemical agents. Another physician, who was present at Wells' presentation in 1811, was John Blackall (1771–1860) of Exeter, quoted by Bright. Blackall, whose book on dropsy (Blackall, 1814) ran through five editions up to 1824 (plus a US edition of 1820) and was widely influential, also noted a few diseased kidneys but ignored them. Blackall was also unclear as to whether the serum in the urine represented the relief of the dropsical accumulation (as Cotugno had suggested).

References

Blackall J (1814). *Observations on the Nature and Cure of Dropsies and Particularly on the Presence of the Coagulable Part of the Blood in Dropsical Urine*. Longman, Hurst, Rees, Orme and Brown, London.

Brande WT (1812). An account of some changes from disease in the composition of the urine. *Trans Soc Improve Med Chir Knowl* **3**, 187–193 (delivered 3 February 1807).

George CRP (1996). William Charles Wells (1757–1815)—a nephrologist of the Scottish enlightenment. *Nephrol Dial Transplant* **11**, 2513–2517.

Neild GH (1996). William Cruickshank (FRS-1802) clinical chemist. *Nephrol Dial Transplant* **11**, 1885–1889.

Wells W (1812). Observations on the dropsy, which succeeds scarlet fever. *Trans Soc Improve Med Chir Knowl* **3**, 167–185 (read 4 November 1806).

5.3 Reports of medical cases, vol. 1

Author

R Bright

Reference

Published by Longman Green, London, UK (1827).

Summary

The concept that diseases 'of the kidneys' existed was exposed for the first time: '… I have never yet examined the body of a patient dying of dropsy attended by coagulable urine in whom some obvious derangement was not discovered in the kidneys'. The kidney section contains 24 detailed case reports. Many patients had complications of kidney failure such as fits, pericarditis, and anaemia, all carefully recorded. All but five had died, and the appearances of their kidneys are illustrated in full-colour mezzotints, prepared from sketches taken at the post mortem examination. Bright was wealthy and an artist himself—he could afford the best-quality illustrations, as well as paper and print for the book. Three broad appearances were noted: an injected red kidney, a large pale kidney, and a smaller, hard contracted kidney. These are carefully described and illustrated, but not named or 'classified'. Their coagulable urine and dropsy was attributed to follow the kidney alterations.

A section on 'Observations on the chemical properties of the urine in the foregoing cases' gives in three letters details of the urine in 28 samples from 13 patients, by John Bostock (1773–1846) a chemist and physician and colleague of Bright's at Guy's (Cameron, 1994), whose reputation was lost in the midst of adulation for Bright's work. In fact, Bostock's chapter is one of the most important contributions of the book. Bostock wrote '… we have therefore an example of the blood exhibiting a very great deficiency of albumin at the same time that we observe the mode in which it passes off from the system by means of the kidney, whilst this organ has its appropriate office of secreting urea nearly suspended'. Although the crude measurement of proteinuria was simple, that of urea required huge quantities of urine—but also 'ounces' of blood.

Importance

This landmark publication almost extinguished the previous work in the area reviewed previously, and within 10 years of its publication, the term 'Bright's disease', used to cover most forms of parenchymatous renal disease but above all that with coagulable urine, emerged first in France. Although only about 250 copies of Bright's magnificent book were sold, and it was never translated into any foreign language, its contents influenced many areas of medicine, but none more than the study of kidney disease. An avalanche of papers appeared during the next decade on renal disease, mostly confirming and extending Bright's work on the post-mortem appearances and chemistry of renal disease (the work of Christison and Rayer is dealt with in subsequent papers). The relationship between three main types of kidney described by Bright in patients with albuminuria and/or haematuria with dropsy (the 'angry' petechial, swollen red kidney, the pale enlarged kidney, and the smaller, hard granular kidney) was central to this debate. Some suggested distinct diseases, others the evolution of a single form through stages. Contrary ideas on prognosis emerged, however, that the outlook of patients with coagulable urine could be much better than the very poor prognosis suggested by Bright's initial findings, or that remission might even occur. Bright himself acknowledged this in 1840 in a further 'memoir' (Bright, 1840) and a patient of his (also a doctor), who was given by Bright at most 2 years of life, survived into his

80s. Principally, however, Bright then studied and recorded the cardiac affects of kidney disease, and published two further classic papers in 1836 (Bright, 1836a,b) on this subject, which laid the foundation for the early understanding of hypertension. By 1840, the new improved apochromatic, apomorphic microscopes were coming into clinical use and would revolutionize histopathology; one of Bright's many students, Joseph Toynbee published his work with Bright in this area (Toynbee, 1846), using microdissection—sectioning using a double-bladed knife invented by Gabriel Valentin (1810–1883), had still to come to Britain from Europe.

References

Bright R (1836a). Cases and observations illustrative of renal disease accompanied by the secretion of albuminous urine. *Guy's Hosp Rep* **1**, 38–379.

Bright R (1836b). Tabular view of the morbid appearances 100 cases connected with albuminous urine. *Guy's Hosp Rep* **1**, 380–400.

Bright R (1840). Cases illustrative of renal disease accompanied by the secretion of albuminous urine. Memoir the second. *Guy's Hosp Rep* **5**, 101–161.

Cameron JS (1994). John Bostock MD FRS (1773–1846): physician and chemist in the shadow of a genius. *Am J Nephrol* **14**, 365–370.

Toynbee J (1846). On the intimate structure of the human kidney and on the intimate changes in its several parts undergo in Bright's disease. *Med Chir Trans* **29**, 304–326.

5.4 Traité des maladies des reins [Treatise on kidney diseases]

Author

P Rayer

Reference

Published by J.B. Ballière, Paris, France (1839–1841).

Summary

Rayer began studying diseases of the kidney in 1830, and published this near 2000-page book only 9 years later. Unlike the cool elegance of Bright's large design, this book is in small (octavo) pages, with cramped type and many footnote references in a detail unusual for the period. Moreover, almost every section includes a historical review of the literature of the subject. That on albuminous nephritis ('Bright's disease') runs to more than 100 pages, and has been translated, with contexts (Berry *et al.*, 2005). Volume 2 of the book is almost entirely devoted to albuminous nephritis.

Immediately, Rayer's dissatisfaction with existing clinical and anatomical terminology is discussed and the new term '*néphrite albumineuse*' introduced and defended. A classification of Bright's disease into six anatomical forms is described, two acute and four chronic, and all are illustrated in the atlas. He suggests that his third form corresponds to Bright's first, his fourth to Bright's second, and his sixth to Bright's third. This does not appear to be how we would now allocate them (Berry *et al.*, 2005), and Rayer's extra subtypes now appear somewhat superfluous. Then the varied relationships to clinical findings such as albuminuria and dropsy are described in detail. Rayer was by this time using routine microscopy of the urine, which is recorded throughout the 99 cases discussed under this heading. He did not, however, apply it to renal tissue. Bright had carefully avoided naming his three main forms, and in his paper of 1840, 'Memoir the second' cited in our discussion of paper 5.3, he declined to speculate on whether the relationship between them was three distinct diseases or evolutionary appearances of a single form. Rayer also seems to have been in doubt as to the relationship: 'Nevertheless, [these six forms] may be joined or mixed in a single case …'.

Importance

Rayer has the distinction of publishing two landmark specialist textbooks with atlases, the first on diseases of the skin in 1823 and the second on nephrology (Richet *et al.*, 1991). Rayer's book was the first textbook on renal disease and was a landmark in the beginning of specialism in medicine. Although translated into German, it never appeared in English, and as a result was then—and has been since—undervalued by Anglophone authors and historians. It was also criticized by some influential British physicians at the time, for example Robert Graves of Dublin (Graves, 1964).

Nevertheless, the book covers every aspect of the kidneys, from the size and weights of neonatal kidneys in the first volume to injuries of the urinary tract and diseases of the prostate in the third. Each section has a historical introduction or appendix, and the text references alone make the book invaluable. Rayer was certainly the first historian of nephrology. The section on what the British called Bright's disease and Rayer called '*néphrite albumineuse*' was the dominant description of this topic in Francophone countries, at least until that of Charcot in the 1870s. Rayer distinguished six anatomical forms of Bright's disease, in a fashion similar to Christison (see paper 5.5). He had a microscope installed on the ward so as to be available 24 h a day, and he more or less invented urine microscopy with his pupils, especially Eugène Vigla (1813–1872) (Cameron, 2009).

Given his vast accumulation of knowledge, busy metropolitan practice (he was physician to Louis Philippe and Napoleon III) and his team of active pupils at the Charité Hospital, it is sad to record that in 1842 Rayer was offered, as he already had a number of veterinary contacts and interests, an appointment as Professor in the Faculty of Rural Economy in return for withdrawing from the post of Professor of Medicine. He accepted this possibly political appointment, and published nothing more except two papers on glanders in horses until his death 25 years later.

References

Berry D, Cameron JS, Booker M, Mackenzie C (2005). The history of albuminous nephritis by Pierre-Francois Olive Rayer. *Medl Hist* (Suppl.) **24**, 1–114.

Cameron JS (2009). Historical introduction. In: Fogazzi G, Pontcelli C, Ritz E. *The Urinary Sediment. An Integrated View*, 3rd edn, pp. 1–16. Elsevier-Masson, Milano.

Graves R (1864). *Clinical Lectures on the Practice of Medicine*. Fannin, Dublin, p. 265.

Richet G (1991). Séance consacré à Pierre Rayer (1793–1867). *Histoire des Sciences Mèdicales* **25**, 261–307.

5.5 On granular degeneration of the kidneys and its connexion with dropsy, inflammations, and other diseases

Author

R Christison

Reference

Published by Adam and Charles Black, Edinburgh, UK (1839).

Summary

The first 164 pages of this small book are devoted to a general discussion of the subject, followed by 124 pages devoted to the histories of 'illustrative cases', including a section boldly entitled 'Cases with recovery', which he, unlike Bright, had often observed. Then come sections on the pathogenesis and morbid appearances of the kidney, in which seven forms of disease are described, followed by the symptoms and clinical history. The causes of granular kidney are then explored, the prognosis discussed with particular attention to answering the question of whether the disease is curable, and lastly a section on treatment (Cameron, 2007).

Much of this text on dropsy confirms and little extends Bright's observations. However, the acute phase(s) were scarcely covered by Bright in his book of 1827 (although discussed in his papers of 1836; see paper 5.3), but Christison knitted into the spectrum of what he preferred to call granular kidneys this *acute* phase of congestion, drawing on other work from the 1831 Edinburgh epidemic of scarlatina (Hamilton, 1833). Next, Christison presented new observations on the nature of the disease in the chronic phase. He made also many chemical observations, noting that in these patients the specific gravity of the serum was generally low and confirmed as resulting from a lowered serum albumin. The neurological consequences of granular disease of the kidney remained a puzzle. Christison reached the important conclusion that, in the state of uraemia, '… ultimately its intrinsic result is to overwhelm the functions of the brain, probably the consequence of the blood…being (on the one hand) poisoned by the accumulation of urea, and deprived on the other hand of its colouring matter (haematosine)'.

His detailed observations on anaemia in advanced disease of the kidneys were a landmark. Despite technical inadequacies, he quantitated anaemia in patients with granular kidneys and established normal values identical to those used today.

Importance

Writing just after Christison's book had appeared, Rayer quotes it profusely and with obvious admiration. Richet has called Bright, Rayer, and Christison 'the three musketeers of Nephrology's beginnings' but Christison is the least recognized today. Christison published a long, adulatory review of Bright's 1827 book the following year, and then reported 28 of his own cases of the disease in 1829 (Christison, 1829), followed by a paper identifying the milky serum of a dropsical patient as fat (Christison, 1830). Nine years later came his book on nephritis with further cases, after his standard text on poisonings had appeared, and much more work in forensic science. A main clinical advance by Christison was to establish that the granular kidney was indeed common in all classes of people (which had been hotly disputed), that the acute form was part of the spectrum, and that recovery and relapse could be seen.

Fourcroy and Vauquelin had already speculated as early as 1808 that urea might be the toxic agent, in an extraordinary leap of imagination (Fourcroy and Vauquelin, 1808)—even though incorrect! Completely new, however, were Christison's observations on the anaemia of chronic renal failure. Chevreul in Paris had described 'Hematosine' (haemoglobin) in 1814 as the colouring matter of the blood, and it had been noted by Bright (see paper 5.3) that, in patients with chronic disease, 'after a time, the healthy colour of the countenance fades'. His detailed observations of the anaemia were confirmed by Owen Rees in London, but interest then waned, and many observers in the second half of the century (such as George Johnson and Samuel Wilks) fail to mention anaemia at all in relation to renal disease.

Christison largely used the text of his book to create the sections on kidney disease he contributed the following year to the popular 20-author, six-volume book, *A System of Practical Medicine Composed in a Series of Original Dissertations*, edited by Alexander Tweedie (1794–1884), the second of his two multi-author texts. In this compendium, a new feature is Christison's description of '*suppression of urine*'—acute kidney injury—not related to stones, which is one of the first accounts of this condition and as a clinical description of the untreated state could not be bettered. Christison relates this to acute nephritis and to poisonings, on which he was an expert.

References

Cameron JS (2007). Sir Robert Christison (1797–1882): the man, his times, and his contributions to nephrology. *J R Coll Phys Edin* **37**, 155–172.

Christison R (1829). Observations on the variety of dropsy which depends upon diseased kidney. *Edin Med Surg J* **32**, 262–291.

Christison R (1830). On the cause of the milky and whey-like appearances sometimes observed in the blood. *Edin Med Surg J* **33**, 274–280.

Fourcroy AF, Vauquelin N (1808). Nouvelles expériences sur l'urée. *Ann Mus Hist Nat* **11**, 226.

Hamilton G (1833). On the epidemic scarlatina and dropsical affection which prevailed in Edinburgh in the autumn of 1831. *Edin Med Surg J* **39**, 54–94.

5.6 Lectures on the pathology, diagnosis and treatment of Bright's disease

Author

G Johnson

Reference

Published by Smith Elder, London, UK (1873) (also by Putnam, New York, USA, 1874).

Summary

Johnson, almost forgotten today, published a dozen or more papers on Bright's disease from 1846 (Johnson, 1846) through to this 1873 magnum opus of lectures running serially from 4 January to 28 June in the *British Medical Journal* and also published as a monograph. In 1852, he had also summarized his thoughts in a book (Johnson, 1852). His work started in the mid-1840s, when he first examined urine with a microscope using the new instruments, but kidney tissue was still 'torn with needles' to demonstrate for the first time the fatty infiltration of the kidney accompanying the fatty casts in the urine. He also observed the thickening of the arteriolar walls, as well as confirming Bowman's then recent description of the Malpighian corpuscle, which he concentrated on in a further paper (Johnson). His scientific output continued during studies of many hundreds of patients, the introduction of vegetable and chemical staining in the 1850s and 1860s, proper section cutting (although even in 1873 he was still using Valentin's primitive double-bladed knife of 1837), and finally and most importantly, paraffin embedding of tissue for cutting (introduced by Klebs in 1870). Johnson remained decidedly of the opinion throughout that several distinct separate forms of 'Bright's disease' (defined more or less as proteinuric renal disease) co-existed, separate from each other. One was the acute form of blood-engorged nephritis often seen after scarlatina. Apart from his emphasis on the fatty nature of the large pale kidney, more and more he focused on the microscopic changes in the blood vessels with hypertrophied muscular walls in chronic forms, and related them to the hardened pulse of chronic Bright's disease but through a tortuous—and erroneous—mechanism.

Importance

Johnson (1818–1896), unusually for a doctor at that time, was of humble (farming) stock. He made a number of important contributions but was chronically obstinate in his opinions, and also argumentative, which overshadowed his career to some extent. His first discovery in renal disease was his description of fatty infiltration of the kidney in large, pale dropsical kidneys in 1846. He was an early (although not a pioneer) advocate of urine microscopy, although seemingly ignorant of German work on the urinary sediment in the early 1840s. As he also ignored Traube's work on blood pressure, it is possible that he could not read German. He viewed Bright's disease as three principal and separate disorders—acute, fatty, and granular (not his terminology), with benign albuminurias comprising another category. Despite his pioneering and long-term microscopic studies of arteries from 1850, Robinson makes little mention of high intra-arterial pressure, as advocated by Traube and Senhouse Kirkes in the mid-1850s as a cause of arterial and cardiac hypertrophy, although he does mention it in 1850 with reference to a protective thickening of the capillaries in the corpora Malpighiana. His theories that the muscular arteriolar hypertrophy he so carefully observed and quantitated had a propulsive effect on the blood proved erroneous. He used an ophthalmoscope from the late 1860s, and described fundal appearances in Bright's disease, as did Clifford Allbutt. In 1873, when Johnson's 'lectures' appeared, Akbar Mahomet's use of the sphygmograph to detect 'essential' hypertension was just being described, and Johnson's battle with William Gull and Henry Sutton over their description of 'arteriocapillary fibrosis' in hypertensives was imminent. In his dying year, he published a further book on hypertension and vessel changes to state his and refute others' views (Johnson, 1896).

Johnson was arguably the leading clinician in the field of renal medicine in Britain in the second half of the nineteenth century, his only rival perhaps being Samuel Wilks.

References

Johnson G (1846). On the minute anatomy and pathology of the kidney in Bright's disease of the kidney and on the relation of the renal disease to those of the liver, heart and arteries with which it is associated. *Med Chir Trans* **29**, 1–23.

Johnson G (1850). On the proximate cause of albuminous urine and dropsy, and on the pathology of the blood-vessels in Bright's disease. *Med Chir Trans* **33**, 106–120.

Johnson G (1852). *On the Diseases of the Kidneys with their Pathology, Diagnosis and Treatment, with an Introductory Chapter on the Anatomy and Physiology of the Kidney.* John W. Parker, London.

Johnson, G, (1896). *The Pathology of the Contracted Granular Kidney and the Associated Cardio-arterial Changes.* J&A Churchill, London.

5.7 Pathogénie de certains oedèmes Brightiques: action de chlorure de sodium ingéré [Pathogenesis of certain Bright's oedema: the action of ingested sodium chloride]

Authors

F Widal and A Lemierre

Reference

Bulletins et Mémoires de la Société Médicale des Hôpitaux de Paris 1903, **12**, 678–699; and *Semaine Médicale* 1903, **3**, 199.

Summary

Widal (1859–1929) and his pupil Lemierre (1875–1956) (who later had a major role in the founding the Société de Pathologie Rénale in 1949, renamed as the Société de Néphrologie from 1960) studied nine patients in great detail, submitting each to carefully conducted and sequential balance studies involving augmentations or reductions in their salt intake. The experiments, which lasted up to 3 months, were designed and executed with great care (de Wardener, 1993). All measurements of salt were in the form of chloride, as only this could be measured at that time. A 'sodium-free' diet (1.5 g NaCl over 24 h) led to the disappearance of oedema accompanied by weight loss, whilst a sodium-rich diet (15.5 g NaCl over 24 h) resulted in the reappearance of oedema.

Importance

Most early observers of oedema concentrated on the idea of simple failure of renal excretion of water as its genesis. Carl Ludwig (1816–1893) (Ludwig, 1885, cited by de Wardener, 1993) was the first to pioneer the idea of sodium balance in humans, suggesting renal perception and regulation of the amount of salt by a mechanism then unknown. As it was almost impossible to measure sodium before flame photometry was introduced in the late 1940s, chloride was measured laboriously by a gravimetric method as an alternative until about 1950. Widal's name is still familiar because of his typhoid test developed in 1896, but then he turned his mind to even more important work, generally much less well known today, on sodium in health and renal disease. Widal went on to study nitrogen intake and consequent urea excretion, using similar depletion and equilibrium balance studies to this previous work on chloride (Widal and Javal, 1904), showing the two (chloride and nitrogen) to be independent. This work of Widal was part of a wave of interest in Paris in chemistry applied to renal diseases. Other Parisians involved were Léon Ambard (1876–1962), who developed a urea ratio test of function (see discussion of paper 5.9), and Charles Achard (1869–1944), who in 1900 introduced the first exogenous test of renal function using subcutaneous injection of methylene blue with a measurement of excretion over 24 h, which was used by Widal. This was replaced by the similar phenolsulfonthalein excretion test of Rowntree and Geraghty in 1911, which reigned for half a century. At the same time, in Berlin, Hermann Strauss (1868–1944) also studied salt balance and retention in cardiac and renal diseases as part of comprehensive clinical studies of Bright's disease (Strauss, 1903). Strauss' needle allowed safe and easy withdrawal of blood samples for study from 1903 onwards and greatly facilitated metabolic studies.

Although Widal advocated salt restriction as a rational treatment of oedemas (Widal and Javal, 1903), the difficulties of maintaining low-salt intakes in free-ranging outpatients rather than long-term patients in hospital began to emerge; much later (Sir) George Pickering visited Volhard in Frankfurt and learned his patients had a saying 'to lie like someone on a salt-free diet' ('Lügen *wie ein Salzlёser*'). Nevertheless, salt and oedema were now irreversibly entwined, and the story of salt and hypertension would follow. Only in the past few decades have we learned that the retention and accumulation of salt in nephrotics depends principally upon enhancement of an intrarenal mechanism, dependent mainly on increased distal tubular sodium reabsorption through the amiloride-sensitive apical channel, ENaC. These ideas have largely replaced the concept of a response to hypovolaemia, in turn resulting from hypoalbuminaemia ('underfilling'), thought from the 1940s onwards to be the major mechanism of oedema. Nevertheless, sodium restriction in clinical practice still suffers neglect today, as Scribner and others have pointed out.

References

de Wardener HE (1993). Histoire des méfaits rénaux du sodium. *Néphrologie d'Hier et d'Aujourd'hui* **1**, 6–10. [The figures in this paper show the details of Widal's experiments.]

Ludwig CFW (1885). Manuscript notes of lectures 1869–1870. In: *A Textbook of Pharmacology, Therapeutics and Materia Medica*. Edited by TL Brunton. Lea Brothers and Co., Philadelphia, Pennsylvania, p. 503.

Strauss H (1903). Zur behandlung und Verholung der Nierenwassersucht. In: *Therapie der Gegenwart*. Urban & Schwarzenberg, Berlin, Germany, pp. 193–200.

Widal F, Javal A (1903). La cure de déchloruration: son action sur l'oedème, sur l'hydratation et sur la'albuminurie – certaines périodes de la néphrite epithééliale. *Bull Mem Soc Med Hop Paris* 26 June, 219.

Widal F, Javal A (1904). Le méchanisme regulateur de la rétention de l'urée dans le mal de Bright. *Compt Rend Soc Biol* **56**, 301–304.

5.8 Die Bright'sche Nierenkrankheit. Klinik, Pathologie und Atlas [Bright's kidney disease: clinic, pathology and atlas]

Authors

F Volhard and T Fahr

Reference

Published by Springer, Berlin, Germany (1914).

Summary

Pathologists and clinicians had argued over the divisions of Bright's disease for half a century, usually returning to the antithesis between acute and two chronic forms (see paper 5.3). However, the realization that high blood pressure could result from but also damage the kidney required incorporation into any schema. This was done authoritatively by two brilliant German investigators, the clinician Volhard (1872–1950) and pathologist Fahr (1877–1945). Their book was published at the outbreak of World War I, but still dominated thinking until the next global conflict 25 years later. The book was notable as one of the last major books to be beautifully illustrated by coloured drawings of the microscopic and macroscopic pathology, before photography and microphotography took over. By 1925, Addis (see paper 5.9) was using photomicrographs. (An idea of the hand-coloured illustrations of Volhard and Fahr can be seen in reference Fogazzi and Ritz, 1998). The classification of Volhard and Fahr was comprehensive:

1. Nephrosis
   - Genuine
   - Necrotizing
2. Nephritis
   - Diffuse glomerulonephritis
     - o Acute
     - o Subacute
     - o Chronic
   - Focal nephritis
     - o Focal glomerulonephritis
     - o Interstitial nephritis
     - o Embolic focal nephritis
3. Nephrosclerosis
   - Simple (benign)
   - Combined (malignant)

They adopted Möller's term 'nephrosis'. 'Genuine' nephrosis was the large white proteinuric kidney of Bright, Johnson and Wilks, but toxic and other nephropathies were also included so that the term 'nephrosis' generated more and more confusion.

Importance

During the latter third of the nineteenth century, two advances affected our understanding of nephritis: the relationship between high blood pressure and renal disease was advanced and explored, and better histological techniques allowed the potential of the fine microscopes already available to be exploited. Whilst many of the advances in clinical hypertension were in Britain, and also France through Kirkes, Mahomet, Gull, Allbutt, Huchard and others, microscopic pathology was supreme in Germany. Edwin Klebs (1834–1913), who introduced paraffin embedding in 1869 and coined the name 'glomerulonephritis', described hypercellularity in the patients dying in the acute nephritic phase in 1875 (Klebs, 1870), and Theodor Langhans (1839–1915) in Bern 4 years later confirmed these observations and also described extracellular proliferation—the cellular proliferative and later (1885) the leukocytic infiltrative component of nephritis, to add to the desquamative/degenerative tubular processes already described (Langhans, 1879). The role of the interstitium and fibrosis had remained controversial, ever since Virchow and Frerichs in the 1850s. Finally, there was the rediscovery of the fatty nature of some patients with 'pure nephrosis' by Möller and Munk, using histology and polarized light. Clearly, a new, broader synthesis was needed, incorporating the benign and more malignant vascular lesions. This was amply supplied by Volhard and Fahr in their beautiful book, whose ideas more or less dominated thinking worldwide until the advent of renal biopsy. It is worth noting that they did not pay much regard to the physiological work on the role of chloride retention (as a surrogate for sodium, which then could not be measured easily) in the genesis of oedema by Achard and others in Paris (Achard, 1905), and nearer home, Hermann Strauss (Strauss, 1902). All the histological forms of nephritis that we still recognize today are described by Volhard and Fahr, some for the first time such as focal segmental glomerulosclerosis, crescentic glomerulonephritis, and mesangiocapillary (membranoproliferative) glomerulonephritis. But perhaps their most important work was in the area of hypertension and nephrosclerosis. They described the difference between 'benign' nephrosclerosis and 'malignant' nephrosclerosis, in which the vicious circle of renal and arterial damage first described by Akhbar Mahomet in the 1870s was present. 'Benign nephrosclerosis' remains a controversial topic today in its relation to glomerulosclerosis, proteinuria, and above all renal failure.

References

Achard C (1905). Le role du sel en pathologie et en thérapeutique. *J Med Chir Prat* **76**, 241–247.

Fogazzi GB, Ritz E (1998). Novel classification of glomerulonephritis in the monograph of Franz Volhard and Theodor Fahr. *Nephrol Dial Transplant* **13**, 2965–2967.

Klebs TAE (1870). *Handbuch der pathologischen Anatomie*. Hirschwald, Berlin, Germany, pp. 644–648.

Langhans T (1879). Ueber der Veraenderungen der Glomeruli bei nephritis nebst einigen Bemerkungen ueber die Einstehung der Fibrincylinder. *Virchows Arch Pathol* **76**, 85–118.

Strauss H (1902). *Die chronische Nierenzudungen in ihrer Einwirkung auf die Blutflussigkeit und deren behandlung*. Hirschwald, Berlin, Germany.

5.9 Glomerular nephritis: diagnosis and treatment

Author

T Addis

Reference

Published by Macmillan, New York, USA (1948).

Summary

Addis's rather quirky, rambling book summarized in an everyday, almost non-technical style his nearly 100 papers on renal physiology and disease, and also his life's philosophy (Piccoli, 2010). Ironically, he died from complications of an infarcted kidney a year after its publication. He attempted to measure the extent of renal damage in life using functional, histological, and uroscopical measurements. Perhaps his sceptical attitude to function tests derived from his first work on the kidney around 1915–1917 attempting to standardize a test of overall renal function, based on Ambard's 1900 work in Paris on blood and urinary urea concentrations (see paper 5.7). This test of the volume of urea 'freed' (the term suggested by his colleague George D. Barnett) over 12 h led to the 'clearance' concept of Rehberg and Van Slyke a decade later. Addis accepted that creatinine gave superior results, and abandoned urea. Next, he tackled the disease of the kidney itself, and, as histology was available only at autopsies from incidental or uraemic death, he emphasized a *clinical* classification (Addis, 1925). This followed nevertheless the triple division based on histopathology advocated by Volhard and Fahr. Finally he attempted to make urinalysis quantitative, measuring proteinuria and quantitating the urinary sediment—which became known as an 'Addis count'. He described broad 'renal failure' urinary casts for the first time. In 1931, he collaborated with Jean Oliver in an analysis of 78 patients with all types of nephritis whose kidneys became available for histology and microdissection (Addis and Oliver, 1931). Addis's other main contribution was the effect of low-protein diets in humans with renal disease and in animals with partial nephrectomies. He emphasized the work of the kidneys in excreting urea, and related this to hypertrophic growth, ideas still currently of interest. His animal work led him to recommend restriction of both protein and salt intake as treatments, which still resonate today.

Importance

The first North American (if we except Wells) cited in this chapter might well have been the Canadian–American William Osler (1849–1919), who had a major interest in the kidney and in his textbook on medicine (Osler, 1893) gave crisp, concise, and influential descriptions and classifications of Bright's disease, hypertension, and renal failure. Addis was born and trained in Scotland and then in Heidelberg, where he did crucially important work on haemophilia, and then was invited directly by Dean Wilbur to Stanford, California, in 1911. There he remained, isolated from the East coast group of renal physician scientists, despite later being invited to join them by Donald van Slyke. He preferred to stay with his rats and his long-term patients in Stanford for a second and then a third decade of follow-up. He was the leading American clinician in the renal field in the 1930s and 1940s, and the first American nephrologist to achieve an international reputation. Thereafter, advances in renal disease swung heavily towards the USA, as, in parallel with Addis's work in the clinical field, Homer Smith (1895–1962) in New York was working out the physiological basis of renal function. Addis did important work on clearance, on the classification and diagnosis of nephritis, and, above all, on the management of patients with the various forms of renal disease still referred to as Bright's disease. Addis's advocacy of a low-protein diet persisted after his death, at first mostly in Europe during the 1950s, but re-emerging worldwide as a major theme of investigation and treatment during the 1970s and 1980s. In contrast, the 'Addis count', his careful but laborious quantification of urine microscopy, had faded away as a clinical tool by 1960, despite the posthumous popularity in the USA of the book on the urinary sediment by Richard W. Lippman (1916–1959), a pupil of Addis and Oliver (Lipmann, 1952). Addis was active politically as a lifelong anti-fascist and supported the Spanish republican movement with money and assistance in the 1930s. He was in fact a communist but perhaps fortunately died just before the McCarthy witch hunts. He emphasized repeatedly that work from their laboratory was the result of a team, which he selected and nurtured with great care.

References

Addis T (1925). A clinical classification of Bright's disease. *J Am Med Soc* **85**, 163–167.

Addis T, Oliver J (1931). *The Renal Lesion in Bright's Disease*. Paul Hoeber, New York.

Lipmann RW (1952). *Urine and the Urinary Sediment*. Charles C. Thomas, Springfield, Illinois.

Osler W (1893). *Principles and Practice of Medicine*. Appleton, New York.

Piccoli G (2010). Patient-based continuum of care in nephrology: why read Thomas Addis' 'Glomerular nephritis' in 2009? *J Nephrol* **23**, 164–167.

5.10 Natural history of Bright's disease. Clinical, histological and experimental observations

Author

A Ellis

Reference

Lancet 1942, **i**, 1–7, 34–36, 72–76.

Abstract

There are two varieties of nephritis, differing in their aetiology, mode of onset and course. Recovery is the rule in one and the exception in the other. We have designated these two types of nephritis type 1 and type 2. Type 1 nephritis commonly has a history of preceding infection (84%). Its onset is abrupt, blood is usually present in the urine, complete recovery normally occurs (82%). Type 2 nephritis has a history of preceding infection in less than 5% and even in these it is often indefinite. Its onset is insidious, blood is rarely present in the urine, the disease is progressive and recovery is rare. We include nephrosis in type 2 nephritis. The course of the two types of nephritis is different. Type 1 may run a rapid or a very chronic course; type 2 nephritis runs a continuously progressive course. The histological pictures in the two types of nephritis is different, especially in the late stages. Until further evidence is available it is best to regard essential hypertension as non-renal in origin. It is seen in two forms—benign hypertension, which comprises more than 90% of all patients with hypertension, and malignant hypertension. In benign hypertension there is usually no evidence of renal impairment, and renal failure only very rarely occurs. In malignant hypertension renal involvement is always present in the late stages, and death in renal failure is common. The condition is rapidly progressive, the patient dying within a year of the first symptom. The pathognomonic sign of malignant hypertension is papilloedema…So-called chronic interstitial nephritis is a hotch-potch of various renal disorders on which [a] vicious circle [of hypertension and renal damage] has been superimposed. The expression should therefore be discarded…and replaced by 'chronic hypertensive Bright's disease'…They are best separated by a study of their natural history.…[Adapted.]

Importance

For a lecture that was never given (because of 'enemy action' in the London Blitz in 1942), on data that were never published in detail, and probably not refereed, this paper had a remarkable influence and impact, although this was confined principally to the English-speaking world. Ellis (1883–1966), in his written Croonian lecture to the Royal College of Physicians of London, wrote also on behalf of his younger colleagues Clifford Wilson (1906–1997) and Horace Evans (1903–1963). Wilson went on to have an influential career in nephrology, with diabetic nephropathy (see paper 9.2) and experimental malignant hypertension (Wilson and Byrom, 1941) two notable discoveries. They had studied together some 600 patients since 1924, when Ellis came via the armed forces from Canada to head the London Hospital academic medical unit. They returned to the brutal simplification of Samuel Wilks (Wilks, 1853), separating off the various acute nephritic patients (type 1) and then rolling up all the chronic patients as a usually progressive, proteinuric, frequently oedematous 'type 2', avoiding all the arguments about nephrosis, parenchymatous, or desquamative nephritis, granular and large fatty kidney. A retrospective justification is that prognosis in all forms of persistently proteinuric nephritis depends much more upon the degree of proteinuria and the presence or absence of hypertension than the details of the glomerular histology, other than in those with no visible glomerular changes. Ellis presented details of 318 patients with type 1 ($n = 173$) or type 2 ($n = 145$) nephritis in the lecture. Rapidly, this simple and appealing idea of type 1 and 2 nephritis caught on and was widely used. It disappeared when renal biopsy revealed five or six histological classes in 'type 2'. A possible response to corticosteroid treatment now required prediction, principally in those with minimal change disease, as well as some with focal segmental sclerosis or membranous nephropathy. Ellis and colleagues excluded a group of 35 haematuric patients from type 1, whose haematuria was immediate, with recurrence in 11; persistent albuminuria was rare. Today, they would almost certainly be classified as IgA nephropathy, but Ellis and colleagues used the term 'acute focal nephritis', following Volhard and Fahr. Of their 103 patients with malignant hypertension, only seven survived, and 76 were known to have died. Ellis regarded this as a different disease from essential, 'benign' hypertension, although admitting with Fishberg that a few went on to renal failure with glomerulosclerosis.

References

Wilks S (1853). Cases of Bright's disease, with remarks. *Guy's Hosp Rep* **9**, 232–315.

Wilson C, Byrom FB (1941). The vicious circle in chronic Bright's disease. Experimental evidence from the hypertensive rat. *Quart J Med* **10**, 65–93.

Chapter 6

Primary glomerular disease—since 1950

Richard J. Glassock

Introduction

As elegantly described by Stewart Cameron in the preceding chapter, the 180-year period from 1770 to 1950 was pre-occupied with establishing the connection between clinical findings (including the examination of urine and the beginnings of clinical chemistry) and the presence of kidney diseases, specifically those involving the glomerulus. The discoveries of Richard Bright in 1827 (see papers 3.1 and 5.3) represented a turning point, with classification and nomenclature proceeding incrementally from then, but often bringing with them vagueness and confusion. The introduction of percutaneous renal biopsy in the prone position by Brun and Iversen in 1951 (see paper 3.6) handed to clinicians a new tool for examining the pathology of glomerular disease, previously relegated to the post-mortem room. Now clinicians could relate bedside observations in *living* patients with the morphological appearances of the glomeruli. Very soon the methods of fluorescence tagging of antibodies for the detection of antigens in tissues (introduced by Coons and Kaplan) and electron microscopy (introduced and popularized by deDuve, Palade, and Farquhar, among others) expanded the field greatly. Great interest in linking morphology to pathogenesis was stimulated by the experimental work of Germuth and Dixon, who led the development of a new field—renal immunopathology. A panoply of immunological and non-immunological pathways for the production of glomerular injury exploded onto the scene. Treatments for glomerular disease, other than diet and life style, began to emerge after 1950 [first with adrenocorticotropic hormone (ACTH) and cortisone] and gradually took on a new importance as anecdotes gave way to randomized controlled trials. New entities also emerged, as older classifications of disease were revised, divided, and subdivided. Finally, the revolution in molecular biology (ushered in by the discovery of the structure of DNA by Watson and Crick in 1953) created a second wave of reductionist inquiry delving even deeper into the origins of glomerular disease. All of these advances were properly documented in a growing cadre of books and monographs devoted to nephrology and nephron pathology, echoing the past classics of Rayer, Volhard, and Fahr and Addis. Thus, the post-1950 era of glomerular disease was dominated by technological advances, a focus on mechanisms, delineation of new entities, and increasingly detailed expositions of the natural history of the disease and its therapeutic modification. The excitement that attended these advances was pivotal in attracting clinicians and scientists to become students of glomerular disease.

Chapter 6 covers the so-called primary glomerular diseases—loosely defined as those in which the clinical manifestations are the consequence of the glomerular injury itself and where all non-renal aspects of the disorder can ultimately be traced to an effect of disordered glomerular structure and/or function. Chapter 7 deals with those entities in which organs or organ systems, in addition to the kidneys, are involved, often due to participation of systemic disease processes, so-called secondary glomerular diseases.

The selection of these landmark papers is both personal and arbitrary. Many influential papers and reviews have been set aside, but this should not negate or diminish their importance.

6.1 Cortisone treatment of nephrosis

Authors

GC Arniel, HE Wilson

Reference

Archives of Disease in Childhood 1952, **27**, 322–328.

Abstract

Six cases of nephrosis were treated with large doses of cortisone, the treatment being stopped abruptly. In four of the cases a dieresis with loss of oedema and albuminuria followed the termination of therapy. Two of these cases have had no recurrence of pedema or albuminuria and their blood chemistry has remained normal.

It is suggested that the oedema in nephrosis is not primarily due to a diminution in the plasma proteins. Furthermore the low level of blood proteins is not satisfactorily explained by loss of albumin in the urine. It appears probable that there is a reduced synthesis in nephrotic patients.

Cortisone is considered to be a useful method of provoking dieresis in nephrotic patients.

Importance

This paper was selected to highlight the transition to an interest in treatment of glomerular disease in the mid-twentieth century. This pivotal study carried out at the Royal Hospital for Sick Children in Glasgow, UK, followed the course of six children (ages 17 months to 7 years) with nephrotic syndrome treated with cortisone in doses of 100–300 mg/day (roughly equivalent to prednisone 20–60 mg/day) for 5 days. Dramatic remission of oedema, hypoalbuminaemia, and albuminuria were seen in most (four out of six) children, but only 36–72 h after stopping the cortisone. oedema, hypoalbuminaemia, and albuminuria actually worsened during the periodic of drug administration. An earlier preliminary one-page report by Barnett and colleagues (Barnett *et al.*, 1950) in New York and Philadelphia also described the effects of ACTH and cortisone on what we would now call 'minimal change disease' in children with nephrotic syndrome aged 2–4 years. A dramatic diuresis, remissions of oedema, and elevations of inulin clearance were observed in eight out of ten children with intramuscular doses of ACTH equal to 50–100 mg/day for 7–12 days. Cortisone in doses of 100 mg/day for 10 days was not effective in five children. Similar findings were reported simultaneously by Riley in the same edition of the same journal (Riley, 1950). Taken together, these early observational studies demonstrated that drug treatment of nephrotic syndrome (in children) was possible with cortisone-like drugs or ACTH, a major breakthrough, although the mechanism responsible for the benefit was obscure and remains so to this day. These studies signified a beginning for the field of therapeutics in glomerular disease. Their focus was more on the diuresis and disappearance of oedema than on the alteration of the natural course of the disease. ACTH appeared more effective, although the use of too low a dose of cortisone could explain the difference between the Arneil and Barnett studies. The 'delayed' effects of ACTH and cortisone on diuresis are interesting and most likely reflect the time lag in reconstitution of the glomerular barrier to protein. Although the focus of therapy since the 1950s has been mainly on the use of oral corticosteroids, we now recognize that ACTH may have direct effects on the podocyte to improve permselectivity independent of an effect to increase adrenal steroidogenesis.

Others, at about the same time, began to explore other novel ways of treating glomerular disease, including nitrogen mustard (Chasis *et al.*, 1949).

References

Barnett HL, McNamara, H, McCrory W, Forman C, Rapaport M, Michie A, Barbero G (1950). The effects of ACTH and cortisone on the nephrotic syndrome. *Am J Dis Child* **80**, 519–520.

Chasis H, Goldring W, Baldwin DS (1949). Effect of febrile plasma, typhoid vaccine and nitrogen mustard on renal manifestations of human glomerulonephritis. *Proc Soc Exp Biol Med* **71**, 565–567.

Riley CM (1950). The effect of adrenocorticotrophic hormone on salt and water excretion in children with the nephrotic syndrome. *Am J Dis Child* **80**, 520–521.

6.2 An electron microscopic study of the glomerulus in nephrosis, glomerulonephritis and lupus erythematosus

Authors

MG Farquhar, RL Vernier, RA Good

Reference

Journal of Experimental Medicine 1957, **106**, 649–660.

Abstract

Renal biopsies from 16 patients with nephrosis, 7 patients with glomerulonephritis, and 3 patients with disseminated lupus erythematosus were studied with the electron microscope.

The observations presented indicate that early in the course of each of these diseases alterations occur in the fine structure of the glomeruli which serve to distinguish one disease process from another.

In nephrosis, some distortion of the organization of the epithelial foot processes was seen in all patients. These epithelial changes constituted the early, consistent lesion of the disease. There was frequently also a swelling of the endothelium.

In glomerulonephritis, pronounced proliferative changes involving the endothelium and to a lesser extent the epithelium, together with the laying down of a basement membrane-like material, represented the predominate pathologic processes. There was also a swelling of both endothelial and epithelial cytoplasm. The epithelial foot processes generally appeared normal.

In patients with a clinically "mixed" picture of nephrosis and nephritis, the glomerular changes were likewise "mixed," for various combinations of epithelial, endothelial, and basement membrane abnormalities were present.

In disseminated lupus erythematosus, a more or less generalized thickening of the basement membrane proper associated with a variable degree of endothelial proliferation was seen. It is suggested that an accentuation of the process of basement membrane thickening results in the "wire loop" appearance sometimes seen by light microscopy.

Although the earliest alterations in glomerular fine structure were characteristic for each of the disease processes, at later stages the changes were not always distinctive. The resulting scarred or "hyalinized" glomeruli, composed of relatively homogeneous, basement membrane-like material, and a few atrophic cells, appeared quite similar.

Although the functional implications of the structural changes observed remain obscure at this time, it is believed that insight into mechanisms may stem from such observations.

Importance

This paper exemplifies the impact of newly developed technology on the field of glomerular disease—this one dealing with the new technique of electron microscopy—but it is hard to choose whether electron microscopy or immunofluorescence microscopy, both emerging nearly simultaneously in the late 1950s, had a greater impact on the study of glomerular disease. Coupled with percutaneous renal biopsy, introduced in 1951, they both provided a powerful engine for change in the field, one that persists to the present time. The study by Farquhar and her colleagues selected here was among the first to explore systematically the newly developed technique of electron microscopy in the area of human glomerular pathology. They studied patients with 'nephrosis', glomerulonephritis, and lupus nephritis. They described the fine-structural alterations (effacement or fusion) of podocyte (visceral epithelial cells) in 'nephrosis' and the basement membrane alterations in glomerulonephritis and lupus nephritis. Interestingly, the term 'electron-dense deposits' does not appear in the paper—rather, they described 'accumulations of material resembling basement membranes in density and general appearance'. Inspection of the figures in the publication definitely indicates that 'electron-dense' deposits were present in the material they studied.

At nearly the same time, Mellors and Ortega (1956) utilized the methods of Coons and Kaplan (1950) for preparing fluorescein-tagged reagents to track the deposition of specific proteins (including immunoglobulin). They applied them in renal disease studying frozen tissue (from autopsies) exposed to UV light. They were among the first to demonstrate immunoglobulin deposition in acute and chronic glomerular diseases of various types, including membranous nephropathy (then mistakenly called lipoid nephrosis).

Taken together, these papers on the pathology of glomerular disease illustrate the powerful influence of the new technology on the development of the field of inquiry into glomerular diseases. Whilst they did not provide great insights into pathogenetic mechanism or have much immediate influence on the ability of pathology to classify disease or to elaborate on prognosis, they did initiate a new paradigm in which examination of renal tissue was a means of exploring aetiological and pathogenetic pathways. What was then novel is now routine. Immunofluorescence and electron microscopy became widely employed, both clinically and experimentally, and contributed to the discovery of several new clinico-pathological entities [most notably IgA nephropathy (see paper 6.5) and the fibrillary glomerulopathies (see paper 6.7)]. Subsequent refinements, for example freeze–fracture, scanning, and electron autoradiography, and immunogold, and immunoperoxidase methods, have added additional power to the techniques.

References

Coons AH, Kaplan MH (1950). Localization of antigen in tissue cells. II. Improvements in a method for detection of antigen by means of fluorescent antibody *J Exp Med* **91**, 1–13.

Mellors RC, Ortega LG (1956). Analytical pathology III. New observations on the pathogenesis of glomerulonephritis, lipoid nephrosis, periarteritis nodosa and secondary amyloidosis in man. *Am J Pathol* **32**, 455–499.

6.3 Nephrotic glomerulonephritis

Author

DB Jones

Reference

American Journal of Pathology 1957, **33**, 313–329.

Abstract

This study was based on the examination of the kidneys of 20 cases of nephrotic glomerulonephritis which were divided into four groups: 6 cases presented minimal glomerular lesions; 6, moderate glomerular lesions; 3, the lesion of chronic lobular glomerulonephritis; and 5, chronic membranous glomerulonephritis.

The basic histologic procedure of this study was the use of the periodic acid silver methanamine sequence which reveals the fine structures of the glomerular connective tissue in health and disease better than any other technique. Certain new observations of these lesions have been discussed.

On clinical, pathologic, and natural historical grounds, nephrotic glomerulonephritis and nephritic glomerulonephritis have similarities and differences. It appears that a peculiar auto-antibody injury is present in both processes but the trigger mechanism has not been discovered for nephrotic glomerulonephritis.

It is hoped that future presentations of clinical material on nephrotic glomerulonephritis will make use of 5, 10, and 20 year survival statistics so that a better concept of ultimate prognosis may be reached. [Adapted.]

Importance

This paper has been selected as it gives the seminal observations that led to the description of one of the most common forms of primary nephrotic syndrome seen in adults—namely, membranous glomerulonephritis, now called membranous nephropathy. And it resulted in membranous nephropathy acquiring a new status as a distinct clinico-pathological entity.

David Jones of Syracuse University, New York, applied a special stain (the periodic acid–silver methenamine stain) to 20 cases of glomerulonephritis with nephrotic syndrome. Based on light microscopic morphology alone, he clearly separated membranous nephropathy from minimal change disease, focal segmental glomerulosclerosis, and lobular glomerulonephritis, all of which had previously been considered together under the term 'lipoid nephrosis' and classified as 'Ellis type II disease'. The description of the lesion of membranous nephropathy is remarkably complete and emphasizes the basement membrane alterations (spikes and domes) so characteristic of the more advanced forms of this disorder.

This paper also illustrates how the classifications and nosology of nephritis were changing from one dominated by clinical manifestations to a blend of pathological and clinical features. The work of Jones presaged much of the subsequent morphological and pathogenetic investigation, studies that continue to evolve. Membranous nephropathy was staged subsequently by electron micros-copy and immunofluorescence studies, which identified its signature subepithelial electron-dense deposits and granular capillary wall deposits of IgG attesting to its immune origins. Autopsy stud-ies, as shown here, gradually gave way to studies based on renal biopsy. The latter allowed for much more detailed examination of the natural history of these lesions, but the history of such studies really began with this pioneering investigation.

6.4 A hitherto undescribed vulnerability of the juxtamedullary glomeruli in lipoid nephrosis

Author

AR Rich

Reference

Bulletins of Johns Hopkins Hospital 1957, **100**, 173–186.

Abstract

The glomeruli situated at the cortical-medullary junction of the kidney (the so-called juxtamedullary glomeruli) are strikingly more susceptible to the process which produces obliterative glomerulosclerosis in lipoid nephrosis than are the glomeruli in the other regions of the cortex. They are the first to be visibly altered by the sclerotic process, and the first to become obliterated by it. An adequate understanding of the pathogenesis of the glomerulosclerosis should account for this peculiar susceptibility of the juxtamedullary glomeruli to the injurious process responsible for the destructive glomerular damage; and a more detailed understanding of the normal differences between the juxtamedullary glomeruli and the other cortical glomeruli may be helpful toward the understanding of the at present obscure nature and mechanism of the process that produces the life-threatening glomerulosclerosis of lipoid nephrosis. [Adapted.]

Adapted with permission from The Alan Mason Chesney Medical Archives of the Johns Hopkins Medical Institutions, Rich AR (1957)
A hitherto undescribed vulnerability of the juxtamedullary glomeruli in Lipoid Nephrosis. *Bulletins of Johns Hopkins Hospital*, **100**, 173–186.

Importance

Arnold Rich of Johns Hopkins University, Baltimore, studied 20 fatal cases of 'pure lipoid nephrosis', nine of whom died of infection (commonly pneumococcal peritonitis) and 11 of whom died of 'uremia'. He noted a process of 'obliterative glomerulosclerosis' predominantly affecting the juxtamedullary (deep cortical) nephrons, especially among those dying of 'uremia'. He suggested that the initial injury was in the juxtamedullary area with later spread to the entire cortical nephron population. The obliterative lesion had all the characteristics that we now call focal and segmental glomerulosclerosis with hyalinosis (FSGS). A dozen years later, this observation was confirmed in biopsy studies of similar patients in another 'landmark' paper of comparable significance (Churg *et al.*, 1970).

These studies of Rich provoked a re-examination of the pathology underlying children and adults with nephrotic syndrome, resulting in the establishment of the lesion of FSGS as a real clinico-pathological entity. The recognition that some glomeruli undergo a process of progressive sclerosis beginning in only a portion of the glomerular tufts created a conundrum. Was this merely a more severe form of damage in patients with so-called 'minimal change disease', or was it an entirely separate entity, with a different (but obscure) pathogenesis, easily mistaken in its earliest stages for 'minimal change disease', especially as the focal distribution of the lesions might easily allow them to be missed in a biopsy?

Studies of monogenetic forms of the disease, recurrences in the renal allograft, and examination of lesions in patients with haemodynamic or toxin-induced alterations of glomerular function have amply demonstrated the characteristics of the lesion of FSGS, which separate it from 'minimal change disease', but the pathogenesis of both of these lesions remains incompletely understood today, except that both seem to be the result of podocyte injury (D'Agati *et al.*, 2011).

References

Churg J, Habib R, White RHR (1970). Pathology of the nephrotic syndrome in children. A report from the International Study of Kidney Disease in Children. *Lancet* **760**, 1299–1302.

D'Agati VD, Kaskel FJ, Falk RJ (2011). Focal segmental glomerulosclerosis. *N Engl J Med* **365**, 2398–2341.

6.5 Les dépôts intercapillaires d'IgA-IgG [IgA–IgG intercapillary deposits]

Authors

J Berger, N Hinglais

Reference

Journal de Urologie et Nephrologie (Paris) 1968, **74**, 694–695.

Abstract

In the renal biopsies of 25 patients there was evidence by immunofluorescence of intercapillary deposits which stained with anti-IgA serum, and less intensely with sera against IgG and β_1C-globulin. On the other hand, there was no staining with antisera to IgM, fibrinogen, albumin, caeruloplasmin, α_2-macroglobulin and β-lipoprotein. The intercapillary deposits were present in all glomeruli.

The intercapillary deposits could not be identified by light microscopy except in 3 cases. In half the cases, the histological diagnosis was focal glomerulonephritis: some glomeruli having focal lesions which were hyaline or sometimes necrotic. In the remaining cases, the diagnosis included unclassified glomerulonephritis, chronic nephritis, isolated arteriolar changes, or normal kidney.

The presence of dense and finely granular deposits situated between the basement membrane and the intercapillary cells was confirmed by electron microscopy in the 10 cases studies with that technique.

All patients had moderate proteinuria and microscopic haematuria. In half the cases there were episodes of macroscopic haematuria, typically following a throat infection. Renal function was normal in the great majority of cases. Three patients were hypertensive.

The time from first presentation to renal biopsy varied from a few months to twelve years.

It appears that in the majority of cases of chronic focal glomerulonephritis, there are diffuse intercapillary deposits as well as focal lesions. This observation, regardless of its theoretical interest, has a practical utility: immunofluorescence facilitates the diagnosis of this type of glomerulonephritis in cases where the light microscopy may suggest the kidney is normal, or is affected by other lesions. [Translated.]

Importance

This seminal one-page paper in French launched a revolution in glomerular disease. It was a simple observational study, conducted at the Hôpital Necker in Paris, of 25 subjects with recurrent bouts of gross haematuria (with moderate proteinuria) or microscopic haematuria, often following an upper respiratory infection. Immunofluorescence performed on the renal biopsy material by Jean Berger showed extensive mesangial deposition of both IgA and IgG (with IgA predominant in many). Electron microscopy (carried out by Nicole Hinglais) in ten subjects showed mesangial electron-dense deposits. The patients in this report all had normal renal function and the follow-up was too short to determine whether the findings had prognostic significance, but a larger study including 55 patients published a year later (Berger, 1969) seemed to indicate a benign outcome for most subjects. The observations in Paris were quickly confirmed in many other countries, and the new disease, for a time called Berger's disease but now called simply IgA nephropathy, was found to have a global distribution and is the commonest primary glomerular disease in most developed countries. Unfortunately, many patients (at least 50%) have a slowly progressive course and the disease can recur in the transplanted kidney, also shown by Berger and colleagues.

It is hard to overestimate the significance of this short paper. It is the closest that clinical nephrology has to a 'Watson–Crick' moment. It was the first description of a specific renal disease identified by its immunofluorescence pattern. Although the initial reaction was sceptical, by 1975 the entity of Berger's disease or IgA nephropathy was well established. Over time, IgA nephropathy has changed from being regarded as a mild disorder with relatively innocuous clinical presentation to being understood as an immensely varied condition (both clinically and morphologically) with an uncertain but sometimes poor prognosis. Mesangial IgA deposition can also be found in other diseases, including the closely related entity, Henoch–Schönlein purpura. The discovery of IgA nephropathy spawned an intense search for underlying mechanisms of mesangial IgA deposition that has only recently begun to yield results with broad explanatory power. Despite optimism about promising, reliable, non-invasive diagnostic tests, IgA nephropathy today remains a disease requiring renal biopsy for diagnosis. Among young adults undergoing a renal biopsy for suspicion of a primary glomerular disease, IgA nephropathy ranks at the very top in frequency in most parts of the world. If one adds the number of apparently normal subjects who have 'innocent' IgA deposits in the glomeruli, as many as 300 million individuals may have 'IgA nephropathy'. When Berger and Hinglais conducted their original study, the reagents were crude and often troubled by non-specific reactions. They were fortunate to have access to pure anti-IgA antibody prepared by a colleague, Maxime Seligmann. IgA had only been discovered as a distinct immunoglobulin in 1959 by Heremans and colleagues. Berger and Hinglais were fortune to be in the right place at the right time, with access to these newer techniques and reagents, but they added to this the scientific insight required for a truly groundbreaking discovery.

Reference

Berger J (1969). IgA glomerular deposits in renal disease. *Transplant Proc* **1**, 939–944.

6.6 Evidence for *in vivo* breakdown of β_{1c} globulin in hypocomplementemic glomerulonephritis

Authors

CD West, S Winter, J Forristal, JM McConville, NC Davis

Reference

Journal of Clinical Investigation 1967, **46**, 539–548.

Abstract

Evidence has been obtained for the presence *in vivo* of alpha$_{2D}$-globulin, a breakdown product of serum β_{1c}-globulin, in patients with acute and persistent hypocomplementemic glomerulonephritis. The protein has been identified by immunoelectrophoretic analysis, and the amounts present have been determined by direct measurement of specific antigenic determinants present on alpha$_{2D}$. β_{1A}-Globulin, another breakdown product of β_{1c}-globulin, may also be present *in vivo* in severely hypocomplementemic patients, but its levels are much lower than those of alpha$_{2D}$-globulin...

Measurement of specific antigenic determinants has been carried out in both fresh EDTA plasma and aged serum. In the fresh plasma, the concentration of D antigen, found on both β_{1c}- and alpha$_{2D}$-globulins, has been related to that of B antigen, found only on β_{1c} and taken as a measure of the concentration of this protein. In the hypocomplementemic patients, the concentration of D antigen, in comparison to that of B, was greater than in the normal subjects. Similarly, in aged serum, the level of alpha$_{2D}$ was greater than would be expected from the amount of β_{1c} that had been broken down *in vitro*, measured by the concentration of β_{1A}.

...The levels tended to be lower in less severely hypocomplementemic patients, and none could be detected in normal plasma.

Only small quantities of A and D antigens are detectable in the urine of patients with hypocomplementemic nephritis. The rate of excretion is about equal to that of the normal subject.

The study indicates that the low serum levels of β_{1c}-globulin that may be present over long periods in patients with persistent hypocomplementemic glomerulonephritis can be ascribed, in part, to *in vivo* breakdown of this protein as a result of reaction with immune complexes. The contribution of β_{1c} deposition on immune complexes and of diminished synthesis to the depressed serum levels cannot be assessed by the present study. [Extract.]

Importance

This landmark study is selected to exemplify the advances in pathobiological investigations in human renal disease that occurred in the 1960s, when the role of aberrations in the complement system in renal disease was the subject of intense investigation. This was stimulated by elegant biochemical studies (by Müller-Eberhard and others) that elucidated the complex nature and multiprotein components of the complement system. Clark West and his colleagues at the Children's Hospital in Cincinnati, Ohio, were intrigued by observations that some children with persistent glomerulonephritis had low serum complement (β_{1c} globulin, the C3 component of complement) (West *et al.*, 1964, 1965; Gotoff *et al.*, 1965). They sought to understand this better by conducting studies to ascertain whether C3 was being synthesized at a slower rate, being deposited in tissue (as a part of an 'immune complex') or broken down at an accelerated rate in the circulation. The investigation included 94 subjects (some normal, some nephritic with low serum C3, and some nephritic with normal C3 levels). By examining the serum concentration of fragments of the native C3 protein, they demonstrated conclusively that *in vivo* breakdown of C3 is at least in part a mechanism for the low C3 levels seen in some children (and adults) with persistent glomerulonephritis. They designated this group of children and adults with persistent (chronic) glomerulonephritis and continually low C3 levels 'hypocomplementemic glomerulonephritis'. West and his colleagues remained at the forefront of this work characterizing the clinical, morphological, and biochemical features of this unique group of patients. Very soon, it became apparent that this pattern of low serum C3 was tightly associated with a form of glomerular disease known as lobular or membranoproliferative glomerulonephritis, one of the first renal diseases to be linked to a biochemical disturbance in complement metabolism. Since then, this has become an expanding category of renal disease, which now encompasses genetic, infection-related, and auto-immune disorders affecting any one of the multitude of active protein and regulatory factors within the complement cascade, including the classical, alternative, lectin, and fibrin-related pathways. The work illustrated here by the pioneering studies of West and colleagues is but one example of the evolving story of complement and its role in kidney disease. Sometime in the not too distant future, treatment modalities will emerge that are directed to modifying the deleterious influence of disturbed complement activation and its regulation on kidney structure and function.

References

Gotoff SP, Fellers FX, Vawrter GF, Janeway CA, Rosen FS (1965). The beta1c globulin in childhood nephrotic syndrome. Laboratory diagnosis of progressive glomerulonephritis *N Engl J Med* **273**, 524–560.

West CD, Northway JD, Davis NC (1964). Serum levels of beta1C globulin, a complement component, in the nephritides, lipoid nephrosis and other conditions. *J Clin Invest* **43**, 1507–1515.

West CD, McAdams AJ, McConville JM, Davis NC, Holland NH (1965). Hypocomplementemic and normocomplementemic persistent (chronic) glomerulonephritis: clinical and pathologic characteristics. *J Pediatr* **67**, 1089–1098.

6.7 Fibrillary renal deposits and nephritis

Authors

JL Duffy, E Khurana, M Susin, G Gomez-Leon, J Churg

Reference

American Journal of Pathology 1983, **113**, 279–290.

Abstract

The authors have studied 8 patients whose glomeruli contain abundant fibrils in their mesangial matrix and basement membranes. Although the location of these fibrils is very similar to that of amyloid, they are about twice the size of amyloid fibrils, averaging 20 nm in width, and fail to react as amyloid does with special stains. Immunofluorescence-microscopic studies are usually positive with antiserums to IgG, often IgM, and in some cases IgA, and also kappa and lambda light chains, C3, and C4. The fibrils are associated with diffuse mesangial widening and increased mesangial matrix strands. Although peripheral glomerular capillary walls appear to be spared initially, their eventual involvement leads to glomerular capillary collapse and glomerular obsolescence. Crescent formation occurred in 5 cases, focally in 3 and diffusely in 2. Tubular basement membrane involvement was seen in 1 case. These patients exhibit hematuria, and proteinuria, and often hypertension and renal insufficiency. Proteinuria was in the nephrotic range in 3 patients in whom involvement of glomerular capillary basement membranes was extensive. Unless electron microscopy is applied to renal biopsies, these cases may be considered to represent mesangiocapillary or rapidly progressive glomerulonephritis, or amyloidosis. The nature of these fibrils is as yet not determined. It is likely that they have been called 'atypical amyloidosis' in the past.

Importance

This paper by Duffy and colleagues exemplifies the expansion in our knowledge of renal disease that came about through the 'routine' application of sophisticated light, immunofluorescence, and electron microscopy to material obtained by percutaneous renal biopsy in patients with renal disease of uncertain causation. New clinico-pathological entities were described. These workers described an entity of non-amyloid fibrillary deposits containing immunoglobulin in a case series of eight patients with nephritis. Similar findings in a single case had been described by Rosenmann and Eliakim in 1977 (Rosenmann and Eliakim, 1977). These observations created a new and distinct entity of non-amyloid fibrillary nephritis. A twist on this entity was described by Korbet *et al.* (1985), who reported 11 patients with organized, immunoglobulin-containing, non-amyloid fibrillary deposits that were microtubular structures; they designated them 'immunotactoids' to distinguish them from the organized deposits seen in cryoglobulinaemia and other disorders. The 'immunotactoids' were different in morphology from the fibrillary deposits first described by Duffy and colleagues, but the clinical and light microscopic features were similar, except that immunotactoid glomerulopathy was more frequently associated with a monoclonal immunoglobulin disorder.

This paper of Duffy and colleagues highlights the rapidly evolving knowledge being derived from detailed analysis of renal biopsy material, and in particular stresses the importance of electron microscopy, which was critical in delineation of the non-amyloid fibrillary glomerulopathies.

There were many other fresh insights into glomerular disease, and novel clinico-pathological entities were rapidly being discovered. Another example is IgA nephropathy, which was defined following the introduction of immunofluorescence to renal biopsy analysis (see paper 5.5). A further striking example, still being debated, was the separation of 'collapsing glomerulopathy' within the spectrum of FSGS (see paper 5.4), which gave much impetus to the concept that many primary (and secondary) glomerular diseases arise from diffuse injury to the podocyte. Weiss *et al.* (1986) were the first to recognize what is now called 'collapsing glomerulopathy', which is believed by some to be a variant of FSGS, whilst others regard it as a distinct clinico-pathologic entity in it own right. As this entity can occur with or without infection with human immunodeficiency virus and can also develop consequent to a variety of toxic exposures and immune diseases, it most probably represents an extreme example of diffuse podocyte injury (Detweiler *et al.*, 1994).

References

Detweiler RK, Falk RJ, Hogan SL, Jennette JC (1994). Collapsing glomerulopathy: a clinically and pathologically distinct variant of focal segmental glomerulosclerosis. *Kidney Int* **45**, 1416–1434.

Korbet SM, Schwartz MM, Rosenberg BF, Sibley RK, Lewis EJ (1985). Immunotactoid glomerulopathy. *Medicine (Baltimore)* **64**, 228–243.

Rosenmann E, Eliakim M (1977). Nephrotic syndrome associated with amyloid-like glomerular deposits. *Nephron* **18**, 301–308.

Weiss MA, Daquioag E, Margolin EG, Pollak VE (1986). Nephrotic syndrome, progressive renal failure and glomerular 'collapse': a new clincio-pathologic entity? *Am J Kidney Dis* **7**, 20–28.

6.8 Evidence suggesting under-treatment in adults with idiopathic focal segmental glomerulosclerosis. Regional Glomerulonephritis Registry Study

Authors

Y Pei, D Cattran, T Delmroe, A Katz, A Lang, P Rance

Reference

American Journal of Medicine 1987, **82**, 938–944.

Abstract

During the past 11 years, the Metro Toronto Glomerulonephritis Registry has prospectively followed all cases of glomerulonephritis starting from the time of biopsy. Focal segmental glomerulosclerosis was diagnosed by strict histologic criteria in 103 patients. Exclusion of patients with follow-up of less than 12 months reduced the number to 93 (55 adults and 38 children). Mean length of follow-up from the time of biopsy was 61 months. Ninety percent of children, but only 33 percent of adults received treatment with steroids, with or without cytotoxic drugs (p <0.001). Complete remission, defined as daily proteinuria of less than 250 mg, was not different in adults (39 percent) from that in children (44 percent), with a mean remission duration for all patients of 38 months. Chronic renal insufficiency, defined as a creatinine clearance of less than 0.8 ml/second/1.73 m^2 for more than 12 months, was similar in adults (40 percent) and children (34 percent). Five-year renal actuarial survival, defined as the absence of chronic renal insufficiency, was 96 percent for patients with a history of complete remission, and 55 percent for those without (p <0.0002). Logistic regression analysis showed treatment to be the only significant factor for complete remission (p <0.001). Complete remission, in turn, was important for renal preservation, defined as the absence of chronic renal insufficiency (p <0.001). Age did not affect the treatment response or long-term renal outcome in focal segmental glomerulosclerosis. Yet, the percent of adults treated was much lower than that of children, despite the fact that the majority of the untreated adults had the same clinical parameters as the treated adults and children. Thus, a judicious course of treatment is as much indicated in adults as in children with this disorder.

Importance

This short report utilized information collected prospectively by a glomerular disease registry in Metropolitan Toronto, Canada, the first of many similar registries (usually basing case ascertainment on renal biopsy findings). This report explored treatment of idiopathic FSGS with corticosteroids, evaluating whether the data suggested undertreatment of this condition in adults compared with that of children: 90% of children but only 33% of adults received corticosteroid treatment for FSGS. However, the compete remission rate was similar in adults (39%) and children (44%), and, as expected, such a complete remission was a significant factor in determining freedom from end-stage renal disease after long-term follow-up. Whilst descriptive and observational in nature, this study served to stimulate great interest in treatment of this condition, which had previously been regarded as 'untreatable,' at least in adults.

This has been selected as a landmark paper for two reasons. Firstly, it is one of the first reports to emanate from a registry of glomerular disease, and demonstrated the value and richness of data that can be derived from such registries. And secondly, because it was 'practice changing'. Registries have played an important role in the evolution of our knowledge about glomerular disease and have often provided hypothesis-generating observational data that provide the rationale for the subsequent development of randomized controlled clinical trials of treatment. This paper is an exception as it did not stimulate a randomized clinical trial of corticosteroid therapy for FSGS in adults.

Nevertheless, it did provoke a re-examination of the possible benefits of corticosteroids (particularly in more prolonged treatment regimens) and subsequently, based largely on detailed studies of observational data, has led to prolonged corticosteroid therapy becoming standard clinical practice.

6.9 A randomized trial of methylprednisolone and chlorambucil in idiopathic membranous nephropathy

Authors

C Ponticelli, P Zucchelli, P Passerini, L Cagnoli, B Cesana, C Pozzi, S Pasquali, E Imbasciati, C Grassi, B Redaelli, M Sardelli, F Locatelli

Reference

New England Journal of Medicine 1989, **320**, 8–13.

Abstract

We conducted a controlled trial to investigate the long-term effects of treatment with methylprednisolone and chlorambucil in patients with idiopathic membranous nephropathy. We have previously reported that after a mean of 31 months, treated patients did better. We now report the results of a longer follow-up.

Eighty-one patients with proteinuria ($\geq$3.5 g per day) and biopsy-proved membranous nephropathy were randomly assigned to receive either supportive therapy alone or a six-month course of corticosteroids alternated with chlorambucil (0.2 mg per kilogram of body weight per day) every other month. Methylprednisolone was first given intravenously in three pulses (1 g per day) and was then given orally (0.4 mg per kilogram per day) for 27 days.

The patients were followed for 2 to 11 years (median, 5). Two patients in the control group and one in the treatment group died. At the last follow-up visit, 9 of 39 patients assigned to the control group (23 percent) and 28 of 42 patients assigned to the treatment group (67 percent) did not have the nephrotic syndrome. At five years there were more remissions of the nephrotic syndrome in treated patients than in controls (22 of 30 vs. 10 of 25; P = 0.026). Compared with base-line values, the mean reciprocal of the plasma creatinine level declined significantly in the control group (33 percent; P = 0.0002) but not in the treatment group (6 percent; P not significant). Plasma creatinine increased by 50 percent or more in 19 controls (49 percent) and in 4 treated patients (10 percent).

We conclude that a six-month course of methylprednisolone and chlorambucil can bring about sustained remission of the nephrotic syndrome and help to preserve renal function in patients with idiopathic membranous nephropathy.

Importance

This paper epitomizes the application of randomized controlled trial (RCT) methodology to the treatment of glomerular disease. Ponticelli and his colleagues concentrated on idiopathic membranous nephropathy with full-blown nephrotic syndrome and well-preserved renal function. In this open-label but controlled study, 42 subjects were randomized to a protocol of monthly cycles of intravenous methylprednisolone, oral prednisone, and oral chlorambucil for 6 months (now known as the 'Ponticelli regimen') and 39 were allocated to 'supportive' therapy alone (not including renin–angiotensin system blockade). At 5 and 10 years after enrolment, those treated with the Ponticelli regimen were more likely to be in complete or partial remission and to have better preserved renal function. These findings were later confirmed in another long-term study (Jha *et al.*, 2007).

The value of RCTs has improved greatly over the years, not least because of higher standards required for publication of such trials and better appreciation of the intricacies of their design, including the necessary numbers of randomized subjects for adequate statistical power and careful attention to drop-out rates. For example, one of the earliest RCTs in glomerular disease, the Medical Research Council study of nephrotic syndrome by Black *et al.* (1970) may well have been rejected for publication in the current era as underpowered and of inadequate design by today's more rigorous standards. The Medical Research Council trial had a very limited effect on practice, quickly being made obsolete by studies in larger numbers of better characterized patients. On the other hand, the Ponticelli trial selected here had an immediate and lasting effect on treatment of membranous nephropathy, although not without lingering controversy, not least the question of whether this regimen should be reserved only for patients with membranous nephropathy who, after a period of observation, are shown to have persistent or deteriorating renal disease.

RCTs in glomerular disease are to this day hampered by the relative infrequency of many diseases, as well as their clinical, morphological, and pathogenetic heterogeneity. Furthermore, their often prolonged course means that outcomes may need to be based on surrogates, such as a change in proteinuria or renal function rather than on patient-centred 'hard' events, such as death or end-stage renal disease. Nevertheless, RCTs, such as the one by Ponticelli and co-workers, have the capacity to change practice, receive independent confirmation, and stand the test of time, after appropriate challenge of their findings and implications. It is highly likely that well-done RCTs in the field of glomerular disease in the future will be strong candidates for 'landmark' status in the next 50 years.

References

Black DAK, Rose G, Brewer DB (1970). Controlled trial of prednisone in adult patients with the nephrotic syndrome. *Br Med J* **3**, 421–426.

Jha V, Ganguli A, Saha TK, *et al.* (2007). A randomized, controlled trial of steroids and cyclophosphamide in adults with nephrotic syndrome caused by idiopathic membranous nephropathy. *J Am Soc Nephrol* **18**, 1899–1904.

6.10 M-type phospholipase A$_2$ receptor as target antigen in idiopathic membranous nephropathy

Authors

LH Beck, RGB Boneigo, G Lambeau, DM Beck, DW Powell, TD Cummins, JB Klein, DJ Salant

Reference

New England Journal of Medicine 2009, **361**, 11–21.

Abstract

Background: Idiopathic membranous nephropathy, a common form of the nephrotic syndrome, is an antibody-mediated autoimmune glomerular disease. Serologic diagnosis has been elusive because the target antigen is unknown.

Methods: We performed Western blotting of protein extracts from normal human glomeruli with serum samples from patients with idiopathic or secondary membranous nephropathy or other proteinuric or autoimmune diseases and from normal controls. We used mass spectrometry to analyze the reactive protein bands and confirmed the identity and location of the target antigen with a monospecific antibody.

Results: Serum samples from 26 of 37 patients (70%) with idiopathic but not secondary membranous nephropathy specifically identified a 185-kD glycoprotein in nonreduced glomerular extract. Mass spectrometry of the reactive protein band detected the M-type phospholipase A$_2$ receptor (PLA$_2$R). Reactive serum specimens recognized recombinant PLA$_2$R and bound the same 185-kD glomerular protein as did the monospecific anti-PLA$_2$R antibody. Anti-PLA$_2$R autoantibodies in serum samples from patients with membranous nephropathy were mainly IgG4, the predominant immunoglobulin subclass in glomerular deposits. PLA$_2$R was expressed in podocytes in normal human glomeruli and colocalized with IgG4 in immune deposits in glomeruli of patients with membranous nephropathy. IgG eluted from such deposits in patients with idiopathic membranous nephropathy, but not in those with lupus membranous or IgA nephropathy, recognized PLA$_2$R.

Conclusions: A majority of patients with idiopathic membranous nephropathy have antibodies against a conformation-dependent epitope in PLA$_2$R. PLA$_2$R is present in normal podocytes and in immune deposits in patients with idiopathic membranous nephropathy, indicating that PLA$_2$R is a major antigen in this disease.

Importance

It would be hard not to select this seminal paper with broad transformative power as the bookend to a chapter of landmark papers in primary glomerular disease appearing in the last 60 years. Beck and his colleagues tackled a mystery that has lingered unsolved since the original definition of idiopathic membranous nephropathy as an immune-mediated disease in the late 1950s: what is/are the antigen(s) and antibody/antibodies? In a series of elegant studies, they solved the mystery and in the process created a whole other series of questions needing answers. In concept, the study was simple: to identify the molecular nature of an extract of kidney that reacted with serum or renal tissue eluates from subjects with membranous nephropathy. In practice, the challenge was more difficult and had eluded a solution for many decades, despite the existence of a very reproducible laboratory model in rats of membranous nephropathy, partly because the human and rodent antigen were different. But the problem yielded to a sophisticated protein chemistry and immunological approach. An M-type phospholipase receptor (PLA$_2$R), presumably a constituent of normal human podocyte, was identified as the pathogenetic antigen, and circulating IgG4 (and possibly IgG1) auto-antibodies were identified as the vector of injury in idiopathic membranous nephropathy but very uncommonly in other forms of membranous nephropathy. The observations were quickly confirmed, and allowed for the first time measurement of the 'activity' of the immunological processes directly responsible for the disease.

This paper has overtones of a Sherlock Holmes or Hercule Poirot novel. A victim was identified (a patient with idiopathic membranous nephropathy), the weapon was known (IgG4 auto-antibodies) but the exact target and the perpetrator were a mystery. This paper solved the target issue (PLA2R on podocyte) but the perpetrator still remains in the shadows. What causes the victim to make these auto-antibodies to a constituent of normal tissue in the first place? The answer to this fundamental question probably lies in the genetic make-up (immune-response genes) of the victim and subtle changes in the three-dimensional structure of the target antigen (neo-epitopes). Nevertheless, this study provided powerful new tools to analyse the natural history of this disease and its response to varying forms of treatment, including its well-known tendency to undergo spontaneous remissions and to recur in renal allografts. Based on preliminary data, other diseases of mysterious pathogenesis may also yet yield to studies exploring mechanisms of kidney injury, such as FSGS (Wei *et al.*, 2011). Time will tell.

Reference

Wei C, El Hindi S, Li J, *et al.* (2011). Circulating urokinase receptor as a cause of focal segmental glomerulosclerosis. *Nat Med* **17**, 952–960.

Chapter 7

Secondary glomerular disease—since 1950

Richard J. Glassock

7.1 Lupus nephritis: a clinical and pathologic study based on renal biopsies

Authors

RC Muehrcke, RM Kark, CL Pirani, VE Pollak

Reference

Medicine (Baltimore) 1957, **36**, 1–145.

Summary

Observations were made on 33 living patients with lupus nephritis seen at the Presbyterian and Cook County Hospitals in Chicago over a 2-year period, supplemented by pathological findings in 21 autopsied patients with lupus nephritis overseen at these institutions over an extended period. The purpose of this retrospective observational study was to characterize the pathophysiology and natural history of lupus nephritis. Detailed clinical examination, serial renal biopsies (and autopsy material) were used to create a composite picture of the diversity of lupus nephritis and its evolution over time.

Importance

This seminal paper is a monumental treatise 133 pages long (one of the longest ever published in a first-line journal). The study was carried out as the authors recognized an increased frequency of patients with systemic lupus erythematosus who were developing overt manifestations of renal disease and surviving for longer due to better general management (e.g. antibiotics, antihypertensive drugs) and perhaps as a consequence of the treatment with adrenocorticotropic hormone (ACTH) and corticosteroids.

The clinical description of the patients included in the analysis anticipates many of the descriptions of lupus nephritis that were to follow. Although the nomenclature and classification of lupus nephritis evolved after this publication, many of the fundamental findings of lupus nephritis are contained within the text and photomicrographs. It must be remembered that renal biopsy had been introduced into clinical use only about 5 years earlier, and immunofluorescence and electron microscopy were not yet part of the routine examination of renal biopsy material. In addition, the lupus erythematosus cell phenomenon was described only 7 years before the authors began this study.

Several 'firsts' were presented in this paper: (i) The 'pseudo-nephrotic syndrome' in lupus nephritis, wherein marked proteinuria and hypoalbuminaemia were present but the serum cholesterol was reduced rather than elevated; (ii) conversion of the pathological findings over time; (iii) glomerular injury in the presence of normal urinalyses; and (iv) presentation of lupus nephritis with a paucity of clinical features of systemic lupus. The authors were struck with the relentlessly progressive nature of the disease and the common occurrence of renal failure, which was invariably fatal at that time. In their experience, 'if they live long enough almost all patients with progressive lupus nephritis will pass though an edematous stage of nephritis associated with hypoalbuminemia, hypercholesterolemia and much proteinuria'. While these manifestations of lupus nephritis have been altered dramatically by the introduction of more effective therapy, it is useful to recall, using the prism of history, how devastating the renal disease was, and still can be, in patients with lupus.

7.2 Effect of large doses of prednisone on the renal lesions and life span of patients with lupus glomerulonephritis

Authors

VE Pollak, CL Pirani, RM Kark

Reference

Journal of Laboratory & Clinical Medicine 1961, **57**, 495–511.

Abstract

In 1957 we reported on ten patients with lupus glomerulonpehritis who had been studied by percutaneous renal biopsy. They had been treated with an average of 50 mg of cortisone daily. All died at an average of 13.8 months after they were first studied; eight died in renal failure. Subsequently, sixteen patients with lupus glomerulonephritis were treated with large doses of prednisone—an average of 47.5 mg daily for 6 months. Only seven have died, five in renal failure. The other nine are living now, an average of 34.2 months after they were first studied.

The two groups of patients were compared in detail at the time of the initial biopsy study and before treatment began. They were comparable both clinically and in terms of renal function. Detailed histologic analyses of the initial renal biopsy showed comparable severity and activity of the renal lesions. Serial histologic studies showed progression and continued activity of the renal lesions in the group treated with small doses of prednisone. In the high steroid group, the active lesions decreased or disappeared in most patients; glomerular basement thickening and adhesions were the main residua in the glomeruli.[Adapted.]

Importance

This seminal paper describes the benefits of larger doses of prednisone on the renal lesions and outcomes of lupus nephritis followed in an observational manner. The two groups were comparable clinically and histologically at the onset of treatment, but the 'low-dose' group were all treated in 1953–1955 and the 'high-dose' group were treated in 1956–1958. Eight patients received 'low doses' of cortisone (averaging 50 mg/day of cortisone) and 16 patients 'high doses' of prednisone (averaging 47.5 mg/day of prednisone, equivalent to approximately 225 mg/day of cortisone). All of the low-dose group died after an average of 13.5 months with or of renal failure. Seven of the high-dose group died, five in renal failure. The life expectancy was prolonged in the high-dose group. Serial biopsies showed improvement in the renal lesions only in the high-dose group. Severe Cushing's syndrome was noted in 15 of the 16 patients treated with high-dose prednisone, and viral and bacterial infections (including reactivation of tuberculosis) were common. Peptic ulcer disease, diabetes mellitus, osteoporosis, myopathy, and psychiatric disturbances were also noted. The level of renal function (as assessed by blood urea nitrogen) predicted the outcomes in the high-dose group. This paper exemplifies the interest that emerged in the late 1950s in treating severe lupus nephritis aggressively after the ominous outcome of renal involvement in systemic lupus was well characterized (see paper 7.1). The design of this study was flawed in contemporary terms (historical controls, low numbers studied, and short term follow-up) and the side-effects of treatment were considerable. Nevertheless, this study did generate the hypothesis that lupus nephritis was a treatment-modifiable disease. It had a significant impact on thinking about lupus nephritis and its management, and indirectly spawned other attempts to manage this disease, many of which were designed to obviate the serious side effects of prolonged 'high-dose' prednisone therapy so evident in this initial study (see papers 7.4 and 7.10).

7.3 The role of anti-glomerular basement membrane antibody in the pathogenesis of human glomerulonephritis

Authors

RA Lerner, RJ Glassock, FJ Dixon

Reference

Journal of Experimental Medicine 1967, **126**, 989–1004.

Abstract

These observations established the presence of anti-GBM antibodies in the sera and/or kidneys of six humans with glomerulonephritis. Further, it seems clear that these antibodies do combine with the host's glomeruli *in vivo* and with GBM antigen of several species *in vitro*.

Transfer of acute glomerulonephritis to normal recipient monkeys was possible with serum or renal eluate IgG from the three patients with anti-GBM antibodies in whom sufficient material was available. Based on this transfer of nephritis and on the presence of these antibodies at the site of injury in the nephritic kidneys of both the patients and the recipient monkeys, it seems likely that they are at least a contributing, if not primary, cause of the glomerular injury.

The frequency of anti-GBM antibodies in human nephritis is not certain, but on the basis of preliminary observations it would appear that they are present in all cases of Goodpasture's nephritis and somewhat less than half of the cases of subacute and chronic glomerulonephritis of adults.

The nature and source of immunogen stimulating the production of anti-GBM antibodies is not known, but the presence of potentially nephritogenic GBM antigens in normal urine raises the question of possible autoimmunization.

From a practical point of view, it appears that patients forming anti-GBM antibodies may not be good candidates for renal transplantation since they are likely to produce in the transplants the nephritic changes already suffered by their own kidneys.

Importance

This paper was the first to describe an auto-immune glomerular renal disease. It describes the detection of an IgG anti-antibody to native constituents in the glomerular basement membrane (GBM) evoking a severe glomerular injury, often with crescents. The anti-GBM auto-antibody could be detected in serum and eluted from diseased kidneys with 'linear' deposits of IgG along the capillary wall. Eluted antibody could induce nephritis in monkeys, and renal transplantation of patients with circulating anti-GBM antibody showed a recurrence of linear deposits of IgG in post-transplant renal biopsies. Thus, for the first time, Koch's postulates (as modified by Witebsky) were successfully applied to a human auto-immune glomerular disease.

This discovery of anti-GBM nephritis depended on several antecedent observations and developments: (i) the technique of immunofluorescence microscopy, described by Coons and Kaplan in 1950, that allowed the tracing of proteins (such as IgG antibodies) deposited in tissues; (ii) the recognition that 'linear' staining of IgG by immunofluorescence in glomerular disease was a hallmark of a disease mediated by binding of circulating antibody to native GBM antigens; this knowledge emanated from studies on nephrotoxic serum nephritis (Masugi nephritis) and other forms of experimental nephritis such as Steblay's nephritis (in sheep immunized with heterologous GBM antigens); (iii) the recognition that tissue deposits of IgG (representing anti-GBM antibody) could be eluted intact from diseased tissue specimens [kidneys removed at the time of transplantation in patients with end-stage renal disease (ESRD)]; and (iv) the discovery that the native antigen in GBM could be solubilized to serve as detecting antigen for assays of circulating and eluted antibody in *in vitro* systems. The studies of anti-GBM nephritis paid many dividends, as the reagents developed were subsequently used to characterize the native GBM collagen moieties involved in hereditary disease of Alport syndrome (the Goodpasture antigen) (Pedchenko *et al.*, 2010). Sensitive and specific immunochemical assays for anti-GBM antibody were subsequently developed and its presence was associated with the clinical presentation of pulmonary haemorrhage and glomerulonephritis (Goodpasture disease). The presence of circulating anti-GBM antibody served as a rationale for the development of successful therapy (plasma exchange and immunosuppression) (Lockwood *et al.*, 1976) for anti-GBM antibody disease, a true 'bench-to-bedside' evolution.

References

Coons AH, Kaplan MH (1950). Localization of antigen in tissue cells; improvements in a method for the detection of antigen by means of fluorescent antibody. *J Exp Med* **91**, 1–13.

Lockwood CM, Rees AJ, Pearson TA, Evans DJ, Peters DK, Wilson CB (1976). Immunosuppression and plasma-exchange in the treatment of Goodpasture's syndrome, *Lancet* **i**, 711–715.

Pedchenko V, Bondar O, Fogo AB, *et al.* (2010). Molecular architecture of the Goodpasture autoantigen in anti-GBM nephritis. *N Engl J Med* **363**, 343–354.

7.4 Treatment of lupus nephritis with cyclophosphamide

Authors

JS Cameron, M Boulton-Jones, R Robinson, C Ogg

Reference

Lancet 1970, **ii**, 846–850.

Abstract

Six patients with glomerulonephritis associated with systemic lupus erythematosus were treated with cyclophosphamide for an average of 9 months to date. Four of the patients showed some resistance to treatment with corticosteroids; all were cushingoid and three had severe hypertension. Renal biopsies were done in all six, and showed lupus glomerulonephritis, active in three. Three patients showed considerable improvement, proteinuria disappearing in two, and becoming trivial in the third. The nephrotic syndrome present in all three remitted, and two showed an increase in glomerular filtration-rate. The condition of another two patients remained unchanged, although reduction of corticosteroids and disappearance of toxic signs was achieved in both with continuing control of the disease. One patient anuric when treatment was started with haemodialysis, heparin, prednisolone and cyclophosphamide, had an active necrotizing renl lesion which was uncontrolled and resulted in death. It is concluded that if a controlled trial of cytostatic agents is set up to evaluate their usefulness in patients with the nephritis of systemic lupus, then cyclophosphamide should be one of the drugs considered for examination.

Importance

This paper launched the use of cyclophosphamide (CYC) to manage severe lupus nephritis. The authors described a small uncontrolled study of six patients with lupus nephritis (five with proliferative lupus nephritis and one with membranous lupus nephritis) all of whom had active extra-renal disease, and four of whom had proved 'resistant' to steroid treatment. Nephrotic syndrome, present in three cases, remitted in all. Improvements in clinical features accompanied by lower doses of steroid were observed commonly. Only one of the six patients treated with CYC was considered to be a 'failure'. The authors concluded that a controlled trial was needed to resolve the issue of efficacy and safety of CYC in lupus nephritis. The authors also noted that such an assessment would need to take into account the appearance of the disease on renal biopsy and the clinical stage of the disease when treatment is commenced. Both were prescient comments indeed about the proper design of trials in lupus nephritis.

The use of CYC in renal disease can be traced to the seminal paper of Chasis *et al.* in 1949 describing the use of nitrogen mustard in glomerulonephritis. However, experience with such agents remained very limited, and at the time that this landmark paper from Guy's Hospital, London, appeared, 'high-dose' prednisone was still the mainstay of therapy for severe lupus nephritis with unsatisfactory results, and a marked adverse effect profile of the corticosteroids was still stimulating great interest in alternative strategies, including the concomitant use of 'immunosuppressive' chemical agents such as azathioprine, 6-mercaptopurine, thioguanine, and alkylating agents. This landmark paper, although reporting experience in only six patients, was instrumental in promoting the need for effective treatment trials of alkylating agents, which eventually came to fruition with the National Institutes of Health trial of 1986 (Austin *et al.*, 1986). This latter randomized controlled trial helped established the long-term efficacy of combined CYC and prednisone regimens in severe lupus nephritis and demonstrated the ineffectiveness of a steroid-only regimen for the long-term outcome of the disease. This paper, although its conclusions were highly preliminary, had a material impact on bringing alkylating agents to the fore in the management of severe lupus nephritis.

References

Austin HA III, Klippel JH, Balow JE, *et al.* (1986). Therapy of lupus nephritis. Controlled trial of prednisone and cytotoxic drugs. *N Engl J Med* **314**, 614–619.

Chasis H, Goldring W, Baldwin DS (1949). Effect of febrile plasma, typhoid vaccine and nitrogen mustard on renal manifestations of human glomerulonephritis. *Proc Soc Exp Biol Med* **71**, 565–567.

7.5 Manifestations of systemic light chain deposition

Authors

RE Randall, WC Williamson Jr, F Mullinax, MY Tung, WJ Still

Reference

American Journal of Medicine 1976, **60**, 293–299.

Abstract

In two patients with terminal renal failure, manifestations of disease developed in multiple organ systems. One had a previous diagnosis of multiple myeloma with kappa light chain proteinemia and proteinuria. The other had idiopathic lobular glomerulonephritis. Hepatic and neurologic abnormalities developed in both; in the latter gastrointestinal, cardiac and endocrine disease developed as well. Clinical and pathologic correlations suggest that the retention and tissue deposition of light chains produced the organ dysfunction, inasmuch as free kappa light chain determinants were demonstrated histologically in the clinically affected organs. The deposition in these patients may be an extreme example of a common but previously unrecognized form of plasma cell dyscrasia.

Importance

Although this is only a 'case report', it is a landmark paper as it established the existence of a new entity, now called light-chain deposition disease, and described the amorphous, non-fibrillar character of the deposits of κ light chain, which are now referred to as 'Randall-type' deposits after the senior author of the paper.

This paper described two cases presenting with advanced renal failure and manifestations of disease in multiple organ systems (primarily liver, heart, and kidneys). One had multiple myeloma and κ light-chain proteinuria. The other had a picture of 'lobular' glomerulonephritis. Both were seen to have extensive tissue deposits of κ light chain in many organs by electron microscopy. The deposits were of an amorphous or flocculent character and were negative by Congo Red and silver methenamine staining. The reporting of these two cases established that monoclonal light chains (particularly κ light chain) could be deposited in many organs in the absence of typical amyloid light-chain fibrils and provoke clinically recognizable disease.

We now recognize that lambda light chains can evoke a similar pattern (although much less commonly) and we also recognize that many other non-amyloid deposition diseases also exist, consisting of whole or fragments of immunoglobulins. We remain ignorant of the fundamental mechanisms responsible for their affinity for certain tissues. Light-chain deposition disease is rare, and it has not yet been possible to define properly the best therapeutic strategies, although therapy directed against monoclonal plasma cell proliferation can be effective, including the use of melphalan, dexamethasone, thalidomide or lenalinomide, bortezomib, and autologous stem-cell transplantation.

7.6 Crescentic glomerulonephritis without immune deposits: clinicopathologic features

Authors

MM Stilmant, WK Bolton, BC Sturgill, GW Schmitt, WG Couser

Reference

Kidney International 1979, **15**, 184–195.

Abstract

Of 46 patients with acute crescentic glomerulonephritis involving 20 to 90% of glomeruli, 16 had no definable systemic disease and no significant glomerular immune deposits by immunofluorescent or electron microscopy. Anti-GBM antibody and circulating immune complexes were further excluded by radioimmunoassay and Raji cell assay in all patients tested. Clinical features included a 10:6 male:female ratio, mean age of 58 years (range, 13–77), disease duration of less than 3 months, rapidly deteriorating renal function, and frequent pulmonary manifestations. Nine patients had oliguria, serum creatinine concentrations over 6 mg/100 ml, and required dialysis, but three of these patients subsequently recovered renal function. These three patients and seven patients with creatinine concentrations of less than 6 mg/100 ml have not progressed to chronic renal failure. In this series, idiopathic acute crescentic glomerulonephritis without immune deposits was more common than was immune complex or anti-GBM nephritis. The clinical, laboratory, and pathologic characteristics of these patients were similar to those reported in anti-GBM and immune-complex-induced glomerulonephritis. These observations expand the spectrum of rapidly progressive crescentic glomerulonephritis. They suggest that glomerular immune deposits may be less important than other factors in determining the extent of renal injury and subsequent clinical course in crescentic glomerulonephritis.

Importance

This paper made the original observations that 16 of 46 patients (35%) with acute necrotizing and crescentic glomerulonephritis lacked significant glomerular immune deposits by both immunofluorescence and electron microscopy. There was a male predominance and the average age of the patients was 58 years. All had rapidly deteriorating renal function and many had pulmonary manifestations, including pulmonary haemorrhage. Nine of the 16 patients (56%) required dialysis but one-third of these eventually recovered sufficiently to stop dialysis. Anti-GBM and immune complex forms of crescentic glomerulonephritis were less common in this series. This form of crescentic glomerulonephritis resembled the form of renal vasculitis associated with anti-neutrophil cytoplasmic antibodies (ANCA), although of course ANCA were not described until 1982.

This paper therefore gives the first description of what subsequently became known as 'pauci-immune' necrotizing and crescentic glomerulonephritis, and the observations were quickly confirmed in many pathology laboratories throughout the world. Soon after the seminal paper by van der Woude and colleagues in 1985 (see paper 7.9), it became evident that many (but not all patients) with 'pauci-immune' crescentic glomerulonephritis had circulating ANCA (most often anti-myeloperoxidase) and that the disease was most likely a 'renal-limited' form of microscopic polyangiitis. This was a major conceptual advance in our understanding of crescentic glomerulone-phritis and more or less completed the immunopathological dissection of crescentic disease into three parts: anti-GBM disease, ANCA-associated (often 'pauci-immune') disease, and immune-complex deposition disease. Many refinements in the diagnosis of this disease have occurred sub-sequently, but the fundamental behaviour of the disease is unchanged from that described in this original report.

7.7 Mixed cryoglobulinemia: clinical aspects and long-term follow-up of 40 patients

Authors

PD Gorevic, HJ Kassab, Y Levo, R Kohn, M Meltzer, P Prose, EC Franklin

Reference

American Journal of Medicine 1980, **69**, 287–308.

Abstract

The clinical course of 40 patients with significant quantities of mixed cryoglobulins, but without lymphoproliferative, collagen-vascular or chronic infectious diseases, is presented. These cases comprise 51.3 percent of all mixed and 31.7 percent of all types of cryoglobulins evaluated by us over the period 1960–1978. A characteristic clinical syndrome, consisting of recurrent palpable purpura (100 percent), polyarthralgias (72.5 percent) and renal disease (55 percent), was seen. Biopsy specimens of skin lesions showed cutaneous vasculitis, and half had immune reactants in vessel walls. Seventy percent of patients had evidence of hepatic dysfunction, often subclinical, and more than 60 percent of those tested had serologic evidence of prior infection with hepatitis B virus. Hepatic lesions ranged from minimal triaditis to chronic active hepatitis and/or cirrhosis. All 22 patients in whom clinical renal disease developed had significant proteinuria; 63.6 percent had diastolic hypertension, 77.3 percent edema, 45.5 percent renal failure and 22.7 percent were nephrotic. Glomerular disease associated with deposition of immunoglobulin G, immunoglobulin M and complement, often with coexistent renal arteritis, was confirmed pathologically in 15 cases.

All cryoglobulins had rheumatoid factor activity and consisted of IgM and polyclonal IgG; five also contained IgA. Thirteen had a monoclonal IgM kappa component. Serum protein electrophoresis was unremarkable or showed diffuse hyperglobulinemia. Striking depression of early complement components was noted but did not correlate well with the cryoprotein concentration, renal involvement or clinical course.

Follow-up for periods up to 21 years from onset of symptoms revealed that renal involvement has a deleterious effect on prognosis. Postmortem examinations of nine patients demonstrated widespread vasculitis in addition to renal involvement. Preterminal infection was found in eight.

Importance

This landmark paper was the first substantial description of the clinical syndrome associated with circulating 'mixed' IgG/IgM cryoglobulinaemia In 40 cases, up to then the most extensive experience with this disease to date, they documented a characteristic 'mixed cryoglobulinaemia syndrome' consisting of recurrent palpable purpura, polyarthralgia, and renal disease. Many patients had hepatic disease (thought then to be due to hepatitis B virus infection), and those with renal disease were commonly nephrotic with impaired renal function. Serum complement components were commonly decreased and striking depression of C4 levels to <5 mg/dl seen in 63% of patients tested. The cryoglobulins were mixed IgM κ/IgG in 30% and mixed polyclonal IgM and IgG in 58%. Rheumatoid factor was positive in 68% of those tested. Renal disease had a profound deleterious effect on survival, and vasculitis and crescentic glomerulonephritis were frequently observed at autopsy. Treatment with corticosteroids and CYC seemed to be beneficial, but the effects of plasma exchange were equivocal.

The recognition of the syndrome of mixed IgM/IgG cryoglobulinaemia and its relationship to renal disease was an important development, and the findings elaborated by these authors still hold true today but with some significant embellishments. This paper combined mixed IgM κ (monoclonal)/polyclonal IgG cryoglobulinaemia and mixed polyclonal IgM/polyclonal IgG cryoglobulinaemia under a single heading. We now know that the former is commonly associated with hepatitis C virus (HCV) infection, a viral disease not recognized in 1980. Recognition of the importance of a membranoproliferative pattern of glomerular injury in the sequence of HCV-associated mixed cryoglobulinemia also came later. The tropism of HCV for B cells explains many of the clinical manifestations of HCV-associated mixed cryoglobulinaemia. We now have more effective and specific treatment strategies for this condition: treatment of the HCV infection (ribavarin and interferon), removal of cryoglobulin (plasma exchange), and reduction of cryoglobulin production (rituximab). Nevertheless, the efficacy of CYC and corticosteroids has been supported by subsequent studies, and can still be helpful in some circumstances, especially with very severe vasculitis and crescentic glomerulonephritis.

7.8 Effect of cyclophosphamide upon the immune response in Wegener's granulomatosis

Authors

AS Fauci, SM Wolff, JS Johnson

Reference

New England Journal of Medicine 1971, **285**, 1493–1496.

Abstract

Nine patients with Wegener's granulomatosis were studied before and after treatment with cyclophosphamide alone. The study was undertaken to determine any immunologic abnormalities associated with the disease, to observe the effect of cyclophosphamide on the clinical course, as well as on the immune response in man, and to observe any correlation between clinical response and immunosuppression. Untreated patients had elevated mean serum IgA levels of 470 as compared with 200 mg per 100 ml in normal controls and elevated mean-parotid-fluid secretory IgA levels of 4.7 as compared with 1.8 mg per 100 ml in normal controls. Seven of the nine patients receiving cyclophosphamide had undetectable humoral and delayed hypersensitivity response to a new antigenic stimulus, and five of the seven retained previously established delayed hypersensitivity. A favorable clinical response seemed to be correlated.

Importance

This paper, and its companion by the same authors 2 years later (Fauci and Wolff, 1973) are landmarks in the therapy of Wegener's granulomatosis (WG) (also known in a recently proposed nomenclature as granulomatous polyangiitis; Falk *et al.*, 2011). Up to that time, WG had a dismal prognosis and the only available therapy, corticosteroids, was unable to control either the renal or extrarenal vasculitis. With these papers, an effective therapy emerged for the first time, and treatment regimens were built on this basis from the early 1970s onwards. This paper describes in detail the response of only nine patients with WG to treatment with CYC. Five of the nine patients had renal disease and seven of the nine developed a complete or partial remission, some of which were long lasting. Encouraged by this dramatic response, the authors extended their studies into a larger series (Fauci and Wolff, 1973) that generally confirmed these preliminary observations. Treatment with CYC had significant effects on immune function and caused transitory leukopenia but it was not possible to determine whether these changes were responsible for the observed beneficial effects on the course of the disease in this early study. Prolonged treatment with CYC could result in a long-term remission (a 'cure') but at the expense of significant complications (such as bone marrow hypoplasia, infections, non-bacterial hemorrhagic cystitis and bladder cancer, and haematological neoplasia). Cyclophosphamide-based regimens were then extended to other forms of systemic polyangiitis with good success. However, long-term complications of prolonged CYC, often used for a year or more, generated great concern. Subsequently, randomized controlled trials using prolonged CYC therapy as the standard of care have supported the shorter-term use of CYC as an 'induction' regimen followed by long-term maintenance with better tolerated agents (such as azathioprine) (Jayne *et al.*, 2003). Nevertheless, CYC (intravenously or orally) for a short course has remained at the core of therapy, and can result in long-term relapse-free control of the disease in the majority of patients. Progressive renal failure can also be avoided provided treatment is started early enough, before too much irreversible renal damage has occurred. Only recently is the possibility emerging that CYC may not be needed at all for some patients, as the anti-CD20 monoclonal antibody rituximab is also very effective for inducing remission in selected cases of granulomatous polyangiitis and microscopic polyangiitis (Jones *et al.*, 2010), although the long-term outcomes of rituximab therapy are still not well known.

References

Falk RJ, Gross WL, Guillevin L, *et al.* (2011). Granulomatosis with polyangiitis (Wegener's): an alternative name for Wegener's granulomatosis. *Arthritis Rheum* **63**, 863–864.

Fauci AS, Wolff SM (1973). Medicine (Baltimore) Wegener's granulomatosis: studies in eighteen patients and a review of the literature. *Medicine (Baltimore)* **52**, 53–61.

Jayne D, Rasmussen N, Andrassy K, *et al.* (2003). A randomized trial of maintenance therapy for vasculitis associated with antineutrophil cytoplasmic autoantibodies. *N Engl J Med* **349**, 36–44.

Jones RB, Tervaert JW, Hauser T, *et al.* (2010). Rituximab versus cyclophosphamide in ANCA-associated renal vasculitis. *N Engl J Med* **363**, 211–220.

7.9 Autoantibodies against neutrophils and monocytes: tool for diagnosis and marker of disease activity in Wegener's granulomatosis

Authors

FJ van der Woude, N Rasmussen, S Lobatto, A Wiik, H Permin, LA van Es, M van der Giessen, GK van der Hem, TH The

Reference

Lancet 1985, **i**, 425–429.

Abstract

Immunoglobulin G (IgG) autoantibodies against extranuclear components of polymorphonuclear granulocytes were detected in 25 of 27 serum samples from patients with active Wegener's granulomatosis and in only 4 of 32 samples from patients without signs of disease activity. In a prospective study of 19 patients these antibodies proved to be better markers of disease activity than several other laboratory measurements used previously. The autoantibodies were disease specific and the titres were related to the results of an in-vitro granulocyte phagocytosis test, in which 7S IgG antibodies were internalised after specific binding to the cell, resulting in gradual formation of ring-like cytoplasmic structures. This autoantibody may have a pathogenetic role in Wegener's granulomatosis. The detection of this antibody is valuable for diagnosis and estimation of disease activity.

Importance

This paper describes IgG auto-antibodies directed to extranuclear (cytoplasmic) components of polymorphonuclear granulocytes in subjects with active systemic polyangiitis of the type usually known as Wegener's granulomatosis (WG) or, as in a recently proposed nomenclature, granulomatous polyangiitis (Falk *et al.*, 2011). These antibodies were detected in an indirect immunofluorescence test using ethanol-fixed granulocytes and monocytes as a substrate. The association with active disease was striking: 93% of patients with clinically active WG had such antibodies in the serum, whereas only 13% of serum samples from patients with WG and no signs of clinical activity were positive for antibody, nor were these antibodies found in any normal control sera. The titres of the antibody fell as disease activity subsided. The authors speculated that these auto-antibodies might play a pathogenetic role in the disease and that they might be helpful in the diagnosis and prognosis of WG.

Although similar if not identical auto-antibodies had been described previously by Davies *et al.* (1982) and Hall *et al.* (1984), this report was the first to investigate systematically the diagnostic and prognostic utility of an indirect immunofluorescence-based assay. It can be considered as the seminal paper introducing the concept of 'anti-neutrophil cytoplasmic antibodies' (ANCA) and the association of these antibodies with systemic polyangiitis. Subsequently, these antibodies were shown to be directed against constituents of the azurophilic granules of leukocytes, either proteinase 3 or myeloperoxidase. Sensitive and antigen-specific assay systems were developed and a pathogenetic role for such antibodies proven by studies in animals with experimentally induced disease. The original observations of these authors were confirmed on multiple occasions and laboratory testing for ANCA is now a mainstay for the diagnosis and subsequent clinical management of both systemic and renal-limited forms of polyangiitis.

References

Davies DJ, Moran JE, Niall JF, Ryan GB (1982). Segmental necrotising glomerulonephritis with antineutrophil antibody: possible arbovirus aetiology? *Brit Med J* **285**, 606.

Falk RJ, Gross WL, Guillevin L, *et al.* (2011). Granulomatosis with polyangiitis (Wegener's): an alternative name for Wegener's granulomatosis. *Arthritis Rheum* **63**, 863–864.

Hall JB, Wadham BM, Wood CJ, Ashton V, Adam WR (1984). Vasculitis and glomerulonephritis: a subgroup with an antineutrophil cytoplasmic antibody. *Aust N Z J Med* **14**, 277–278.

7.10 Mycophenolate mofetil *versus* cyclophosphamide for induction treatment of lupus nephritis

Authors

GB Appel, G Contreras, MA Dooley, EM Ginzler, D Isenberg, D Jayne, LS Li, E Mysler, J Sánchez-Guerrero, N Solomons, D Wofsy, and the Aspreva Lupus Management Study Group

Reference

Journal of the American Society of Nephrology 2009, **20**, 1103–1112.

Abstract

Recent studies have suggested that mycophenolate mofetil (MMF) may offer advantages over intravenous cyclophosphamide (IVC) for the treatment of lupus nephritis, but these therapies have not been compared in an international randomized, controlled trial. Here, we report the comparison of MMF and IVC as induction treatment for active lupus nephritis in a multinational, two-phase (induction and maintenance) study. We randomly assigned 370 patients with classes III through V lupus nephritis to open-label MMF (target dosage 3 g/d) or IVC (0.5 to 1.0 g/m^2 in monthly pulses) in a 24-wk induction study. Both groups received prednisone, tapered from a maximum starting dosage of 60 mg/d. The primary end point was a prespecified decrease in urine protein/creatinine ratio and stabilization or improvement in serum creatinine. Secondary end points included complete renal remission, systemic disease activity and damage, and safety. Overall, we did not detect a significantly different response rate between the two groups: 104 (56.2%) of 185 patients responded to MMF compared with 98 (53.0%) of 185 to IVC. Secondary end points were also similar between treatment groups. There were nine deaths in the MMF group and five in the IVC group. We did not detect significant differences between the MMF and IVC groups with regard to rates of adverse events, serious adverse events, or infections. Although most patients in both treatment groups experienced clinical improvement, the study did not meet its primary objective of showing that MMF was superior to IVC as induction treatment for lupus nephritis.

Importance

This study was chosen to illustrate the advances made in the design and conduct of randomized controlled trials (RCTs) in secondary glomerular diseases, and to illustrate how far the field of treatment of lupus nephritis has advanced since the days described in the paper 7.1 in 1957. Appel and colleagues reported on an open-label, single-blinded RCT comparing intravenous CYC (the standard of care) with oral mycophenolate mofetil (MMF) in patients with moderately severe lupus nephritis (both regimens included tapering steroid treatment). It was one of the largest RCTs ever conducted in lupus nephritis, with 370 patients randomized and followed for 6 months for end points of a response to treatment, defined as a reduction in proteinuria to subnephrotic levels and a stabilization of renal function. The randomized patients had mean serum creatinine levels of approximately 1.1 mg/dl (100 μmol/l) at baseline and the average 24 h urine protein was approximately 4.0 g/day. There was no difference in response rates at the end of follow up: 56% of those receiving MMF and 53% of those receiving CYC. The complete remission rate at 6 months was also similar in the two groups (approx. 8%). MMF seemed to be somewhat more effective in subjects of non-white ancestry. Adverse events were somewhat more common with CYC, but deaths were numerically slightly more common with MMF (9/184 with MMF versus 5/180 with CYC). The characteristics of the adverse events were different in the two groups, as expected. Thus, MMF was shown to be approximately equal (but not superior) to CYC in the short-term management of lupus nephritis. Subjects who responded were subsequently randomized to a maintenance regimen of MMF or azathioprine. This follow-on study showed that MMF was superior to azathioprine for maintenance of a remission in lupus nephritis (Dooley *et al.*, 2011).

Whilst many similar RCTs could have been selected as landmark papers, this study stands out as exemplary due to its rigorous design and large size. Even though it failed to meet its primary end point, it has had a significant impact on practice, as many physicians were loath to use CYC in the management of young women with lupus nephritis and sought possible alternative strategies for short-term management. Combined with the follow-on maintenance trial, it appears that many patients with lupus nephritis (of moderate severity) can be effectively treated with MMF for both induction of remission and maintenance for a prolonged relatively relapse-free interval. The shortcoming of this otherwise highly significant study is that the follow-up was relatively short. It has been known for decades that the evolution of lupus nephritis to ESRD may take many years; thus, we still do not know if these regimens will forestall the development of ESRD. However, we have come along way since the cortisone treatment era of the 1950s.

Reference

Dooley MA, Jayne D, Ginzler EM, *et al.* (2011). Mycophenolate versus azathioprine as maintenance therapy for lupus nephritis. *N Engl J Med* **365**, 1886–1895.

Chapter 8

Infection and renal disease

Trevor Gerntholtz

Introduction

Over the last century, non-communicable diseases have assumed primacy as the growing cause of death, first in the developed world and now also in the developing world. However, communicable disease has not retreated, and infection remains a major cause of death, especially but not exclusively in the developing world. This remains particularly true of renal disease. Infection remains a key aetiological agent in many types of renal disease, and new infective renal diseases, most notably those associated with human immunodeficiency virus (HIV) infection have emerged.

Furthermore, over the last 50 years or so, the interruption of the natural history of both acute kidney injury (AKI) and end-stage renal disease (ESRD) by renal replacement therapy has led to a multitude of iatrogenic infective problems, which continue to challenge nephrologists.

The landmark papers selected in this chapter reflect the changing interface between the emerging specialty of nephrology and infectious disease over the last 50 years. The papers are presented in chronological order. The chapter starts with the first application of modern dialysis technology to a tropical cause of AKI, acute malaria, and ends with papers addressing the infectious challenges of using dialysis and transplantation for the treatment of ESRD. These include the dialysis patient who is prone to infection because of unnatural skin breach by a percutaneous haemodialysis catheter, the transplant patient put at risk for opportunist infection by immunosuppressive therapy, and finally the challenge of renal transplantation when there is ongoing HIV infection.

In between, we see the impact of modern diagnostic and research techniques on our understanding of the aetiology, pathogenesis, and treatment of infection-related glomerular disease. This impact began with the introduction of renal biopsy in 1951 (see paper 3.6) and the progressive sophistication of immunopathogenic investigative techniques, whose application to glomerular disease is also demonstrated in Chapters 6 and 7.

Infection as a primary cause of renal disease will not disappear for the foreseeable future. Furthermore, it seems likely that iatrogenic, opportunistic infective disease will remain as challenging as ever, particularly as nephrologists seek to push the boundaries of immunosuppressive therapy in both transplantation and primary renal disease.

8.1 The artificial kidney in malaria and blackwater fever

Authors

RC Jackson, AW Woodruff

Reference

British Medical Journal 1962, **i**, 1367–1372.

Abstract

Of four patients (one civilian and three Service men) who developed acute renal failure complicating *P. falciparum* malaria and blackwater fever, two had severe cerebral malaria, from which one recovered. Of the remaining two, one died during transit a few hours before admission and the other patients survived.

Haemodialysis was performed on three of the patients. One patient, a civil airline pilot, became ill in the United Kingdom; the other three were evacuated by air from Bahrein, Aden, and West Africa via Las Palmas.

The dangers of inadequate malaria prophylaxis and delay in starting treatment on malaria are stressed. Tubular necrosis is confirmed by renal biopsy and necropsy as the lesion causing the renal failure which follows severe *P. falciparum* malaria and blackwater fever. Attention is drawn to its reversibility and to the importance of its early recognition.

The concept that patients with blackwater fever should not be moved must be revised if those with renal failure are to have every chance of survival. If acute renal failure is present for three days arrangements should be made for transfer to a centre with facilities for haemodialysis. The possibility of patients with malaria developing acute renal failure in the United Kingdom or temperate climates should be borne in mind.

It is probable that this is the first record of patients with malarial renal failure being managed with the aid of an artificial kidney.

Importance

This landmark article is extraordinary for many reasons. Written in the UK 50 years ago, it gives many insights into the evolving therapeutics of the time. The language of the article itself is also a refreshing change from the prosaic scientific monologues of today's journals.

The clinical problem being addressed was well known. Acute malaria due to *Plasmodium falciparum* was and remains a major cause of AKI in endemic malaria areas. The term blackwater fever of course refers to malaria accompanied by dark urine due to haemoglobinuria provoked by severe intravascular haemolysis. The mortality rate for this condition was 20–25%; untreated uraemia accounted for about half of these deaths, the others dying because of cerebral malaria and multi-organ failure due to anoxia.

Kolff had first used his rotating drum dialysis machine in 1943 to treat acute kidney injury (see paper 12.1). His twin coil dialyser was used in the first dialysis treatment programme for AKI in the UK established in Leeds in 1956 (Turney *et al.*, 2011) and by the early 1960s was being used in a small number of renal units in the UK, of which one of the most prominent was run by the Royal Air Force, the unit that published this landmark paper. Thus, this is the first published description of an interface between modern dialysis technology and a type of AKI hitherto confined to the developing world.

The authors relied on urine output and rises in blood urea to evaluate clinical progress, and make no mention of serum creatinine levels. This is perhaps surprising, as the measurement of creatinine, by the Jaffe reaction, had been available since the 1890s, although in the 1960s creatinine assays were still being improved for speed and accuracy (see paper 3.2).

Another interesting aspect is the pathological descriptions of the necropsy material in two of the patients and the renal biopsy in a third (performed because of persistent renal failure after 3 months). The description of tubular necrosis as the dominant renal lesion is especially noteworthy, as tubular occlusion had been regarded previously as most important. What is also apparent is the occurrence of secondary bacterial infections in these patients, often requiring the use of additional antibiotics.

The importance of early evacuation to a specialist centre is emphasized, perhaps self-evident to the modern reader, but the crucial context was the prevailing dogma at that time that those with malaria and blackwater fever were 'too ill to move'.

The authors also make a plea for the use of prophylaxis in those who are travelling to malaria areas ('the continent of Africa'). None of the patients reported here took effective malaria prophylaxis despite it being prescribed. Three of those reported here were young servicemen, but the fourth, a civil airline pilot, who became ill in the UK, reminds us that the age of modern air travel that was beginning to open up in the 1960s would bring to hospitals in countries such as the UK a range of important diseases hitherto familiar only in the tropics.

Reference

Turney JH, Blagg CR, Pickstone JV (2011). Early dialysis in Britain: Leeds and beyond. *Am J Kidney Dis* **57**, 508–515.

8.2 Glomerulonephritis with deposition of Australia antigen-antibody complexes in glomerular basement membrane

Authors
B Combes, J Shorey, A Barrera, P Stastny, EH Eigenbrodt, AR Hull, NW Carter

Reference
Lancet, 1971, **ii**, 234–237.

Abstract

A patient with persistent Australia (Au) antigenæmia after post-transfusion hepatitis developed membranous glomerulonephritis. Immunofluorescent staining of kidney tissue revealed glomerular deposits of IgG, complement C3, and Au antigen in a pattern characteristic of immune complex deposition. These findings suggest that Au antigen was involved in the formation of immune complexes whose glomerular deposition initiated the pathologic process leading to the development of diffuse membranous glomerulonephritis.

Importance

This landmark article was the first demonstration of the presence of hepatitis B virus (HBV) in the glomerular basement membrane deposits in a patient with membranous nephropathy. The surface antigen of HBV had first been isolated in the serum of an Australian aboriginal patient, hence the term 'Australia antigen'. This paper was therefore written prior to a full understanding of the protein structure of HBV, including its surface and core antigens.

The patient, a 53-year-old male, developed acute hepatitis with the eventual appearance in the circulation of the Australia (Au) antigen 4 months after a blood transfusion following a motor vehicle accident. It should be noted in passing that he received corticosteroids, the treatment of choice in the 1970s for 'acute hepatitis'. The patient had generalized swelling and ascites, which was presumed to represent renal as well as hepatic disease, when the new onset of proteinuria was confirmed. The authors went on to perform both a liver and a kidney biopsy, the latter showing the characteristic changes of membranous nephropathy, including capillary wall staining for IgG and C3, and on electron microscopy subepithelial electron dense deposits. The authors sought evidence of the Au antigen in the basement membrane deposits using a specific guinea pig antibody against Au antigen, which was in turn visualized using rabbit anti-guinea pig antibodies. The biopsy of a patient with lupus nephritis who was Au antigen negative was used as an appropriate control.

The unequivocal presence of Au antigen in the glomerular basement membrane deposits together with the proteinuria led the authors to deduce that the Au antigen was the aetiological agent, provoking the antibody and complement response and leading to the characteristic features of membranous nephropathy. Whilst not perhaps fully satisfying Koch's postulates, this was nevertheless one of the first convincing demonstrations of the direct involvement of an infective agent in immune-mediated glomerular disease and is a beautiful demonstration of the potential power of a carefully studied single index patient to inform clinical practice.

8.3 Associated focal and segmental glomerulosclerosis in the acquired immunodeficiency syndrome

Authors

TK Rao, EJ Filippone, AD Nicastri, SH Landesman, E Frank, CK Chen, EA Friedman

Reference

New England Journal of Medicine 1984, **310**, 669–673.

Abstract

Of the 92 patients with the acquired immunodeficiency syndrome (AIDS) who were seen at our institution over a two-year period, 9 acquired the nephrotic syndrome (urinary protein >3.5 g per 24 hours) and 2 had azotemia with lesser amounts of urinary protein. Five of these 11 patients had a history of intravenous-heroin addiction, but in the remaining six, there were no known predisposing factors for nephropathy. In nine patients (including the six non-addicts) the course of renal disease was marked by rapid progression to severe uremia. Renal tissue examined by biopsy in seven patients and at autopsy in three revealed focal and segmental glomerulosclerosis with intraglomerular deposition of IgM and C3. In the 11th patient, renal biopsy revealed an increase in mesangial matrix and cells, with deposition of IgG and C3 consistent with a mild immune-complex glomerulonephritis, and severe interstitial nephritis. We conclude that focal and segmental glomerulosclerosis may be associated with AIDS and suggest that rapid deterioration to uremia may characterize this renal disease.

Importance

In 1984, when this article was published, patients were presenting to hospitals with signs and symptoms indicating severe immune deficiency, resulting in the use of the acronym AIDS (acquired immunodeficiency syndrome). The precise aetiology (HIV) was still unknown.

This landmark report is the first clinico-pathological description of 11 patients with AIDS who presented with kidney disease at a hospital in Brooklyn, New York, between 1981 and 1983.

The authors described the archetypical glomerular lesion of what was later to be named HIVAN (HIV-associated nephropathy). The characteristic lesions of focal segmental glomerulosclerosis are described together with the interstitial inflammation and tubular dilatation (later referred to as 'microcysts'). The clinical correlate was that nine out of the 11 patients presented with nephrotic syndrome. Deterioration of renal function was rapid: from presentation to severe uraemia took 8–16 weeks. Ten patients had died, and the 11th was receiving maintenance dialysis at the time of writing, emphasizing the aggressive nature of the disease, both renal and extrarenal. The high incidence of opportunistic infections was also noted.

Heroin use is a well-established cause of focal segmental glomerulosclerosis, so this needed to be considered as the cause of the renal disease rather than AIDS. However, six of the 11 patients were not drug users, and later reports soon confirmed that the HIVAN lesion was regularly seen in those who were not drug users.

One patient, however, did not have what is now regarded as typical HIVAN, but instead showed evidence of mesangial proliferation with marked interstitial inflammation. Granular mesangial deposition of C3 and IgG was also seen, and electron microscopy revealed both mesangial and subendothelial electron dense deposits. Although this patient also had a poor clinical outcome, these different histological features suggested immune complex-mediated glomerulonephritis. Today, this form of immune complex mediated HIV-associated kidney disease is regularly seen as well as typical HIVAN, and is usually known as HIVICK (HIV immune complex kidney).

Since this landmark report, much has been learnt about the mechanisms by which HIV injures the glomerulus (see paper 8.6). However, still lacking is a consensus on how best to classify HIV-associated renal disease. Nor, despite the passage of more than a quarter of a century since this report, are there substantial prospective randomized controlled trials (RCTs) investigating treatment options for the various forms of HIV-related kidney disease.

8.4 Treatment of hepatitis B virus-associated membranous nephropathy with recombinant alpha-interferon

Author

CY Lin

Reference

Kidney International 1985, **47**, 225–230.

Abstract

An open, randomized trial study on the therapeutic effect of recombinant alpha-interferon (IFN alpha) in 40 patients with hepatitis B virus membranous nephropathy (HBVMN) was conducted. All were pathologically proven to have HBVMN which showed no response to corticosteroid treatment represented by persistent heavy proteinuria. Both HBeAg and HBsAg were positive in all. Group 1 was composed of 20 patients who were treated with recombinant IFN alpha (5 subjects, body wt < 20 kg; 8 subjects, body weight 20 kg) by subcutaneous (s.c.) injection three times a week for 12 months. In group 2 there were 20 patients who received supportive treatment only. At the end of the third month of treatment, all patients in Group 1 were free of proteinuria. In contrast, 10 patients (50%) in Group 2 had persistent heavy proteinuria and another 10 patients (50%) had light proteinuria with exacerbation during respiratory tract infection. At the end of the twelfth month, 8 patients (40%) in Group 2 still had persistent heavy proteinuria and 12 patients (60%) had light proteinuria with frequent relapses. Eight patients (40%) in Group 1 had HBeAg seroconversion between the fourth and sixth months and HBsAg seroconversion between the tenth and twelfth months. HBe seroconversion only [HBeAg (−)/HBsAg (+)] was found in four patients. Four patients had no change in HBV serological markers [HBeAg (+)/HBsAg (+)]. The remaining 4 patients had HBeAg (−)/ HBeAb (+) HBsAg (−)/HBsAb (−) at the end of the twelfth month. In contrast, there was no seroconversion of HBeAg (+)/ HBsAg (+) in Group 2 patients. These results suggest that IFN alpha therapy is of value in complete resolution of heavy proteinuria, and provides some benefit in seroconversion of HBeAg (+)/HBsAg (+) in children with HBVMN.

Importance

Although there had been previous observational studies of the use of interferon in treating patients with HBV membranous nephropathy, this is a landmark paper because it the first RCT of such therapy, indeed it is the first RCT of any antimicrobial therapy in patients with infection-associated glomerulonephritis. Remarkably, the single author claims sole responsibility for all the work described in the paper, which was conducted on Chinese children in Taipei, Taiwan. Forty children with proteinuria and biopsy-proven HBV membranous nephropathy were enrolled. Patients had to be HBV surface antigen (HBsAg) positive (in peripheral blood) and to have evidence on renal biopsy of either hepatitis B core antigen, HBsAg, or HBV e antigen (HBeAg) deposits in the glomerular basement membranes. Patients were randomized either to receive treatment with either alpha interferon (IFN-α) by subcutaneous injection three times a week for a year, or to a control arm using 'supportive' treatment only. Corticosteroids and other immunosuppressive treatments were not allowed.

All patients were followed up at monthly intervals for a year. The results were remarkable in that all patients in the IFN-α treatment group showed a decrease in their proteinuria within 3 months, and by 9 months all 20 patients were free of proteinuria, which continued to the end of the 1-year study. This contrasted markedly with only seven of 20 in the control group being free of proteinuria at the end of the year. Renal function was initially normal in both groups and remained so through the trial. Eleven of the patients in the treatment group lost seropositivity for HBsAg and HBeAg, but none did in the control group. It should be noted that, even in those whose serum was not cleared of HBV antigens in response to IFN-α, there was none the less a dramatic improvement in proteinuria.

This is an important RCT of treatment for a deep-seated kidney infection with very good clinical response rates. The high doses of IFN-α had some adverse effects but overall were remarkably well tolerated. It would have been most interesting to know of any correlation between clinical response, resolution of the membranous lesion, and clearance of virus from the deposits, and perhaps most especially to have seen the renal lesions in those with persistent viraemia but loss of proteinuria. However, practical realities and ethical concerns would both no doubt have prevented a second biopsy in these children.

8.5 Membranoproliferative glomerulonephritis associated with hepatitis C virus infection

Authors

RJ Johnson, DR Gretch, H Yamabe, J Hart, CE Bacchi, P Hartwell, WG Couser, LL Corey, MH Wener, CE Alpers, R Willson

Reference

New England Journal of Medicine 1993, **328**, 465–470.

Abstract

Background and methods: Hepatitis C virus (HCV) infection causes both acute and chronic liver disease and is also associated with mixed cryoglobulinemia. Whether HCV is also associated with renal disease, as is the hepatitis B virus, is not known. We describe the clinical, pathologic, virologic, and immunologic features of eight patients with HCV infection who were referred to nephrologists for glomerulonephritis. Four patients were treated with interferon alfa.

Results: All eight patients had proteinuria, and seven had decreased renal function. Renal biopsy in all patients revealed membranoproliferative glomerulonephritis, characterized by the deposition of IgG, IgM, and C3 in glomeruli. Electron microscopy of the biopsy specimens showed cryoglobulin-like structures in three of four patients. All eight patients had HCV RNA detected in their serum, elevated serum aminotransferase concentrations, and hypocomplementemia, and the majority had cryoglobulins and circulating immune complexes in their serum. Cryoprecipitates from the three patients who were tested contained HCV RNA and IgG anti-HCV antibodies to the nucleocapsid core antigen (HCVc or c22–3). IgM rheumatoid factors, present in all patients, bound anti-HCV IgG in all six patients tested. Four patients received interferon alfa for 2 to 12 months; all had evidence of decreased HCV replication and improvement of their renal and liver disease

Conclusions: Chronic HCV infection is associated with cryoglobulinemia and membranoproliferative glomerulonephritis. The pathogenesis is unknown, but may relate to deposition within glomeruli of immune complexes containing HCV, anti-HCV IgG, and IgM rheumatoid factors.

Importance

Hepatitis C virus (HCV) was identified only as recently as 1989 as a cause of non-A, non-B hepatitis. It was apparent from the beginning that this infection was associated with many extrahepatic manifestations, usually associated with cryoglobulins. Case reports soon began to emerge describing an association between HCV infection and glomerular disease, including membranoproliferative glomerulonephritis (MPGN) and membranous nephropathy. However, this paper was the first to report a cohort of patients with MPGN, which is now recognized as the main pattern of HCV-induced renal pathology. The authors grouped together five patients from Seattle, USA, and three patients from Hirosaki,Japan. All eight presented with proteinuria but with reasonably preserved renal function.

Renal biopsies were performed, in all cases showing glomerular hypercellularity in the lobulated pattern typical of MPGN. Immunofluorescence demonstrated IgG, IgM, C3, and occasional IgA deposits. Electron microscopy where available showed subendothelial and mesangial electron dense deposits

Although it had for some time been suspected that many cases of MPGN were associated with chronic infection, this had been confirmed definitely in only a few cases. All these eight patients had HCV RNA detected in the serum, and in the three whose serum cryoglobulins were evaluated, anti-HCV antibodies and HCV antigen [demonstrated by polymerase chain reaction (PCR)] were found in the cryoprecipitates. Unfortunately, the authors were unable to find clear evidence that HCV antigens or HCV RNA were deposited in the glomeruli to help unravel the exact aetiology of this disease, but this could perhaps be explained by the insensitivity of the reagents used, especially if the antigen was masked by antibody.

Four of the patients were treated with IFN-α over a period varying from 2 to 12 months. There was a dramatic reduction in the amount of proteinuria in all four patients, together with an improvement in liver function and a loss of circulating HCV RNA. However, this did not always translate into an improvement in glomerular filtration rate.

This paper serves to highlight how difficult it was to prove an infective aetiology in kidney disease despite the demonstration of a consistent histological pattern in eight HCV-infected patients with resolution of some clinical parameters (proteinuria) in four of them following successful eradication of the HCV. Nevertheless, HCV infection has subsequently been confirmed as a major association with MPGN in many parts of the world.

8.6 Nephropathy and establishment of a renal reservoir of HIV type 1 during primary infection

Authors

JA Winston, LA Bruggeman, MD Ross, J Jacobson, L Ross, VD D'Agati, PE Klotman, ME Klotman

Reference

New England Journal of Medicine 2001, **344**, 1979–1984.

Case summary

A 35-year-old man had a six-week history of fatigue, weight loss, abdominal pain, diarrhoea, and night sweats. Several days before admission, he developed a rash and cervical and inguinal lymphadenopathy. He had a negative test for HIV-1 infection 4 months before admission. Serum creatinine concentration was 1.9 mg/dl (168 µmol/l), serum albumin 1.6 g/dl, urine protein 17 g/day; there was microscopic haematuria. HIV-1 antibodies were positive, plasma HIV-1 RNA level > 750,000 copies/ml, CD4 cell count 459/mm³. Serum creatinine rose to 6.3 mg/dl and he temporarily required haemodialysis. After 6 weeks of highly active antiretroviral therapy (HAART), plasma HIV-1 RNA level became undetectable, and there was sustained improvement in renal function—serum creatinine was 1.4 mg/dl, urine protein 1.5 g/day.

Two renal biopsies were performed—one before, and one three months after initiation of HAART. The first biopsy showed typical features of HIVAN with focal segmental glomerulosclerosis and on electron microscopy podocyte hypertrophy and endothelial tubuloreticular structures; there was also marked tubulointerstitial injury with some fibrosis. In the first biopsy the proliferation marker, Ki67, was expressed in podocytes with loss of synaptopodin. After three months of HAART, there was marked improvement in morphology with restoration of podocyte foot processes, loss of tubuloreticular inclusions, loss of Ki67 and restoration of normal synaptopodin expression. Tubular morphology also markedly improved. However the number of renal epithelial cells that expressed HIV-1 mRNA was similar before and during treatment, although circular forms of unintegrated HIV-1 DNA were absent on HAART. [Adapted.]

Importance

Although 'only' a case report, this is nevertheless a landmark paper that challenged a number of currently held views about the pathogenesis and clinical course of HIVAN.

Previous reports had emphasized that HIVAN was a late complication of HIV infection, yet this patient presented with severe nephrotic syndrome, renal impairment, and substantial morphological changes of HIVAN, including some interstitial fibrosis, on the initial renal biopsy very early in the course of the infection.

There was at this time only limited anecdotal evidence that HIVAN might respond to antiretroviral therapy. A rapid and relentless downhill course of renal function once HIVAN was diagnosed was considered typical. However, this patient had an excellent clinical and morphological response to therapy: proteinuria was reduced from 17 to only 1.5 g/day, and serum creatinine, which had risen rapidly during the hospital admission to the point that dialysis was required, improved and stabilized. The morphological response to therapy was even more impressive—marked resolution of the glomerular injury towards normal podocyte architecture, loss of podocyte expression of the proliferation marker Ki67, and restoration of synaptopodin expression, a mature podocyte marker. Against expectation, there was also recovery of the tubulointerstitial injury, including resolution of microcyst formation.

The findings in this case emphasized the value of the early introduction of highly active antiretroviral therapy (HAART) for treatment of HIVAN; this approach has now become the norm. However, the viral studies contained an important warning. Circular forms of unintegrated HIV-1 DNA (considered to indicate recent infection of the cell) were absent from renal epithelial cells following HAART, suggesting that therapy was preventing new infection of cells, but the number of renal epithelial cells, both tubular and glomerular, that expressed HIV-1 mRNA was similar before and during treatment. The implication was that the kidney appears to be an important reservoir for HIV-1 infection, and therefore a prime site for recurrence of active HIV infection if HAART is interrupted for any reason—a warning of importance for both personal and public health strategies designed to achieve adequate provision of HAART in many different socio-economic settings worldwide.

We should continue to rely on prospective RCTs in advancing clinical therapeutics and on observational cohort studies to provide information on disease mechanisms and natural history. Nevertheless, this landmark paper illustrates beautifully how careful observation and thorough evaluation of individual cases with striking clinical features can help lead to important advances.

8.7 Prevention of tunneled hemodialysis catheter-related infections using catheter-restricted filling with gentamicin and citrate: a randomized controlled study

Authors

GK Dogra, H Herson, B Hutchison, AB Irish, CH Heath, C Golledge, G Luxton, H Moody

Reference

Journal of the American Society of Nephrology 2002, **13**, 2133–2139.

Abstract

Tunneled catheters are widely used for the provision of hemodialysis. Long-term catheter survival is limited by tunneled catheter-related infections (CRI). This study assesses the efficacy of catheter-restricted filling with gentamicin and citrate in preventing CRI in hemodialysis patients. A double-blind randomized study was conducted to compare heparin (5000 U/ml) with gentamicin/citrate (40 mg/ml and 3.13% citrate; ratio 2:1) as catheter-lock solutions. A total of 112 tunneled catheters in 83 patients were enrolled at the time of catheter insertion for commencement or maintenance of hemodialysis. The primary end point was CRI. Catheter malfunction, defined as blood flow rate of <200 ml/min for three consecutive dialyses and/or the use of urokinase, was also assessed as a secondary end point. Infection rates per 100 catheter-days were 0.03 in the gentamicin group *versus* 0.42 in the heparin group ($P = 0.003$). Kaplan–Meier survival analyses showed mean infection-free catheter survival of 282 d (95% CI, 272 to 293 d) in the gentamicin group versus 181 d (95% CI, 124 to 237 d) in the heparin group (log rank, 9.58; $P = 0.002$). Cox regression analyses showed a relative risk for infection-free catheter survival of 0.10 (95% CI, 0.01 to 0.92) in the gentamicin group when adjusted for gender, race, diabetes mellitus, catheter malfunction, and hemoglobin ($P = 0.042$). The incidence of catheter malfunction was not significantly different between groups. Predialysis gentamicin levels were significantly higher in patients randomized to gentamicin (gentamicin/citrate: median 2.8 mg/L [range, 0.6 to 3.5 mg/L], $n = 5$; heparin: median <0.2 mg/L [range <0.2 to 0.2 mg/L], $n = 5$; $P = 0.008$). Tunneled hemodialysis catheter-restricted filling with gentamicin and citrate is a highly effective strategy for prevention of CRI. Although citrate as a catheter-lock solution provides adequate anticoagulation for the interdialytic period, gentamicin levels suggest significant risk for chronic aminoglycoside exposure and associated ototoxicity. Before this technique is adopted, these preliminary observations warrant replication in future studies that will examine the efficacy and safety of lower doses of gentamicin or alternative agents with a reduced potential for toxicity.

Importance

It is an unfortunate fact that vascular access in a substantial proportion of patients in most haemodialysis units will be provided by tunnelled central venous catheters. Despite an intensive focus over recent years on the advantages of definitive access, ideally using an arteriovenous fistula, dialysis catheters continue to be used widely. Catheter malfunction is a common complication, but catheter-related infection (CRI) is a more serious, and sometimes life-threatening, problem. Any strategy that effectively reduces the risk of CRI would have a major beneficial impact on patient care in modern haemodialysis units.

The benefit of an antibiotic 'lock' had not been studied systematically. This paper from Australia is a landmark because it is the first prospective randomized clinical trial investigating the use of antibiotic 'locking' solutions for tunnelled catheters in the prevention of CRI. Over a 2-year period, 79 patients receiving 108 catheter insertions were randomized to receive either a lumen 'lock' containing gentamicin and citrate (treatment) versus a standard heparin 'lock' (control). Citrate had to be used as the anti-coagulant with the gentamicin to avoid the risk of precipitation with heparin. There was meticulous follow-up at every dialysis using both clinical assessment and cultures looking for either exit-site infection or bloodstream infection. All patients were already being subjected to the standard of care at that time including nasal installation of mupirocin, chlorhexidine body wash, and intravenous antibiotics at the time of catheter insertion, with continued nasal mupirocin after catheter insertion. Those in the treatment arm had a marked and statistically significant decrease in the incidence of CRI (0.03 per 100 catheter days) versus those in the control arm (0.42 per 100 catheter days). In fact, there was not one case of bacteraemia in the antibiotic locked catheter group and only one exit site infection.

The one cause for concern was that, even though the antibiotic lock was supposed to be confined to the catheter alone, without entry into the systemic circulation, there were detectable gentamicin blood levels indicating that there had been some contamination. The study was not designed to establish whether such gentamicin contamination might lead to ototoxicity, nephrotoxicty, or bacterial resistance. Although investigation to establish the ideal antibiotic 'lock' has continued, this landmark paper shows the virtue of a RCT to answer a apparently simple clinical question but one with major patient benefits.

8.8 Is the nephritogenic antigen in post-streptococcal glomerulonephritis pyrogenic exotoxin B (SPE B) or GAPDH?

Authors

SR Batsford, S Mezzano, M Mihatsch, E Schiltz, Rodríguez-Iturbe B

Reference

Kidney International 2005, **68**, 1120–1129.

Abstract

Background: Acute glomerulonephritis can follow infection by group A streptococci. An immune-complex pathogenesis is accepted, but the causative antigen(s) is still controversial. In recent years, 2 streptococcal antigens, the cationic cysteine proteinase exotoxin B (SPE B) and the plasmin receptor, a glyceraldehyde phosphate dehydrogenase (Plr, GAPDH) have attracted attention because: (1) they were localized in glomeruli in patients with acute post-streptococcal glomerulonephritis (APSGN); and (2) serum antibody to these antigens was associated with nephritogenic streptococcal infections. To date, putative nephritogens were always tested independently. Here, the relevance of SPE B and GAPDH was evaluated in the same renal biopsies and serum samples of well-defined APSGN patients.

Methods: Renal biopsies (17 patients) and serum samples (53 patients) with APSGN and appropriate controls were examined. Immunofluorescent staining of frozen sections was performed using specific antibodies to SPE B and GAPDH. Serum antibodies were investigated by both enzyme-linked immunosorbent assay (ELISA) and Western blot methodology.

Results: Glomerular deposits of SPE B were demonstrated in 12/17 APSGN biopsies, and 2 cases were borderline; circulating antibodies were found in all instances (53/53 patients). Glomerular deposition of GAPDH was detected in 1/17 biopsies, and 2 cases were borderline; circulating antibodies were found in 5/47 patients. In 31 control biopsies, only weak staining for each antigen was found in 2 cases.

Conclusion: In this study, glomerular deposits of and antibody response to zymogen/SPE B are more consistently present in APSGN than deposits and antibody response to GAPDH. Zymogen/SPE B is likely to be the major antigen involved in the pathogenesis of most cases of APSGN.

Importance

The first description of 'nephritis' associated with streptococcal infection was made in a scarlatina epidemic in Edinburgh, UK, in the mid-nineteenth century (see paper 5.5), and an immune-complex pathogenesis for post-streptococcal glomerulonephritis had been accepted from the early 1900s. In spite of this, the exact pathophysiological link to *Streptococcus* has been elusive, and there had been many 'false starts' in the identification of which streptococcal antigen was provoking glomerular injury. There are many possible reasons for this rather slow progress, not least that post-streptococcal glomerulonephritis has become distinctly uncommon in the developed world, resulting in histological evidence being slow to accumulate due to the limited availability of renal biopsy material.

Nevertheless, by the time of this study, the search for the culprit antigen had finally been narrowed to two streptococcal products—a cationic cysteine proteinase, known as zymogen or streptococcal exotoxin B (SPE B), and a plasmin-binding membrane receptor, glyceraldehyde

3-phosphate dehydrogenase (GAPDH). Both of these are capable of binding plasmin, which is probably involved in the mechanism of injury.

In this landmark paper, the authors examined the renal biopsies from 17 adults and children with typical acute post-streptococcal glomerulonephritis from three centres (in Chile, Venezuela, and Switzerland) and the sera of 53 patients. In a series of carefully designed and controlled experiments, the authors sought evidence of SPE B and GAPDH in glomerular deposits and of antibodies to the two streptococcal antigens in convalescent sera. They demonstrated that anti-SPE B antibodies were in all patient sera, whereas the prevalence of anti-GAPDH antibodies did not differ from the general population. They found SPE B in 82% of biopsies, and positivity was even more likely in biopsies taken within 14 days of presumed clinical onset, but GAPDH was found in only one biopsy. In addition, for the first time, they showed SPE B within the subepithelial 'humps' that are virtually pathognomonic of post-infectious glomerulonephritis.

This study did not exclude the possibility that other streptococcal antigens could be the pathogenic agent in patients with differing genetic and environments—perhaps explaining a number of Japanese studies that have supported a role for GAPDH. Nevertheless, in these patients from Latin America and Europe, powerful and definitive evidence was presented for the central role of SPE B.

8.9 Prophylactic versus preemptive oral valganciclovir for the management of cytomegalovirus infection in adult renal transplant recipients

Authors

JA Khoury, GA Storch, DL Bohl, RM Schuessler, SM Torrence, M Lockwood, M Gaudreault-Keener, MJ Koch, BW Miller, KL Hardinger, MA Schnitzler, DC Brennan

Reference

American Journal of Transplantation 2006, **6**, 2134–2143.

Abstract

Prophylaxis reduces cytomegalovirus (CMV) disease, but is associated with increased costs and risks for side effects, viral resistance and late onset CMV disease. Preemptive therapy avoids drug costs but requires frequent monitoring and may not prevent complications of asymptomatic CMV replication. Kidney transplant recipients at risk for CMV (D+/R−, D+/R+, D−/R+) were randomized to prophylaxis (valganciclovir 900 mg q.d. for 100 days, n = 49) or preemptive therapy (900 mg b.i.d. for 21 days, n = 49) for CMV DNAemia (CMV DNA level >2000 copies/mL in ≥ 1 whole blood specimens by quantitative PCR) assessed weekly for 16 weeks and at 5, 6, 9 and 12 months. More patients in the preemptive group, 29 (59%) than in the prophylaxis group, 14 (29%) developed CMV DNAemia, p = 0.004. Late onset of CMV DNAemia (>100 days after transplant) occurred in 11 (24%) randomized to prophylaxis, and none randomized to preemptive therapy. Symptomatic infection occurred in five patients, four (3 D+/R− and 1 D+/R+) in the prophylactic group and one (D+/R−) in the preemptive group. Peak CMV levels were highest in the D+/R− patients. Both strategies were effective in preventing symptomatic CMV. Overall costs were similar and insensitive to wide fluctuations in costs of either monitoring or drug.

Importance

Infection with cytomegalovirus (CMV) following kidney transplantation can be devastating for recipients, with high rates of morbidity and mortality if untreated. In addition, active CMV infection increases the risk of acute rejection episodes. CMV infection rates in new kidney-transplant recipients in the absence of prophylactic therapy have been estimated to be between 20 and 60%.

At the end of the twentieth century, treatment of CMV infection was costly, requiring hospital admission for administration of intravenous ganciclovir.

This landmark paper reports the first prospective RCT comparing two strategies of dealing with CMV after renal transplantation, 'prophylaxis' or 'pre-emptive' therapy using the orally active valyl ester prodrug valganciclovir. Both of these strategies had their clinical proponents, but no study had provided objective comparative evidence of their suitability.

Patients were either given valganciclovir routinely for 100 days after transplantation, or they underwent weekly blood testing for CMV viraemia using PCR and were then treated with valganciclovir if they developed significant viraemia.

Both strategies were effective in reducing the rates of clinical CMV disease in the first 100 days after transplantation to 5%. It is notable that the pre-emptive strategy was associated with significantly more episodes of CMV viraemia than prophylaxis, but that once prophylaxis had been discontinued after 100 days, CMV viraemia occurred in 20% of patients, whereas only one patient who was managed pre-emptively developed late viraemia. It may be that a low-grade CMV DNAemia in the pre-emptive group resulted in the formation of protective antibodies. Only five symptomatic CMV infections occurred in the study, four with prophylaxis and one in the pre-emptive group. All four infections in the prophylactic group occurred after the 100-day tablet-taking period had expired.

This well-designed RCT therefore showed that both strategies are effective in reducing CMV infection, and that there is, despite the convictions of some, no substantial difference between them in efficacy or cost. The one practical issue not really susceptible to measurement, however, is convenience. There can be little doubt that it is more straightforward in busy clinical practice to use routine prophylaxis than to organize testing and pre-emptive therapy in those at high risk of CMV infection post-transplant, and for that pragmatic reason alone, the prophylactic approach has gained popularity. This trial provided the reassurance that the patient is not disadvantaged by this approach.

8.10 Outcomes of kidney transplantation in HIV-infected recipients

Authors

PG Stock, B Barin, B Murphy, D Hanto, JM Diego, J Light, C Davis, E Blumberg, D Simon, A Subramanian, JM Millis, GM Lyon, K Brayman, D Slakey, R Shapiro, J Melancon, JM Jacobson, V Stosor, JL Olson, DM Stablein, ME Roland

Reference

New England Journal of Medicine 2010, **363**, 2004–2014.

Abstract

Background: The outcomes of kidney transplantation and immunosuppression in people infected with human immunodeficiency virus (HIV) are incompletely understood.

Methods: We undertook a prospective, nonrandomized trial of kidney transplantation in HIV-infected candidates who had CD4 + T-cell counts of at least 200 per cubic millimeter and undetectable plasma HIV type 1 (HIV-1) RNA levels while being treated with a stable antiretroviral regimen. Post-transplantation management was provided in accordance with study protocols that defined prophylaxis against opportunistic infection, indications for biopsy, and acceptable approaches to immunosuppression, management of rejection, and antiretroviral therapy.

Results: Between November 2003 and June 2009, a total of 150 patients underwent kidney transplantation. Patient survival rates (± SD) at 1 year and 3 years were 94.6 ± 2.0% and 88.2 ± 3.8%, respectively, and the corresponding mean graft-survival rates were 90.4% and 73.7%. A multivariate proportional-hazards analysis showed that the risk of graft loss was increased among patients treated for rejection (hazard ratio, 2.8; 95% confidence interval [CI], 1.2 to 6.6; P = 0.02) and those receiving antithymocyte globulin induction therapy (hazard ratio, 2.5; 95% CI, 1.1 to 5.6; P = 0.03); living-donor transplants were protective (hazard ratio, 0.2; 95% CI, 0.04 to 0.8; P = 0.02). A higher-than-expected rejection rate was observed, with 1-year and 3-year estimates of 31% (95% CI, 24 to 40) and 41% (95% CI, 32 to 52), respectively. HIV infection remained well controlled, with stable CD4+ T-cell counts and few HIV-associated complications.

Conclusions: In this cohort of carefully selected HIV-infected patients, both patient- and graft-survival rates were high at 1 and 3 years, with no increases in complications associated with HIV infection. The unexpectedly high rejection rates are of serious concern and indicate the need for better immunotherapy.

Importance

Since the initial descriptions of HIV-related kidney disease in the 1980s in the USA (see paper 8.3), it has risen in prevalence to become the third most common cause of ESRD in black Americans. The early experience of HIV-positive patients receiving regular dialysis was dismal, but steadily improved, especially after the introduction of HAART. HIV-positive patients then began to be considered as candidates for transplantation. In this landmark description, a series of 150 kidney transplants in HIV-positive patients were undertaken in 19 US centres. Although all patients needed to be stable on HAART therapy with suppressed viral loads and preserved CD4 counts (>200 cells mm³), the actual HAART regimen used was left to individual investigators, as was the immunosuppressive regimen used at each centre.

The results achieved were remarkably good. Patient and graft survival were broadly comparable with those in the general population. One-year graft survival was 90% compared with 74% at 3 years, which made transplantation in this group of patients feasible. The greatest cause of concern was the high rate of severe acute rejection episodes, often corticosteroid resistant, which was unexpected as these patients were likely to be more immunosuppressed because of the HIV infection. Furthermore, the rejections were associated with a worse outcome. Another cause of concern was the biopsy-proven recurrence of HIV-associated nephropathy in two recipients, in spite of persisting complete viral suppression. It was, however, encouraging to see that there was no evidence of progression of the underlying HIV infection and no increase in infections compared with HIV-negative counterparts.

Whilst follow-up on these patients was relatively short (median 1.7 years), the initial results look very promising, especially recalling that these patients had not long previously been regarded as untransplantable. There is no doubt, however, that the success reported here has been hard won; there are many specific challenges in the clinical management of transplantation in HIV-positive patients, not least in the complex interactions of HAART and immunosuppressive agents.

Chapter 9

Diabetes and renal disease

Eberhard Ritz and John Feehally

Introduction

Diabetic nephropathy has a dominating place in the modern practice of nephrology. In many countries it is the commonest identified cause of end-stage renal disease; and those with diabetes and end-stage renal disease have significantly increased morbidity and mortality compared to those without diabetes. Strategies for preventing or slowing the progression of diabetic nephropathy have been the focus of enormous clinical trial efforts in the last 20 years. But the prevalence of type 2 diabetesis increasing, especially in the developing world, and presents a formidable public health challenge—not least because of the largely unfettered power of the food industry to promote unhealthy eating habits in increasingly sedentary populations. This chapter traces the chronology of this move of diabetic kidney disease to the centre stage of nephrology. Starting from the mid-nineteenth century report of Griesinger, the first to appreciate that the kidney were involved in diabetes; and then leaping almost a century to the introduction of renal biopsy in the 1950s which, as in other glomerular disease, gave the first opportunities to observe earlier phases of the pathology than had before been observable only in autopsy studies.

There were dismal outcomes in the early use of dialysis and transplantation in people with diabetes and ESRD in the 1960s. But gradually experience and determination proved what was possible.

It was a decade later when therapeutic approaches to diabetic nephropathy began to emerge with robust data. First when longtitudinal cohorts were published confirming the powerful predictive value of microalbuminuria (first measured reliably in the early 1960s) in anticipating those destined to develop overt diabetic nephropathy. Then when the debate about the importance of hypertension in diabetic nephropathy was finally decided in favour of tight blood pressure control, and then when the protective role of blocking the renin-angiotensin system was established in controlled trials in both type 1 and type 2 diabetes. And most recently with the recognition that more rounded approaches to management not only slow progression of diabetic nephropathy but also the wider metabolic consequences of diabetes.

The required intensity of glycaemic control continues to be debated to this day, especially in type 2 diabetes. But the success of pancreas transplantation in highly selected patients gave the opportunity to prove that early morphological changes of diabetic nephropathy could be reversed when normal glucose metabolism was restored in patients without uraemia who received a pancreas transplant.

Much has been achieved in the care of diabetic nephropathy, but the diabetes epidemic will bring many more challenges ahead.

9.1 Studien über Diabetes [Studies on diabetes]

Author

W Griesinger

Reference

Published by Ebner und Seubert Verlag, Stuttgart (1859).

Summary

If we take diabetic cases without tuberculosis, there is undoubtedly a transformation of the kidney that corresponds to the general category of 'Bright's disease'. The extraordinary frequency of these abnormalities is in line with the literature: 64 of the 225 cases identified in the literature had autopsies and—as in this series—32 had undoubted changes of the kidney. This may even be an underestimate because, at least in the more distant past, this may have been overlooked, considering four of the seven cases in the present series. In the literature, the authors indicated 'Bright's disease' emphasizing different features, such as swelling, less frequently atrophy, granular atrophy of the cortex, fatty degeneration of epithelial cells, small cysts, frequent scars, and inflammation of the pelvis, markedly also of the ureters. In five cases, substantial hyperaemia was reported and substantial swelling (in one report the kidneys were enlarged threefold and were very hyperaemic). In seven cases, such increased volumes were seen only in one kidney.

Importance

In this monograph entitled *Studien über Diabetes*, Wilhelm Griesinger assembled from the published literature autopsy evidence on 64 cases of diabetes, including seven cases he had so far treated in Tübingen, reflecting the relative rarity of diabetes at that time.

The main intention of Griesinger's monograph was to provide arguments against the hypothesis of Claude Bernard that increased glucose release from the liver played a major pathogenetic role in diabetes; his main counterarguments were normal liver weight and normal liver microscopy.

Instead, he observed macroscopic and microscopic abnormalities of the kidneys, and provided, summarized above, the first description of chronic kidney disease (in Griesinger's terminology, 'Bright's disease') in diabetes: 'The opinion that the kidneys are infrequently affected in this disease and that changes of the kidneys, if any, consist only in "true hypertrophy" was wrong...this is not so: In 4 of 5 cases of mine which came to autopsy considerable changes of kidney morphology were seen.'

From primitive histological examination of unstained sections, he showed that vessels, glomeruli, and tubules could all be involved in diabetes. In seven cases, he noted that renal hypertrophy was unilateral, but in retrospect unfortunately made no mention of any disease of the renal artery in those cases.

He even argued that the underlying pathogenesis of diabetes ('*Grundstörung des Diabetes*') was to be found in the kidney.

Griesinger also mentioned, apparently for the first time, pancreas atrophy in some cases, and he was able to contradict the then popular idea that diabetes was the consequence of traumatic events, which in his series were uncommon.

Two patients had died in what we would now describe as uraemia. Griesinger wrote:

…are these different affections of the kidneys really (as some authors suspected) the result of irritation of sugar containing urine? Are they the result of cachexia and marasm? Or are we here confronted with unclear relations concerning the irritation of the nerves?…In any case, these diseases of the kidneys complicate diabetes in a remarkable fashion and are the trigger for a series of pathological processes in many advanced cases. The frequency of these renal lesions is in line with the frequent finding that many diabetic patients have protein in their urine, mostly not constantly, but often at times copiously…there are, however, cases where—with the onset of albuminuria—sugar disappears from the urine. In these cases usually morbus Brightii takes its known course with generalised hydrops etc. In the majority of cases, moderate albuminuria coexists with glycosuria…

Thus, Griesinger was the first to identify the apparent moderation or even remission in their hyperglycaemia (or today, their insulin requirements), which diabetics may undergo as they enter uraemia.

9.2 Intercapillary lesions in the glomeruli of the kidney

Authors

P Kimmelstiel, C Wilson

Reference

American Journal of Pathology 1936, **12**, 83–98.

Abstract

Cases are described which show a striking hyaline thickening of the intercapillary connective tissue of the glomerulus. Evidence is presented which indicates that the change is degenerative in nature and suggests that arteriosclerosis and diabetes may play a part in its causation. The lesion is therefore termed intercapillary glomerulosclerosis. The characteristic clinical features are a previous history of diabetes, severe and widespread edema of the nephrotic type and gross albuminuria. Hypertension is frequently present, in many cases associated with renal decompensation.

The same histological picture frequently complicates intracapillary glomerulonephritis but in the later stages this condition is differentiated histologically by blurring and splitting of the capillary masement membrane.

In extracapillary glomerulonephritis thickening of the intercapillary connective tissue is relatively insignificant and the basement membrane changes are more pronounced.

Importance

Since the mid-nineteenth century, it had been known that diabetes could be associated with structural damage in the kidneys as well as with albuminuria (Abeille, 1856). Later, hyalinized material in proximal tubular cells of diabetic individuals was described by Armanni and later Ebstein (Armanni–Ebstein bodies) (Ebstein, 1882), a finding we now know is simply the result of hyperglycaemia. Then for decades, there was little further insight on how diabetes damaged the kidneys (Eknoyan and Nagy, 2005), apart from the report of MacCallum (1934), who described glomerular lesions resembling the Kimmelstiel–Wilson lesions—but he failed to make the connection with diabetes and ascribed his findings to 'the ageing process of the glomerulus'.

All this changed with this brilliant description of the intercapillary lesions in diabetic patients by Paul Kimmelstiel and Clifford Wilson in 1936. Their discovery was based on the description of intercapillary connective tissue in the glomerulus by Zimmermann (1929).

They described in great detail the kidneys of eight patients. These cases had presented with massive oedema (out of proportion to the existing cardiac failure), with hypertension of the 'benign' type and with a history of long-standing diabetes—with the exception of one case who had died 3 hours after admission with no history obtainable.

By histology, the centres of the glomeruli were regularly hyalinized (staining for fat only exceptionally yielding double refraction) and the number of capillaries was reduced. Often, a ring of open capillaries surrounded the central hyaline masses. There was a high degree of 'arteriolosclerosis' with fatty degeneration. Although the basement membrane of the capillaries was preserved initially, it changed eventually and capillary walls were thickened homogeneously near the central hyaline masses; the capillaries collapsed and finally merged with the central hyaline. There was no definite proof of an inflammatory process. The glomerular capsules showed deposition of a substance, which turned into hyaline-like material, often containing lipoid, followed later by concentric layers of fibrils and nuclei. Practically all glomeruli were diffusely affected.

Tubular changes were not specific: they presented fat deposition and doubly refracting lipoid but less than in the 'nephrotic syndrome'.

They gave a very detailed account of the differences between this novel lesion and intercapillary glomerulonephritis (described by Fahr) and extracapillary glomerulonephritis.

In their summary, they emphasized the striking hyaline thickening of the intercapillary connective tissue of the glomerulus, and the non-inflammatory degenerative nature of the lesion suggested to them that both arteriosclerosis and diabetes were involved in its causation. They coined the term 'intercapillary glomerulosclerosis' and emphasized the characteristic clinical features: history of diabetes, severe oedema, heavy albuminuria, and hypertension.

They emphasized that these glomerular lesions were different from those seen in glomerulonephritis, were specific for diabetes (presumably in all these cases, despite very little clinical information, this was type 2 diabetes), and were not non-specific consequences of hypertension or ageing, as previously assumed. This concept was a major breakthrough, identifying the kidneys as a target organ of diabetes, and in due course leading to the insight that albuminuria and renal malfunction are indicators and prognostic markers of the severity of the diabetic syndrome.

References

Abeille J (1856). *Des Maladies à Urines Albumineuses et Sucrées—ou de L'albuminurie et du Diabète Sucrée.* J.-B. Baillière, Paris.

Ebstein W (1882). Weiteres über Diabetes mellitus insbesondere über die Komplikation desselben mit Typhus abdominalis. *Dtsch Arch Klin Med* **30**, 1–44.

Eknoyan G, Nagy J (2005). A history of diabetes mellitus or how a disease of the kidneys evolved into a kidney disease. *Adv Chronic Kidney Dis* **12**, 223–229.

MacCallum WG (1934). Glomerular changes in nephritis. *Bull Johns Hopkins Hosp* **55**, 416–425.

Zimmermann, KW (1929). Über den Bau des Glomerulus des menschlichen Niere. *Z Mikrosk Anat Forsch* **18**, 520–552.

9.3 Diabetic nephropathy; kidney biopsy and renal function tests

Authors

C Brun, H Gormsen, T Hilden, P Iversen, F Raaschou

Reference

American Journal of Medicine 1953, **15**, 187–197.

Abstract

Kidney biopsy findings in twelve patients with diabetes mellitus have been compared with the clinical and laboratory findings in these cases, and the results of discrete renal function tests.

In six cases the biopsy specimen revealed solely diffuse glomerular changes; in four cases nodular-diffuse changes; and in one case completely hyalinized glomeruli with remnants of nodules; in one case the biopsy showed normal renal tissue in a patient in whom the further course of the disease showed that the renal symptoms must have been due to cardiac failure.

The kidney biopsy method made possible correction of clinically misdiagnosed diabetic nephropathy in one case, and in four cases which did not show definite clinical signs of diabetic renal disease, it revealed the presence of glomerular changes (diffuse in three cases and nodular-diffuse in one case).

Biopsy of the kidney, therefore, has some diagnostic value in diabetic nephropathy. Its value in the differential diagnosis of chronic pyelonephritis, on the other hand, seems to be very limited.

The present kidney biopsy experience apparently supports the theory that diabetic nephropathy originates as diffuse hyalinization in the basement membranes of the glomerular tufts, and that the nodular changes may be considered a further development of the diffuse form.

The discrete renal function tests, which do not per se permit any safe diagnostic conclusions with regard to the degree and nature of diabetic nephropathy, seem to indicate that glomeruli with rather pronounced changes of diabetic origin, at least in some instances, have a higher filtration capacity than might be supposed from the histologic picture.

Importance

Iversen and Brun had reported their new technique for aspiration biopsy of the kidney in 1951 (see paper 3.6), and in this landmark paper, they presented for the first time data on renal biopsy findings in diabetics with clinical evidence of renal disease. Only 12 cases and only light microscopic analysis was available—no immunofluorescence or electron microscopy, neither of which began to be applied to renal biopsies with any consistency until the end of the 1950s.

Yet in many ways the clinical and pathological spectrum of diabetic nephropathy they displayed is a remarkably complete description of the changes in the kidney with which we are now all too familiar.

First though, it should be noted that one case had a normal renal biopsy, and on clinical re-evaluation, it became clear that the oedema and proteinuria were in fact due to heart failure, resolving with digitalis therapy, a refreshing piece of clinical honesty, which many other authors might have chosen not to declare in a publication.

Recall also the contemporary thinking about diabetic nephropathy. Although it was more than 15 years since Kimmelstiel and Wilson's description of nodular glomerulosclerosis, there was still active discussion about the specifics of the nodular lesions for diabetic nephropathy and whether they were truly pathognomonic of diabetic glomerular injury. Likewise, there was debate about whether clinical features alone could allow the diagnosis of diabetic nephropathy—one comparison of clinical diagnosis with autopsy findings had indicated discordance between the two in 30% of cases.

One patient already mentioned had cardiac failure not renal disease, and another had such advanced glomerulosclerosis that specific features could not be evaluated in the biopsy. Thus, this is in effect a study of only ten biopsies—in patients with a mean age of 54 years and a wide range of duration of known diabetes (median 12 years, range 6 months to 24 years). As only five of the 12 had presented previously with 'diabetic coma', it seems likely that most of these subjects had type 2 diabetes, rather naively described in the paper as 'mild' diabetes. Nine of the ten examined, however, had diabetic nephropathy.

The biopsy findings show a spectrum of injury with which we are now familiar, all ten having diffuse glomerulosclerosis with hyalinization of capillary walls, but only four having superimposed nodular glomerulosclerosis, and none having nodular changes alone. Nodular glomerulosclerosis was in general associated with a longer duration of diabetes, heavier proteinuria, and a greater reduction in inulin clearance, but these clinico-pathological correlates, as is now well recognized, were by no means precise.

9.4 Renal transplantation in patients with insulin-dependent diabetes

Authors

CM Kjellstrand, RL Simmons, FC Goetz, TJ Buselmeier, JR Shideman, B von Hartitzsch, JS Najarian

Reference

Lancet 1973, **i**, 4–8.

Abstract

Forty patients (age 23–48 years) with insulin-dependent diabetes mellitus and end-stage renal failure were accepted for renal transplantation at the University of Minnesota between June 1969, and September 1972. Fifteen patients died: six before transplantation, three within 6 months of transplantation, and six after this period. Infections and myocardial infarctions were the principle causes of death. Age, age of onset of diabetes, electrocardiogram changes, history of angina, or severity of retinopathy were unreliable as prognostic indicators. Women had much better results than men. Rehabilitation and management of the diabetes mellitus in the patients with viable grafts was good. Diabetic nephropathy did not recur and hypertension was easily controlled. Visual acuity, which had rapidly deteriorated in uraemic diabetics, remained stable after transplantation.

Importance

It is difficult with a twenty-first-century perspective to appreciate the nihilism felt in the late 1960s about the fate of diabetics with ESRD. Renal replacement therapy by dialysis and transplantation was expanding rapidly across the developed world, and increasingly good outcomes were being reported in dialysed and especially transplanted patients. However, for people with diabetes, this was not the case—high morbidity and mortality were at first the norm; an early report showed that all diabetics selected for haemodialysis were dead within 2.5 years (Blagg *et al.*, 1971). And for those few deemed fit for transplantation, the outcome for patients and grafts was clearly inferior to people without diabetes.

This report brought new optimism to the field. The patients with diabetes who were given the opportunity of renal transplantation at the University of Minnesota were typical of those presenting late to renal units in the late 1960s. The 14 women and 26 men had an average age of 33.5 years (range 23–48) with a mean 20-year history of diabetes, and 4 years of known kidney disease. Yet only six patients were denied dialysis and transplantation, reflecting the highly selective referral patterns from physicians who knew of the gloomy prognosis for those with end-stage diabetic kidney disease. All except one received haemodialysis before transplantation and, given contemporary approaches to early initiation of dialysis in diabetics, the mean serum creatinine before first dialysis was remarkable high at 14.3 mg/dl (range 5.8–23.6) (1258 μmol/l; range 510–2077). Six died waiting for transplantation and the remaining 34 received 37 kidneys, 27 from living related donors.

Ten other patients received simultaneous kidney and pancreas transplants in the same centre during this period, and are reported elsewhere, testament to the ambitious determination of this innovative and determined team to offer all possible surgical options to patients with diabetic renal failure (Lillehei *et al.*, 1970).

Frustratingly, this report gives no information about the immunosuppressive regimen other than to say that corticosteroids were used. However, contemporary regimens were typically based on corticosteroids and azathioprine as maintenance therapy, with acute rejection being treated with high-dose corticosteroids or, if steroid resistant, by anti-lymphocyte globulin and graft irradiation.

There was no difference in 3-year patient survival between diabetics receiving cadaveric kidneys and non-diabetic transplant recipients. Three-year graft survival of around 40% for diabetic recipients compares unfavourably with 70–80% graft survival achieved for non-diabetics in the same programme, but represented the first evidence that renal transplantation could be considered a viable option for diabetics for whom regular haemodialysis still offered only limited palliation. Unexpectedly, there appeared to be poorer outcomes in diabetics receiving living-donor kidneys but subsequently this has not of course proven to be the case.

Despite corticosteroids, adequate control of diabetes was achieved, and the report of the impact of transplantation on diabetic complications was also very encouraging—visual acuity and also peripheral and autonomic neuropathy were stabilized. Rehabilitation was encouraging, but of course this was a highly selected population: 22 of the 25 surviving to 3 years were reported as partially or totally rehabilitated, including 15 being fully independent as wage-earners or home-makers. In addition, they reported the first successful pregnancy in a transplanted diabetic.

References

Blagg CR, Eschbach JW, Sawyer TK, Casaretto AA (1971). Dialysis for endstage diabetic nephropathy. *Proc Clin Dial Transplant Forum* **1**, 133–135.

Lillehei RC, Simmons RL, Najarian JS, *et al.* (1970). Pancreatico-duodenal allotransplantation: experimental and clinical experience. *Ann Surg* **172**, 405–436.

9.5 Long-term antihypertensive treatment inhibiting progression of diabetic nephropathy

Author

CE Mogensen

Reference

British Medical Journal 1982, **285**, 685–688.

Abstract

Six men aged 26–35 years with proteinuria due to insulin dependent juvenile-onset diabetes were treated for moderate hypertension (mean blood pressure 162/103 mm Hg) and studied for a mean of 73 months for the effect on the progression of nephropathy. All patients were of normal weight. During a mean control period of 28 months before treatment the mean glomerular filtration rate (three or four measurements) was 86·1 ml/min and mean 24-hour urinary albumin excretion (also three or four measurements) 3·9 g (range 0·5–8·8 g).

During antihypertensive treatment the mean systolic blood pressure fell to 144 mm Hg and mean diastolic pressure to 95 mm Hg. In the control period five patients had shown a mean monthly decline in glomerular filtration rate of 1·23 ml/min; with antihypertensive treatment, however, this decline fell to 0·49 ml/min (2p = 0·042). In the remaining patient the glomerular filtration rate was 137 ml/min before treatment and 135 ml/min at the end of the treatment period. In all patients the mean yearly increase in albumin clearance (expressed as a percentage of the glomerular filtration rate) fell from 107% before treatment to 5% during treatment (2p = 0·0099).

This small study indicates that antihypertensive treatment slows the decline in renal function in diabetic nephropathy. Clinical trials beginning treatment in the incipient phase of diabetic nephropathy will define the optimal modality of treatment in this large patient population.

Importance

Before 1980, the life expectancy of a patient with advanced diabetic nephropathy was extremely short and the renal prognosis was dismal. Many diabetologists and nephrologists were of the opinion that hypertension, as stated in 1931 by Paul White, an influential cardiologist, 'may be an important compensatory mechanism which should not be tampered with'. There was a minority view, for example by Volhard in 1923: 'I doubt whether elevated blood pressure serves any reasonable function at all. We are confronted with a vicious circle which is responsible for progression of kidney disease and eventually for the stage of kidney failure.'

Carl Erik Mogensen in Åarhus, Denmark, studied young male diabetics and found that with intermittent proteinuria, there was no deterioration in renal function over 32 months, but with constant proteinuria, the glomerular filtration rate (GFR) decreased and there was a positive correlation between the rate of this decrease and diastolic blood pressure as well as albuminuria. He then showed in a short-term study that a fall in blood pressure over 48 days from 159/101 to 143/93 mmHg was accompanied by lowering of the albumin excretion (Mogensen, 1976).

He then performed this landmark interventional uncontrolled study in only six insulin-dependent juvenile-onset diabetic patients; in these patients aged 26–35 years, the blood pressure was lowered from an average of 162/103 mmHg to a mean level of 144/95 mmHg for a mean of 73 months. In a 'run-in' period, there was a monthly GFR decline of 1.23 ml/min; on antihypertensive treatment, this decreased to 0.49 ml/min. In all patients, albuminuria decreased dramatically.

In this remarkably small study, Mogensen had established 'proof of principle' that anti-hypertensive treatment slowed the decline in renal function in diabetic nephropathy, and proposed that clinical trials should be performed to optimize the treatment in this patient population.

This result was very soon confirmed by other investigators, particularly Hans-Henrik Parving (1983), who showed in ten young insulin-dependent diabetics that anti-hypertensive treatment achieving a mean blood pressure of 128/84 mmHg slowed the rate of decline in GFR with a parallel reduction in urinary albumin.

There are still unresolved issues in the management of hypertension in diabetes. For example, it is not clear which target blood pressure is optimal, whether this is best assessed by patient self-measurement or ambulatory blood pressure monitoring, and whether achieved diastolic and systolic pressure are both important.

Nevertheless, Mogensen's small study, performed against the majority opinion of the rest of the world, introduced the concept that anti-hypertensive treatment is a crucial step in the treatment of progressive diabetic nephropathy in type 1 (and later also shown in type 2) diabetes. This idea was quickly widely adopted (Christlieb et al., 1981) and is the bedrock of today's management of diabetic nephropathy.

References

Christlieb AR, Warram JH, Królewski AS, et al. (1981). Hypertension: the major risk factor in juvenile-onset insulin-dependent diabetics. *Diabetes* **30**, 90–96.

Mogensen CE (1976). Progression of nephropathy in long-term diabetics with proteinuria and effect of initial anti-hypertensive treatment. *Scand J Clin Lab Invest* **36**, 383–388.

Parving HH, Andersen AR, Smidt UM, Svendsen PA (1983). Early aggressive antihypertensive treatment reduces rate of decline in kidney function in diabetic nephropathy. *Lancet* **i**, 1175–1179.

9.6 Microalbuminuria as a predictor of clinical nephropathy in insulin-dependent diabetes mellitus

Authors

GC Viberti, RJ Jarrett, U Mahmud, RS Hill, A Argyropoulos, H Keen

Reference

Lancet 1982, **i**, 1430–1432.

Abstract

The overnight urinary albumin excretion rate (AER) of 87 patients with insulin-dependent diabetes mellitus was measured in 1966–67. 14 years later information was obtained on 63 of the original cohort; those alive were restudied, and for those who had died relevant clinical information and cause of death were recorded. The development of clinical diabetic nephropathy ('Albustix'-positive proteinuria) was related to the 1966–67 AER values. Clinical proteinuria developed in only 2 of 55 patients with AER below 30 µg/min but in 7 of 8 patients with AER between 30 and 140 µg/min. The risk of clinical diabetic nephropathy in the latter group was 24 times higher than in the former. 9·1% of patients with AER below 30µg/min had died, compared with 37.5% with higher AER. The two groups did not differ significantly in age, sex composition, and initial blood pressure. Mean duration of diabetes was longer, but not significantly so, in those with AER above 30µg/min. Thus, elevated levels of microalbuminuria strongly predict the development of clinical diabetic nephropathy. These levels of AER are potentially reversible, and their detection and treatment may prevent diabetic renal disease.

Importance

Proteinuria in type 2 diabetic patients had been described even in the nineteenth century, and before World War I, several reports had noted that albuminuria was predictive of death in diabetes (Gansevoort and Ritz, 2009), but to measure low levels of albuminuria with chemical methods was tedious and unreliable. The renaissance of albuminuria as an indicator of risk started with the advent of immune methods to detect albumin in the urine (Keen and Chlouverakis, 1963).

In 1982, at the time of this landmark report of Viberti and colleagues from Guy's Hospital, London, it was known that overt diabetic nephropathy with proteinuria >0.5 g/24 h was the earliest indicator of the progressive and relentless decline of glomerular function which in those days was still refractory to treatment. On the other hand, it was known that morphological kidney abnormalities developed early in the course of the disease when the urine was negative by Albustix and renal function was normal.

By 1982, Viberti and colleagues were able to report the clinical course over 15 years of 63 out of a cohort of 87 patients with insulin-dependent (presumably mostly type 1) diabetes. Although albuminuria was not correlated with blood pressure, the likelihood of developing clinical overt Albustix-positive proteinuria was markedly higher (87.5 versus 3.6%) in patients whose initial albumin excretion rate had been >30 µg/min compared with those with a rate of <30 µg/min at screening, i.e. the relative risk of clinical nephropathy was elevated by a factor of 24.

While considering that the high albuminuria at baseline may have reflected hyperglycaemia or may have indicated a greater susceptibility to diabetic nephropathy, they also discussed the hypothesis (proven beyond doubt by later studies) that the high initial albuminuria indicated that the nephropathic process had already begun. Furthermore, even in this small cohort, the death rate was also higher with increased albuminuria at baseline, the main causes being uraemia and cardiovascular events.

Soon after, Mogensen (1984) reported that microalbuminuria was similarly predictive of risk in type 2 diabetics, and proposed that 'screening for microalbuminuria in such a population will identify high risk patients with abnormalities that are potentially treatable'. Monitoring of urine albumin excretion is indeed now part of the standard of care for diabetes. This has also done much to increase awareness of the renal complications of diabetes.

The potential significance of albuminuria soon broadened with the 'Steno hypothesis' that 'albuminuria in type 1 diabetes is not only an indication of renal disease, but a new, independent risk-marker of proliferative retinopathy and macroangiopathy' (Deckert *et al.*, 1989). Even in those without diabetes, there is a continuous relationship from the lowest to the highest levels between albuminuria and cardiovascular as well as renal events. It has been argued recently that the concept of 'micro'-albuminuria should be abandoned and urine albumin concentration be treated as a continuous variable that reflects the progressive increase in both cardiovascular and renal risk for progressively higher concentrations of urinary albumin (Ruggenenti and Remuzzi, 2006).

References

Deckert T, Feldt-Rasmussen B, Borch-Johnsen K, Jensen T, Kofoed-Enevoldsen A (1989). Albuminuria reflects widespread vascular damage. The Steno hypothesis. *Diabetologia* **32**, 219–226.

Gansevoort RT, Ritz E (2009). Hermann Senator and albuminuria—forgotten pioneering work in the 19th century. *Nephrol Dial Transplant* **24**, 1057–1062.

Keen H, Chlouverakis C (1963). An immunoassay method for urinary albumin at low concentrations. *Lancet* **ii**, 913–914.

Mogensen CE (1984). Microalbuminuria predicts clinical proteinuria and early mortality in maturity-onset diabetes. *N Engl J Med* **310**, 356–360.

Ruggenenti P, Remuzzi G (2006). Time to abandon microalbuminuria? *Kidney Int* **70**, 1214–1222.

9.7 Similar risks of nephropathy in patients with type I or type II diabetes mellitus

Authors

C Hasslacher, E Ritz, P Wahl, C Michael

Reference

Nephrology Dialysis Transplantation 1989, **4**, 859–863.

Abstract

It is commonly assumed that in patients the risks of developing nephropathy and uraemia are high in type I and low in type II diabetes mellitus. Since type II occurs mostly in elderly individuals with limited life expectancy and high cardiovascular mortality, the true risk may have been underestimated, as many patients do not survive to experience renal complications. To assess renal risk further, we evaluated all patients with type II and type I diabetes mellitus without severe secondary disease who were followed in the outpatient clinic between 1970 and 1985. The cumulative risk of proteinuria after 20 years of diabetes mellitus was 27% in type II and 28% in type I, the findings after 25 years were 57% and 46% respectively. The cumulative risk of renal failure, i.e. serum creatinine greater than 1.4 mg/dl, after 3 years of persisting proteinuria was 41% in both type II and type I, and after 5 years of proteinuria were 63% and 59% respectively. We conclude that the renal risk is similar in patients with type II and type I diabetes mellitus.

Importance

As it was known from autopsy studies that only 5–10% of type 2 diabetics die from renal failure, compared with 30–50% of type 1 diabetics, it was assumed until the late 1980s that the risk of diabetic nephropathy was considerably less in type 2 diabetics, even though there was no difference in the prevalence of another microvascular complication, diabetic retinopathy. Hasslacher and his colleagues set about resolving this uncertainty with a disarmingly simple study, which set out to obtain the first data on the cumulative prevalence of proteinuria in type 2 diabetics. In a single centre they followed cohorts of type 1 ($n = 292$) and type 2 ($n = 464$) diabetics who had no proteinuria and normal serum creatinine at first referral to the hospital clinic; the median follow-up period was 5–6 years. The cumulative prevalence of proteinuria in type 1 diabetics was 44% at 25 years from diagnosis, and in type 2 diabetics was rather higher, 53% at 25 years. Accepting the uncertainty about defining time of onset of diabetes (as opposed to time of detection) in type 2 as opposed to type 1, there was therefore no evidence to support a more favourable renal outcome in type 2 diabetes.

Admittedly, this finding had been hinted at in previous cross-sectional studies. In addition, previous studies had not always defined type 1 and type 2 diabetes rigorously (insulin-treated type 2 diabetics were all too often misassigned as type 1 diabetics), and had not excluded with sufficient accuracy alternative causes of proteinuria. Registry data that might have been informative were also blighted by inaccurate assignment of type 1 and type 2 diabetes. The evidence of lower rates of diabetic nephropathy in type 2 diabetics in autopsy studies was explained by the high burden of macrovascular disease, which resulted in mortality before there had been time for the type 2 diabetics to develop nephropathy.

These results were unexpected, definitive, and changed once and for all our perception of renal risk in type 2 diabetes.

9.8 Reversal of lesions of diabetic nephropathy after pancreas transplantation

Authors

P Fioretto, MW Steffeds, DER Sutherland, FC Goetz, M Mauer

Reference

New England Journal of Medicine 1998, **139**, 69–75.

Abstract

Background: In patients with type I diabetes mellitus who do not have uremia and have not received a kidney transplant, pancreas transplantation does not ameliorate established lesions of diabetic nephropathy within five years after transplantation, but the effects of longer periods of normoglycemia are unknown.

Methods: We studied kidney function and performed renal biopsies before pancreas transplantation and 5 and 10 years thereafter in eight patients with type I diabetes but without uremia who had mild to advanced lesions of diabetic nephropathy at the time of transplantation. The biopsy samples were analyzed morphometrically.

Results: All patients had persistently normal glycosylated hemoglobin values after transplantation. The median urinary albumin excretion rate was 103 mg per day before transplantation, 30 mg per day 5 years after transplantation, and 20 mg per day 10 years after transplantation (P=0.07 for the comparison of values at base line and at 5 years; P=0.11 for the comparison between base line and 10 years). The mean (±SD) creatinine clearance rate declined from 108±20 ml per minute per 1.73 m^2 of body-surface area at base line to 74±16 ml per minute per 1.73 m^2 at 5 years (P<0.001) and 74±14 ml per minute per 1.73 m^2 at 10 years (P<0.001). The thickness of the glomerular and tubular basement membranes was similar at 5 years (570±64 and 928±173 nm, respectively) and at base line (594±81 and 911±133 nm, respectively) but had decreased by 10 years (to 404±38 and 690±111 nm, respectively; P<0.001 and P=0.004 for the comparisons with the base-line values). The mesangial fractional volume (the proportion of the glomerulus occupied by the mesangium) increased from base line (0.33±0.07) to 5 years (0.39±0.10, P=0.02) but had decreased at 10 years (0.27±0.02, P=0.05 for the comparison with the base-line value and P=0.006 for the comparison with the value at 5 years), mostly because of a reduction in mesangial matrix.

Conclusions: pancreas transplantation can reverse the lesions of diabetic nephropathy, but reversal requires more than five years of normoglycemia.

Importance

In the 1990s, it had been shown in type 1 diabetics that progression of renal damage could be attenuated by intensified glycaemic control (The Diabetes Control and Complications Trial/ Epidemiology of Diabetes Interventions and Complications Research Group, 2000), which also reduces accumulation of mesangial matrix and thickening of the glomerular basement membrane in renal allografts (Barbosa *et al.*, 1994; Bilous *et al.*, 1989). However, the question remained unresolved as to whether diabetic lesions might not only be slowed but actually regress.

This landmark study of Paola Fioretto and her colleagues addressed that question by studying renal biopsies in type 1 diabetics with diabetic nephropathy, but not uraemia, who had been insulin independent and euglycaemic for 10 years after pancreas transplantation.

By morphometry, there was no improvement in mesangial matrix volume 5 years after pancreas transplantation, but this was lower by 10 years, as was glomerular basement membrane thickening. The same investigators later reported the disappearance of Kimmelstiel–Wilson nodular lesions (Fioretto *et al.*, 2008), which were previously considered 'end-stage' lesions not susceptible to remodelling.

That reversal takes such a long time is perhaps unsurprising, given the time taken for these lesions to develop after the onset of diabetes, as well as the onset of microalbuminuria—often a decade or more.

These findings were confirmed in a subsequent study: reversal after 10 years occurring despite worsening of interstitial fibrosis and tubular atrophy (the latter perhaps the result of calcineurin inhibitor therapy) (Fioretto *et al.*, 2008).

That the time course is so slow might reflect diminished susceptibility of the extracellular matrix to degradation because of covalent modification or long-lasting effects of hyperglycaemia (the so-called memory effect). Unravelling these mechanisms may open up targets for future clinical intervention.

This key paper showed that, in the very long run, renal lesions are reversible, at least in type 1 diabetes and at least in the relatively early stages of diabetic nephropathy. Whether this also applies to more advanced stages of the disease, where tubulo-interstitial injury as well as injury of the glomerulo-tubular junction (Najafian *et al.*, 2003) drive progression, remains to be seen.

References

Barbosa J, Steffes MW, Sutherland DE, Connett JE, Rao KV, Mauer SM (1994). Effect of glycemic control on early diabetic renal lesions. A 5-year randomized controlled clinical trial of insulin-dependent diabetic kidney transplant recipients. *JAMA* **272**, 600–606.

Bilous RW, Mauer SM, Sutherland DE, Najarian JS, Goetz FC, Steffes MW (1989). The effects of pancreas transplantation on the glomerular structure of renal allografts in patients with insulin-dependent diabetes. *N Engl J Med* **321**, 80–85.

Fioretto P, Caramori ML, Mauer M (2008). The kidney in diabetes: dynamic pathways of injury and repair. The Camillo Golgi Lecture 2007. *Diabetologia* **51**, 1347–55

Najafian B, Kim Y, Crosson JT, Mauer M (2003). Atubular glomeruli and glomerulotubular junction abnormalities in diabetic nephropathy. *J Am Soc Nephrol* **14**, 908–917.

The Diabetes Control and Complications Trial/Epidemiology of Diabetes Interventions and Complications Research Group (2000). Retinopathy and nephropathy in patients with type 1 diabetes four years after a trial of intensive therapy. *N Engl J Med* **342**, 381–389.

9.9 Renoprotective effect of the angiotensin-receptor antagonist irbesartan in patients with nephropathy due to type 2 diabetes

Authors

EJ Lewis, LG Hunsicker, WR Clarke, T Berl, MA Pohl, JB Lewis, E Ritz, RC Atkins, R Rohde, I Raz, for the Collaborative Study Group

Reference

New England Journal of Medicine 2001, **345**, 851–860.

Abstract

Background: It is unknown whether either the angiotensin-II-receptor blocker irbesartan or the calcium-channel blocker amlodipine slows the progression of nephropathy in patients with type 2 diabetes independently of its capacity to lower the systemic blood pressure.

Methods: We randomly assigned 1715 hypertensive patients with nephropathy due to type 2 diabetes to treatment with irbesartan (300 mg daily), amlodipine (10 mg daily), or placebo. The target blood pressure was 135/85 mm Hg or less in all groups. We compared the groups with regard to the time to the primary composite end point of a doubling of the base-line serum creatinine concentration, the development of end-stage renal disease, or death from any cause. We also compared them with regard to the time to a secondary, cardiovascular composite end point.

Results: The mean duration of follow-up was 2.6 years. Treatment with irbesartan was associated with a risk of the primary composite end point that was 20 percent lower than that in the placebo group (P=0.02) and 23 percent lower than that in the amlodipine group (P=0.006). The risk of a doubling of the serum creatinine concentration was 33 percent lower in the irbesartan group than in the placebo group (P=0.003) and 37 percent lower in the irbesartan group than in the amlodipine group (P<0.001). Treatment with irbesartan was associated with a relative risk of end-stage renal disease that was 23 percent lower than that in both other groups (P=0.07 for both comparisons). These differences were not explained by differences in the blood pressures that were achieved. The serum creatinine concentration increased 24 percent more slowly in the irbesartan group than in the placebo group (P=0.008) and 21 percent more slowly than in the amlodipine group (P=0.02). There were no significant differences in the rates of death from any cause or in the cardiovascular composite end point.

Conclusions: The angiotensin-II-receptor blocker irbesartan is effective in protecting against the progression of nephropathy due to type 2 diabetes. This protection is independent of the reduction in blood pressure it causes.

Importance

By the mid-1990s, there was good evidence from randomized controlled trials that angiotensin-converting enzyme (ACE) inhibitors were effective in reducing proteinuria and protecting renal function independent of blood pressure control (Lewis *et al.*, 1993). However, definitive proof that renin–angiotensin system (RAS) blockade would reduce renal failure assessed by hard end points, and would also be effective in type 2 diabetics, had to wait until angiotensin receptor blockers (ARBs) became available, providing the logistic and financial means to organize sufficiently large international multicentre studies. This landmark study using irbesartan, the Irbesartan Diabetic Nephropathy Trial (IDNT), discussed here was confirmed by parallel publication of the RENAAL study using losartan (Brenner *et al.*, 2001).

In the IDNT study, the main outcome was a 20% reduction in time to a composite end point of doubling of baseline serum creatinine, development of ESRD, or death from any cause. This difference was not explained by differences in blood pressure. The IDNT and RENAAL studies were in complete agreement, both showing the benefit of RAS blockade using an ARB in addition to other antihypertensive agents.

Subsequent secondary analysis of the IDNT study indicated that there was higher mortality when systolic pressure was below 120 mmHg (Pohl *et al.*, 2005), and that the risk of myocardial infarction increased progressively with lower diastolic blood pressure, presumably due to reduced coronary perfusion (Berl *et al.*, 2005).

However, it is sobering to note that the addition of ARB in the IDNT study only reduced the median rate of decline of GFR from −6.5 to −5.5 ml/min/1.73 m². The implication being that treatment with ARB should be started in much earlier stages of diabetic nephropathy where more retardation of GFR loss can be achieved.

Although RAS blockade by ACE inhibitors or ARBs has been a huge step forward in the management of diabetic nephropathy, it is not a panacea, and a number of clinical issues remain unresolved. Salt restriction is still required, both directly to increase the efficacy of RAS blockade and because salt stimulates the mineralocorticoid receptor independently of aldosterone. Not all patients respond satisfactorily to RAS blockade, even with doses above those licensed for blood-pressure lowering, and others will have only a transient response (so-called 'escape') (Schjoedt *et al.*, 2004). Therefore 'add-on' therapies are the subject of active investigation. However, it still remains uncertain whether the 'add on' should be the combination of ACE inhibitor and ARB, a direct renin inhibitor, a mineralocorticoid receptor antagonist, an endothelin blocker, or even an activated form of vitamin D.

Undoubtedly, the unequivocal evidence from the IDNT and RENAAL studies of the beneficial impact of RAS blockade on the progression of diabetic nephropathy was a quantum leap forward. However, progressive diabetic nephropathy remains a formidable opponent for the nephrologist, and further quantum leaps are sorely needed.

References

Berl, T., Hunsicker LG, Lewis JB, *et al.* (2005). Impact of achieved blood pressure on cardiovascular outcomes in the Irbesartan Diabetic Nephropathy Trial. *J Am Soc Nephrol* **16**, 2170–2179.

Brenner BM, Cooper ME, de Zeeuw D, *et al.* (2001). Effects of losartan on renal and cardiovascular outcomes in patients with type 2 diabetes and nephropathy. *N Engl J Med* **345**, 861–869.

Lewis EJ, Hunsicker LG, Bain RP, Rohde RD, The Collaborative Study Group (1993). The effect of angiotensin-converting-enzyme inhibition on diabetic nephropathy. *New Engl J Med* **329**, 1456–1462.

Pohl MA., Blumenthal S, Cordonnier DJ, *et al.* (2005). Independent and additive impact of blood pressure control and angiotensin II receptor blockade on renal outcomes in the irbesartan diabetic nephropathy trial: clinical implications and limitations. *J Am Soc Nephrol* **16**, 3027–3037.

Schjoedt, K.J., Andersen S, Rossing P, Tarnow L, Parving HH (2004). Aldosterone escape during blockade of the renin-angiotensin-aldosterone system in diabetic nephropathy is associated with enhanced decline in glomerular filtration rate. *Diabetologia* **47**, 1936–1939.

9.10 Effect of a multifactorial intervention on mortality in type 2 diabetes

Authors

P Gaede, H Lund-Andersen, HH Parving, O Pedersen

Reference

New England Journal of Medicine 2008, **358**, 580–591.

Abstract

Background: Intensified multifactorial intervention – with tight glucose regulation and the use of ren-in-angiotensin system blockers, aspirin, and lipid-lowering agents – has been shown to reduce the risk of nonfatal cardiovascular disease among patients with type 2 diabetes mellitus and microalbuminuria. We evaluated whether this approach would have an effect on the rates of death from any cause and from cardiovascular causes.

Method: In the Steno-2 Study, we randomly assigned 160 patients with type 2 diabetes and persistent micro-albuminuria to receive either intensive therapy or conventional therapy; the mean treatment period was 7.8 years. Patients were subsequently followed observationally for a mean of 5.5 years, until December 31, 2006. The primary end point at 13.3 years of follow-up was the time to death from any cause.

Results: Twenty-four patients in the intensive-therapy group died, as compared with 40 in the conventional-therapy group (hazard ratio, 0.54; 95% confidence interval [CI], 0.32 to 0.89; $P = 0.02$). Intensive therapy was associated with a lower risk of death from cardiovascular causes (hazard ratio, 0.43; 95% CI, 0.19 to 0.94; $P = 0.04$) and of cardiovascular events (hazard ratio, 0.41; 95% CI, 0.25 to 0.67; $P < 0.001$). One patient in the intensive-therapy group had progression to end-stage renal disease, as compared with six patients in the conventional-therapy group ($P = 0.04$). Fewer patients in the intensive-therapy group required retinal photocoagulation (relative risk, 0.45; 95% CI, 0.23 to 0.86; $P = 0.02$). Few major side effects were reported.

Conclusions: In at-risk patients with type 2 diabetes, intensive intervention with multiple drug combinations and behavior modification had sustained beneficial effects with respect to vascular complications and on rates of death from any cause and from cardiovascular causes. (ClinicalTrials.gov number, NCT00320008.)

Importance

Interventions to retard progression of renal disease in diabetic patients had focused on single risk factors such as glycemic control or blood pressure control (DCCT Research Group, 1995; Diabetes Control and Complications Trial/Epidemiology of Diabetes Interventions and Complications Research Group, 2003). Then, in this controlled trial, Gaede and colleagues, from the Steno Memorial Hospital in Copenhagen, introduced the concept of multifactorial intervention aimed at all treatable risk factors in high-risk type 2 diabetic patients identified by persistent microalbuminuria. A hundred and sixty patients with type 2 diabetes were randomized to be treated according to standard guidelines or with intensified target-driven therapy involving a combination of medications using behaviour modification. All patients were on treatment with RAS blockers and received low-dose aspirin.

After a mean follow-up of 7.8 years, glycated haemoglobin (HbA1$_c$), blood pressure, serum lipids, and urinary albumin excretion were all reduced more with intensified therapy. There were also significantly lower risks of cardiovascular disease, nephropathy, retinopathy, and autonomic neuropathy. However, there was no significant difference in mortality.

The randomized trial was followed by a further observation period, during which differences in risk-factor control between the two groups narrowed, probably because at the end of the controlled study, all participants were informed about the benefits of the intensified multifactorial treatment. Nevertheless, a difference in mortality did emerge after a further 8 years, the intensified treatment group having impressive reductions in overall death (20%) and death from cardiovascular causes (14%) and the risk of subsequent diabetic nephropathy being reduced by almost half.

It may seem remarkable that it took so long before the reduced mortality emerged. However, this is in perfect agreement with the Diabetes Control and Complications Trial (DCCT) in type 1 diabetics, in which intensified glycaemic control was compared with standard glycaemic control; after the study had ended, the glycaemic control in the two arms of the study converged, but after 17 years of follow-up, the risk reduction for cardiovascular events in patients who received intensified glycaemic control was 57% (DCCT Research Group, 1995; Diabetes Control and Complications Trial/Epidemiology of Diabetes Interventions and Complications Research Group, 2003). There is also evidence from the UK Prospective Diabetes Study that the quality of glycemic control early after onset of type 2 diabetes determines the patient's long-term outcome (Holman *et al.*, 2008); presumably the result of so-called 'metabolic memory' or a 'legacy effect', perhaps due to persisting epigenetic changes.

Although event rates and mortality were substantially reduced in the Steno-2 study, there still remained a substantial residual risk. What else can be done in addition to such a multifactorial approach?

References

DCCT (Diabetes Control and Complications Trial) Research Group (1995). Effect of intensive therapy on the development and progression of diabetic nephropathy in the Diabetes Control and Complications Trial. *Kidney Int* **47**, 1703–1720.

Holman RR, Paul SK, Bethel MA, Matthews DR, Neil HA (2008). 10-year follow-up of intensive glucose control in type 2 diabetes. *N Engl J Med* **359**, 1577–1589.

Writing Team for the Diabetes Control and Complications Trial/Epidemiology of Diabetes Interventions and Complications Research Group (2003). Sustained effect of intensive treatment of type 1 diabetes mellitus on development and progression of diabetic nephropathy: the Epidemiology of Diabetes Interventions and Complications (EDIC) study. *JAMA* **290**, 2159–2167.

Chapter 10

Acute kidney injury

Dharmvir Jaswal and Adeera Levin

Introduction

Acute kidney injury (AKI) was until recently more commonly called acute renal failure. This chapter describes ten landmark papers, chosen for their contribution to our understanding of AKI, or because they mark specific time points when concepts or issues were articulated in such a manner as to change practice or shift research paradigms. The papers span from 1941 to 2010 and range from small meticulous physiology studies to large epidemiological studies. But all serve to inform some key points in the understanding of AKI: mechanisms of ischaemic damage; the importance of tubulo-glomerular feedback as an adaptive mechanism to preserve volume; the pathophysiology of crush syndrome; the insensitivity of serum creatinine as a marker of early damage, and yet the importance of small changes in serum creatinine for prognosis; the importance and danger of fluid resuscitation; and lastly, the notions of iatrogenic kidney damage, acquired as a consequence of radiocontrast administration or other events during hospital admission. Lastly in assessing best treatment strategies, we have selected two randomized controlled trials (RCTs): one on continuous renal replacement therapy and the other on prevention of contrast-induced nephropathy with N-acetylcysteine. Both studies are important as they have changed the thoughts and actions of many clinicians; none the less, we point out how both are prone to misinterpretation and have been the focus of further discussion and discovery.

In this collection spanning over 70 years study of the science of acute renal failure/AKI, some themes emerge consistently: in particular, the unique physiology of the kidney and the pathophysiological response to injury, and the need to attend to the oliguria and fluid status of patients, within the context of that disturbed physiology. Early identification and prevention remain the clinical 'holy grails' of AKI, and with the perspective of these landmark papers, perhaps we can learn to address these more effectively using a systematic framework that acknowledges the pathophysiology more clearly. There remain key research questions, which, if addressed properly over the next decades, may actually lead to a change in outcomes for those with AKI. The papers all have in common scientific rigour based on physiological principles—an approach that consistently yields thoughtful insights into human disease.

10.1 Crush injuries with impairment of renal function

Authors
EG Bywaters, D Beall

Reference
British Medical Journal 1941, **1**, 427–432.

Abstract

Four cases of crush injury to limbs, producing shock, are described in which after recovery due to replacement of circulatory fluid the patients showed oliguria and pigmented casts. They died in about one week with nitrogen retention. Necropsy revealed degenerative changes in the proximal convoluted tubule and pigment casts in the more distal part of the nephron. The aetiology and possible lines of treatment are discussed.

Importance

In the modern era when large RCTs and complex systematic reviews dominate the clinical literature, this paper by Bywaters and Beall might easily be overlooked by many. Written over 70 years ago, and published at the height of the World War II, this seminal article is important for its contribution to medical knowledge at that time, for the meticulous method in which the clinical course and physiology of just four cases is described, and for the foundation it laid for future research in AKI. Furthermore, this paper demonstrates the capacity to learn from careful observation, even in devastating human situations, so that future generations can benefit. For both political and scientific reasons therefore, this paper is a landmark.

Bywaters and Beall were not the first to formally describe crush syndrome; that accolade goes to Minami, a Japanese investigator working in Berlin, who had published his description in 1923. By using complex cases that reiterated that the tragedy of war has no gender or age preferences, Bywaters and Beall provided a set of case studies, which included intricate descriptions about the physical examination intertwined with drawings, and in so doing described the details of crush syndrome and AKI that occurred as a consequence of the bombings in London during the Blitz. These descriptions of the cases, and the treatments delivered, serve as the basis for current understanding and management of trauma patients.

Although the medical management and physiological explanation for crush syndrome have been refined and redefined since the time of this publication, the paper does highlight the importance of careful observation and detailed documentation as the cornerstone of clinical research: an approach that continues to serve us well (Gonzalez, 2005; Huerta-Alardín *et al.*, 2005).

Four similar but different clinical cases are described with precise details of each aspect of the syndrome. It is this meticulous detailing that led to the identification of patterns and inconsistencies among the cases. Employing the principles of Occam's Razor versus Saint's Triad in a logical and deductive manner, the authors developed the thesis and came to the correct diagnosis (Hilliard *et al.*, 2004). Each clinical observation is related to specific pathological correlates. The work was accomplished by a team of clinicians, surgeons, and pathologists who worked together to understand and treat this syndrome, demonstrating another essential component of research—the importance of collaboration. This landmark paper by Bywaters and Beall not only describes the syndrome of crush injury and AKI but also serves as a historical catalogue of devastation and human tragedy during wartime. None the less, even during these times of tragedy, the role of the physician as healthcare provider, educator, and scientist was maintained.

References

Minami, S (1923). Über Nierenveränderungen nach Verschüttung. *Virchows Arch Pathol Anat* **245**, 247–267.

Gonzalez, D (2005). Crush syndrome. *Crit Care Med* 2005, **33** (Suppl.), S34–S41.

Huerta-Alardín AL, Varon J, Marik PE (2005). Bench-to-bedside review: rhabdomyolysis—an overview for clinicians. *Crit Care* **9**,158–169.

Hilliard AA. Weinberger, SE, Tierney LM, Midthun DE, Saint, S. (2004). Occam's Razor versus Saint's Triad. *N Engl J Med* **350**, 599–603.

10.2 The changes in renal clearance following complete ischemia of the kidney

Author

EE Selkurt

Reference

American Journal of Physiology 1945, **144**, 395–403.

Abstract

Experiments performed on anesthized dogs showed that changes in renal function analogous to those seen in hypotension and shock result from temporary complete renal ischemia produced by clamping the renal artery. These changes occur while the mean blood pressure is maintained at normal levels. It was found that the clearance of creatinine, taken as a measure of glomerular filtration in the normal dog, and the clearance of p-aminohippurate, a measure of effective renal plasma flow, may be markedly reduced following brief periods of complete ischemia, the length and degree of the reduction being in direct proportion to the length of the period of clamping.

The results indicate that prolonged vasoconstriction of the renal arterioles follows the period of ischemia, thus playing a role in the decreased renal clearances. In addition, anoxia resulting from the ischemia produces additional changes in the clearances referable to damage of the renal tubules.

Decreased urine flow after ischemia is associated with the reduced clearances. This is thought to be due to arteriolar vasoconstriction which reduces glomerular filtration, and to renal tubular damage, which modifies the normal tubular water reabsorptive mechanism.

Importance

This paper was seminal in describing the dissociation between glomerular changes, filtration markers, and tubular injury occurring with hypoxic damage. Selkurt describes a series of experiments in which measurement of renal clearance markers was undertaken in the presence of variable anoxic conditions and preserved blood pressure. The mechanisms by which hypoperfusion in the context of preserved blood pressure lead to reduced glomerular filtration rate (GFR) had not been delineated previously. Subsequently, our appreciation of the limitations of serum creatinine as a marker of AKI has been enhanced.

Using anesthetized dogs that underwent cannulation of the renal artery and vein and variable time periods of complete renal ischaemia, Selkurt demonstrated several important clinico-pathological correlates. Firstly, he showed that renal ischaemia for up to 5 min did not correlate directly with a decrease in the renal clearance of creatinine and *p*-aminohippurate, and in fact that renal clearance of these markers was remarkably well preserved. Secondly, he showed that 10 min of complete ischaemia led to an expected significant reduction in the renal clearance of these markers; however, there was a degree of recovery of function, reflecting the intrinsic renal reserve that exists in the face of injury. However, there is a ceiling to that renal reserve in the face of prolonged insult; finally, with complete ischaemia lasting 20 min, anuria and oliguria become clinically relevant surrogate markers of severity of injury. Selkurt's description of the tubular injury in association with the renal vasoconstriction was also a novel observation.

Clarifying the role of serum creatinine as a marker of decreased GFR secondary to prolonged renal arteriolar ischaemia was an important first step in the clinical identification of AKI. Numerous investigators over the subsequent 60 years have built upon that observation. For example, Bonventre and colleagues described the complex interactions between vasoconstriction, endothelial injury, and inflammation in even more detail (Bonventre and Weinberg, 2003; Vaidya *et al.*, 2008). Furthermore, Heyman *et al.* (2002) described the evolution of animal models to mimic human patients more effectively, so that our ability to dissect ischaemic renal injury on a microscopic level improved. Finally, we are now moving to a new era, identifying and assessing biomarkers of AKI such as neutrophil gelatinase-associated lipocalin (NGAL), kidney injury molecule 1 (Kim-1), and cystatin C. This paper by Selkurt reminds us how far we have come and emphasizes how rigorous attention to the scientific method is essential for advancement, but also reminds us about the dissociation between markers of kidney function and damage.

References

Bonventre JV, Weinberg JM (2003). Recent advances in the pathophysiology of ischemic acute renal failure. *J Am Soc Nephrol* **14**, 2199–2210.

Heyman SN, Lieberthal W, Rogiers P, Bonventre JV (2002). Animal models of acute tubular necrosis. *Curr Opin Crit Care* **8**, 526–534.

Vaidya VS, Ferguson MA, Bonventre JV (2008). Biomarkers of acute kidney injury. *Annu Rev Pharmacol Toxicol* **48**, 463–493.

10.3 Acute renal success. The unexpected logic of oliguria in acute renal failure

Authors

Thurau K, Boylan JW

Reference

American Journal of Medicine 1976, **61**, 308–315.

Abstract

The clinical condition known as acute renal failure is recognized by the onset of oliguria, its course is marked by the persistence of oliguria, and recovery is heralded by the advent of diuresis. The dramatic character of oliguria has made it the focus of attention for the physician. Oliguria was viewed as the primary event and therapy was directed to measures to restore urine flow rate to normal. Little thought has been given to the concept that the kidney may be acting appropriately in making a small volume of urine or that oliguria may be the necessary consequence of a functional adaptation protecting the patient from a graver danger.

Importance

AKI is the end result of numerous complex physiological events. Many patients with AKI have multisystem disease making them difficult to study and manage clinically, and there are few appropriate animal models to guide our understanding of the appropriateness of the renal response to injury. This paper by Thurau and Boylan addressed the question of the appropriateness of the renal response in the face of severe injury by describing the teleological foundations and mechanisms of oliguria, with particular attention to the phenomenon of tubuloglomerular feedback. They eloquently described the 'sensibility' of the kidney and the integral role it plays in maintaining homeostasis for the organism. Perhaps most striking is their description of the differential influences on GFR and tubular function, the former being influenced by arterial pressure and the latter by metabolic demand.

The authors described tubuloglomerular feedback, the reduction in GFR that occurs in the face of tubular injury, in elegant detail. This feedback loop is dependent on sensing tubular NaCl as a marker of tubular reabsorptive capacity and translating this to adaptation in the vascular bed wherein the glomerular pole remains responsive to renin as a mediator of vascular tone. Whilst many clinicians regard a reduction in GFR or oliguria, or both, as a maladaptive response, the authors raised the possibility that this very response, if limited in duration, is cardinal to the preservation of volume status and is more appropriately considered as some sign of adaptive capacity in the face of a substantial renal insult.

This concept has significant implications for diagnosis and clinical care, as well as for mechanistic understandings (Vallon, 2003). Oliguria remains one component of current clinical definitions of AKI. The notion of tubular damage has led to attempts to identify tubular damage early as a marker of AKI [e.g. the measurement of circulating neutrophil gelatinase-associated lipocalin (NGAL) and kidney injury molecule 1 (Kim-1) (Devarajan, 2006). This concept has been translated into a clinical paradigm and model of ischaemic AKI, with discrete phases signalled by different levels of 'responsiveness', which may provide a framework for therapeutic interventions and treatments (Molitoris, 2003). The focus on physiological determinants of tubular and glomerular regulation also guides our understanding of the impact of medications including non-steroidal anti-inflammatory drugs, angiotensin-converting enzyme (ACE) inhibitors, and diuretics on kidney function and in the promotion of AKI (Mehta *et al.*, 2002; Abuelo, 2007). This paper is remarkable in its unique approach to the synthesis of complex physiology and clinical implications.

References

Abuelo JG (2007). Normotensive ischemic acute renal failure. *New Engl J Med* **357**, 797–805.

Devarajan P (2006). Update on mechanisms of ischemic acute kidney injury. *J Am Soc Nephrol* **17**, 1503–1520.

Mehta RL, Pascual MT, Soroko S, Chertow GM (2002). Diuretics, mortality, and nonrecovery of renal function in acute renal failure. *JAMA* **288**, 2547–2553.

Molitoris BA (2003). Transitioning to therapy in ischemic acute renal failure. *J Am Soc Nephrol* **14**, 265–267.

Vallon V (2003). Tubuloglomerular feedback and the control of glomerular filtration rate. *News Physiol Sci* **18**, 169–174.

10.4 Hospital-acquired renal insufficiency: a prospective study

Authors

SH Hou, DA Bushinsky, JB Wish, JJ Cohen, JT Harrington

Reference

American Journal of Medicine 1983, **74**, 243–248.

Abstract

Twenty-two hundred sixty-two consecutive medical and surgical admissions were evaluated prospectively to determine the contribution of iatrogenic factors to the development of renal insufficiency in hospital. Of 2,216 patients at risk, some degree of renal insufficiency developed in 4.9 percent. Decreased renal perfusion, post-operative renal insufficiency, radiographic contrast media, and aminoglycosides accounted for 79 percent of the episodes. Iatrogenic factors, broadly defined, accounted for 55 percent of all episodes. Poor prognostic indicators included oliguria, urine sediment abnormalities and, most importantly, severity of renal insufficiency; with an increase in serum creatinine of 3 mg/dl or greater, the mortality rate was 64 percent. Age, admission serum creatinine levels, and the number of episodes of renal insufficiency did not significantly affect outcome. We conclude that there is a substantial risk of the development of renal failure in hospital and that the mortality rate due to hospital-acquired renal insufficiency remains high.

Importance

AKI is a common occurrence in hospitalized patients, although the extent and risk factors have been less well described. The impact of AKI on outcomes in hospitalized patients has become increasingly recognized. This paper was one of the first to describe this entity of 'hospital-acquired' AKI. Whilst clinicians recognize the multiple risk factors that may contribute to the development of an episode of AKI, the importance of this paper lies in its description of factors that can be influenced by physicians during hospitalization.

This prospective cohort study described the prevalence of AKI and described associations of iatrogenic factors to its development. Published 30 years ago, it still provides the foundation for more recent epidemiological concepts in AKI. That AKI occurs in the context of medication administration, contrast-induced injury, and surgical interventions, and that AKI contributes significantly to a patient's risk of mortality, are important observations. AKI, even when rather crudely defined by a rise in serum creatinine, is a potent predictor of patient outcome, and this has been part of the impetus to facilitate earlier identification of AKI using other serum and urinary biomarkers. The paper makes the important point that significant increases in creatinine correlating with severe episodes of AKI are uncommon; however, smaller, incremental increases in serum creatinine are associated with an increased risk of requiring dialysis and death. More recently, this has been validated independently in two studies conducted by Chertow *et al.* (2005) and James *et al.* (2011). The observation in this paper that AKI associated with cardiac disease had worse clinical outcomes is now better understood with the emerging clinical understanding of different aspects of the 'cardio-renal syndrome' (Hobson *et al.*, 2009). Although the definition of AKI used in this study was relatively broad compared with newer refinements, such as the RIFLE ((Risk, Injury, Failure, Loss, and End-stage kidney disease) and AKIN (Acute Kidney Injury Network) definitions, Hou and colleagues were still able to demonstrate that AKI is a common occurrence during hospitalization. There has been much subsequent work on the epidemiology of hospital-acquired AKI, but still lacking are interventional studies to test whether clinical attention to early changes in serum creatinine can actually improve patient outcomes. The EARLI (Early Renal Service Involvement) study would suggest it does, but larger trials are still needed (Balasubramanian *et al.*, 2011).

References

Balasubramanian G, Al-Aly Z, Moiz A, *et al.* (2011). Early nephrologist involvement in hospital-acquired acute kidney injury: a pilot study. *Am J Kidney Dis* **57**, 228–234.

Chertow GM, Burdick E, Honour M, Bonventre JV, Bates DW (2005) Acute kidney injury, mortality, length of stay, and costs in hospitalized patients. *J Am Soc Nephrol* **16**, 3365–3370.

Hobson CE, Sinan Yavas S, *et al.* (2009). Acute kidney injury is associated with increased long-term mortality after cardiothoracic surgery. *Circulation* **119**, 2444–2453.

James MT, Ghali WA, Knudtson ML, *et al.* (2011). Associations between acute kidney injury and cardiovascular and renal outcomes after coronary angiography. *Circulation* **123**, 409–416.

10.5 Early management of shock and prophylaxis of acute renal failure in traumatic rhabdomyolysis

Authors

OS Better, JH Stein

Reference

New England Journal of Medicine 1990, **322**, 825–829.

Abstract

Seismic catastrophes leave in their wake survivors trapped under the rubble who suffer from extensive muscle damage and its devastating sequel of hemodynamic and metabolic disturbances and acute renal failure. We review here the pathogenesis of shock and acute renal failure associated with traumatic rhabdomyolysis and suggest guidelines for early management of shock and the prophylaxis of acute renal failure due to crush syndrome.

Importance

This 1990 review article by Better and Stein is unique in its breadth and depth of discussion. The authors described not only the pathophysiology of AKI secondary to crush syndrome in understandable physiological detail, but also contextualized the syndrome in the setting of disasters, not only describing the optimal treatment of the condition but also suggesting the need for proactive system development for disaster relief. In this way, the authors bridged from bench to bedside to populations and policy. They offered a synthesis of basic and animal experiments into a detailed explanation of crush injury, explored best therapies in the context of a 'natural' RCT and offered insights in 1990 that would go on to form the cornerstone of other key research and observations. Whilst Bywaters, almost 50 years before, had articulately described crush syndrome, and had also described AKI prevention or attenuation with early recognition and intervention, the pathobiological explanation found in this paper and supporting data described extended those observations (Bywaters, 1990).

In considering clinical intervention, Better and Stein actually described what has now come to be known as 'early goal-directed therapy'. This aggressive resuscitation to physiological end points, recently delineated by Rivers *et al.* (2001) and the notion of adverse outcomes linked to a positive fluid balance, described by Bouchard *et al.* (2009) were already clearly articulated here. Interestingly the lessons learned about aggressive volume resuscitation in the presence of AKI from the 1972 experience continue to be forgotten and are being relearned 50 years later.

Within the complex physiology described, Better and Stein remind us of crush syndrome in the context of natural disasters, and the interaction between patients and their environment. The conclusion of this paper is probably one of the first 'blueprints' of what we now call 'disaster planning', articulating the need for organized, well-resourced, response teams. Application of knowledge regarding appropriate prevention and treatment of AKI in these situations forms the basis of present-day guidelines for the management of crush syndromes (Vanholder *et al.*, 2012) Through scientific efforts as well as humanitarian efforts, such as the International Society of Nephrology's

Renal Disaster Relief Task Force and other groups, improved planning, resource allocation, and ultimately better patient outcomes can be achieved.

References

Bouchard J, Soroko SB, Chertow GM, *et al.* (2009). Fluid accumulation, survival and recovery of kidney function in critically ill patients with acute kidney injury. *Kidney Int* **76**, 422–427.

Bywaters EG (1990). 50 years on: the crush syndrome. *Brit Med J* **301**, 1412–1415.

Rivers E, Nguyen B, Havstad S, *et al.* (2001). Early goal-directed therapy in the treatment of severe sepsis and septic shock. *New Engl J Med* **345**, 1368–1377.

Vanholder R, Sever MS (2012). Crush recommendations: a step forward in disaster nephrology. *Nephrol Dial Transplant* **27**, 1277–1781.

10.6 Prevention of radiographic-contrast-agent–induced reductions in renal function by acetylcysteine

Authors

M Tepel, M van der Giet, C Schwarzfeld, U Laufer, D Liermann, W Zidek

Reference

New England Journal of Medicine 2000, **343**, 180–184.

Abstract

Background: Radiographic contrast agents can cause a reduction in renal function that may be due to reactive oxygen species. Whether the reduction can be prevented by the administration of antioxidants is unknown.

Methods: We prospectively studied 83 patients with chronic renal insufficiency (mean [±SD] serum creatinine concentration, 2.4 ± 1.3 mg per deciliter [216 ± 116 µmol per liter]) who were undergoing computed tomography with iopromide, a nonionic, low-osmolality contrast agent. Patients were randomly assigned either to receive the antioxidant acetylcysteine (600 mg orally twice daily) and 0.45 percent saline intravenously, before and after administration of the contrast agent, or to receive placebo and saline.

Results: Ten of the 83 patients (12 percent) had an increase of at least 0.5 mg per deciliter (44 µmol per liter) in the serum creatinine concentration 48 hours after administration of the contrast agent: 1 of the 41 patients in the acetylcysteine group (2 percent) and 9 of the 42 patients in the control group (21 percent; $P = 0.01$; relative risk, 0.1; 95 percent confidence interval, 0.02 to 0.9). In the acetylcysteine group, the mean serum creatinine concentration decreased significantly ($P < 0.001$), from 2.5 ± 1.3 to 2.1 ± 1.3 mg per deciliter (220 ± 118 to 186 ± 112 µmol per liter) 48 hours after the administration of the contrast medium, whereas in the control group, the mean serum creatinine concentration increased nonsignificantly ($P = 0.18$), from 2.4 ± 1.3 to 2.6 ± 1.5 mg per deciliter (212 ± 114 to 226 ± 133 µmol per liter) ($P < 0.001$ for the comparison between groups).

Conclusions: Prophylactic oral administration of the antioxidant acetylcysteine, along with hydration, prevents the reduction in renal function induced by iopromide, a nonioNic, low-osmolality contrast agent, in patients with chronic renal insufficiency.

Importance

The prevention of contrast-induced nephropathy (CIN) has been an area of intense interest for clinicians and researchers. It has been appreciated for decades that elevations in serum creatinine occur after the administration of radiocontrast. There are multiple mechanisms by which the kidney can be damaged after the administration of contrast, including vasoconstriction, insipation of contrast material in tubular fluid, athero-embolic disease, or combinations thereof. The precise definition of CIN has been problematic given these multiple processes. None the less, the search for effective prevention of these changes in serum creatinine after contrast administration has continued, particularly given the relentless growth in the use of contrast for vascular diagnosis and intervention.

This paper is chosen as a landmark as it was the first to excite the clinical world about a possible prevention strategy for CIN. *N*-Acetylcysteine (NAC) is a low-risk intervention without significant adverse effects and its mechanism of action (free oxygen radical scavenger) is logical and appealing.

However, there are many issues with the design of the study, which mean it cannot be interpreted as conclusively supporting the use of N-acetylcysteine to prevent CIN. This was a small randomized prospective placebo-controlled trial that investigated the effect of oral NAC in patients at relatively low risk with stable chronic kidney disease that underwent contrast-enhanced computed tomography scans with a fixed volume of non-ionic low osmolar contrast. Tepel and colleagues found that oral NAC in combination with adequate hydration pre- and post-procedure reduced the incidence of CIN from 21 to 2%. CIN is this study was defined as a 44 μmol/l (0.5 mg/dl) increase in serum creatinine at 48 h post-procedure. The incidence of CIN in this relatively low-risk group was actually quite high. A key finding was that there was a statistically significant reduction in serum creatinine at 48 h in those treated with NAC compared with the controls. However, whilst this was not appreciated at the time of publication, subsequent work has described an interference by NAC in creatinine assays using the Jaffe reaction (Lognard *et al.*, 2008) sufficient to explain the 'outcome' of a rise in serum creatinine of 44 μmol/l in the treatment group and accounting for the significantly positive result. Subsequent large studies have not been able to repeat these findings, albeit in different population groups (Pate *et al.*, 2004). There have been a number of meta-analyses, which on balance, do not support the use of NAC as a preventative agent (Pannu *et al.*, 2004; Gonzales *et al.*, 2007).

Thus, despite the great interest that this paper originally attracted, leading to the widespread clinical use of NAC, it has been selected here to bring attention to the phenomenon of the biochemical interactions of NAC with measurement of creatinine using the Jaffe reaction. It now appears that hydration protocols, which have been tested subsequently in larger studies, offer more substantial protection than NAC alone. Current national and international radiology and AKI guidelines also do not recommend its use.

In the context of increasing awareness of the impact of small increases in serum creatinine on short- and long-term prognosis, it is important to both identify and prevent CIN. Appropriate preparation of patients at risk for CIN (e.g. hydration, cessation of drugs that impair autoregulation) remains the most appropriate therapy (Komenda *et al.*, 2007). The Tepel paper reminds us to pay attention to details of chemical interactions and outcomes, and to understand the true baseline risk of CIN in populations, in order to design trials of sufficient size and rigor to answer clinically important questions.

References

Gonzales DA, Norsworthy KJ, Kern SJ, *et al.* (2007). A meta-analysis of N-acetylcysteine in contrast-induced nephrotoxicity: unsupervised clustering to resolve heterogeneity. *BMC Med* **5**, 32.

Komenda P, Zalunardo N, Burnett S, *et al.* (2007). Conservative outpatient renoprotective protocol in patients with low GFR undergoing contrast angiography: a case series. *Clinical Exp Nephrol* **1**, 209–213.

Lognard M, Cavalier E, Chapelle JP, *et al.* (2008). Acetylcysteine and enzymatic creatinine: beware of laboratory artefact! *Intensive Care Med* **34**, 5973–5974.

Pannu N, Manns B, Lee H, Tonelli M (2004). Systematic review of the impact of N-acetylcysteine on contrast nephropathy. *Kidney Int* **65**, 1366–1374.

Pate G, Humphries KH, Buller CE, *et al.* (2004). A randomized controlled trial of intravenous N-acetylcysteine for the prevention of contrast-induced nephropathy after cardiac catheterization: lack of effect. *Am Heart J* **148**, 422–429.

10.7 Acute kidney injury, mortality, length of stay, and costs in hospitalized patients

Authors
GM Chertow, E Burdick, M Honour, JV Bonventre, DW Bates

Reference
Journal of the American Society of Nephrology 2005, **16**, 3365–3370.

Abstract

The marginal effects of acute kidney injury on in-hospital mortality, length of stay (LOS), and costs have not been well described. A consecutive sample of 19,982 adults who were admitted to an urban academic medical center, including 9210 who had two or more serum creatinine (SCr) determinations, was evaluated. The presence and degree of acute kidney injury were assessed using absolute and relative increases from baseline to peak SCr concentration during hospitalization. Large increases in SCr concentration were relatively rare (*e.g.*, >2.0 mg/dl in 105 [1%] patients), whereas more modest increases in SCr were common (*e.g.*, >0.5 mg/dl in 1237 [13%] patients). Modest changes in SCr were significantly associated with mortality, LOS, and costs, even after adjustment for age, gender, admission *International Classification of Diseases, Ninth Revision, Clinical Modification* diagnosis, severity of illness (diagnosis-related group weight), and chronic kidney disease. For example, an increase in SCr >0.5 mg/dl was associated with a 6.5-fold (95% confidence interval 5.0 to 8.5) increase in the odds of death, a 3.5-d increase in LOS, and nearly $7500 in excess hospital costs. Acute kidney injury is associated with significantly increased mortality, LOS, and costs across a broad spectrum of conditions. Moreover, outcomes are related directly to the severity of acute kidney injury, whether characterized by nominal or percentage changes in serum creatinine.

Importance

AKI is a common complication of hospitalization and an independent risk factor for mortality in critically ill patients. Despite its importance, the true incidence of AKI had been poorly described in the literature, which was largely influenced by the lack of a consensus definition that would enable appropriate recognition, stratification, and management. Although many groups had reported the impact of AKI requiring in-hospital dialysis, the impact of smaller variations of serum creatinine has been reduced to small cohort populations. This paper represents a significant contribution to the understanding of small changes in serum creatinine and the impact on patient outcomes, as well as helping to shape a subsequent consensus definition of AKI.

Chertow and colleagues conducted the largest retrospective single-centre cohort study to date and found that changes in serum creatinine, as small as 0.3 g/dl (26.4 μmol/l) had a statistically significant impact on mortality, length of stay, and cost of hospitalization when adjusted for age, gender, admission ICD-9 (International Classification of Diseases, Ninth Revision) diagnosis, severity of illness (diagnosis-related group weight), and chronic kidney disease. The adjusted odds ratio for mortality with a ≥0.3 mg/dl (26.4 μmol/l) increase in serum creatinine was 4.1 (confidence interval 3.1–5.5). This association between AKI and increased mortality was incremental with increasing severity of AKI as defined by an absolute increase in serum creatinine or a relative change from baseline. Furthermore, AKI carried it with at an increased cost to the healthcare system, in this case in the USA: a serum creatinine increase of ≥0.5 mg/dl was associated with a 3.5-day increase in hospital length of stay ($P<0.0001$) and US$7499 increases in hospital costs (at 2005 rates).

As a result of this paper, there has been a significant change to how AKI is classified with revision of the less stringent RIFLE classification published by Kellum *et al.* (2002), leading to the adoption of the AKIN staging system published by Mehta *et al.* (2007). Although these changes in classification have not been uniformly adopted worldwide, the stricter definition of AKI encompassed within the AKIN staging system may yet translate to better recognition of AKI and earlier intervention in its management. With increasing evidence suggesting that AKI is a risk factor for chronic kidney disease, earlier recognition and intervention of AKI may also have a long-term impact on patient health (Chawla *et al.*, 2011).

References

Chawla, LS, Amdur, RL, Amodeo, S, Kimmel PL, Palant CE (2011). The severity of acute kidney injury predicts progression to chronic kidney disease. *Kidney Int* **79**, 1361–1369.

Kellum JA, Mehta RL, Angus DC, Palevsky P, Ronco C (2002). The first international consensus conference on continuous renal replacement therapy. *Kidney Int* **62**, 1855–1863.

Mehta RL, Kellum JA, Shah SV, *et al.* (2007). Acute Kidney Injury Network: report of an initiative to improve outcomes in acute kidney injury. *Crit Care* **11**, R31.

10.8 Fluid accumulation, survival and recovery of kidney function in critically ill patients with acute kidney injury

Authors

J Bouchard, SB Soroko, GM Chertow, J Himmelfarb, TA Ikizler, EP Paganini, RL Mehta, Program to Improve Care in Acute Renal Disease (PICARD) Study Group

Reference

Kidney International 2009, **76**, 422–427.

Abstract

Fluid accumulation is associated with adverse outcomes in critically ill patients. Here, we sought to determine if fluid accumulation is associated with mortality and non-recovery of kidney function in critically ill adults with acute kidney injury. Fluid overload was defined as more than a 10% increase in body weight relative to baseline, measured in 618 patients enrolled in a prospective multicenter observational study. Patients with fluid overload experienced significantly higher mortality within 60 days of enrollment. Among dialyzed patients, survivors had significantly lower fluid accumulation when dialysis was initiated compared to non-survivors after adjustments for dialysis modality and severity score. The adjusted odds ratio for death associated with fluid overload at dialysis initiation was 2.07. In non-dialyzed patients, survivors had significantly less fluid accumulation at the peak of their serum creatinine. Fluid overload at the time of diagnosis of acute kidney injury was not associated with recovery of kidney function. However, patients with fluid overload when their serum creatinine reached its peak were significantly less likely to recover kidney function. Our study shows that in patients with acute kidney injury, fluid overload was independently associated with mortality. Whether the fluid overload was the result of a more severe renal failure or it contributed to its cause will require clinical trials in which the role of fluid administration to such patients is directly tested.

Importance

Fluid resuscitation has long been a focal point in the early management of critically ill patients. In 2001, Rivers *et al.* (2001) showed that early goal directed therapy that included early recognition of patients with severe sepsis and septic shock, in combination with aggressive and targeted fluid resuscitation in the first 6 h of admission, resulted in a significant reduction in mortality. Although this publication had a substantial influence on clinical practice patterns, the subsequent implications of aggressive fluid resuscitation had been poorly described, and in many cases limited to single-centre observational studies in specialized patient populations.

This paper by Bouchard and colleagues represented the first, prospective multicentre observational study to describe the impact of fluid accumulation on critically ill patients with AKI. Unlike previous single-centre publications by Goldstein *et al.* (2001), which looked at a paediatric intensive care unit (ICU) population, and Payen *et al.* (2008), which looked at patients with AKI and sepsis, this study included a diverse spectrum of adult patients and contrasted outcomes in patients who did not require dialysis with outcomes in patients who required some form of renal replacement therapy. They showed that being fluid overloaded, defined as a 10% increase in body weight relative to baseline, was associated with increased mortality, irrespective of the use of renal replacement therapy. Furthermore, this paper was unique in clarifying the impact of the duration of fluid overload on survival in a dose–response manner. Interestingly, other studies describing the 'under-recognition' of the severity of AKI as measured by serum creatinine extend concepts put forth by the authors of this paper: volume overload impedes organ function and may also impair the clinicians' ability to identify organ dysfunction, especially in the kidney (Waikar and Bonventre, 2009). This paper also showed that volume status at the time of diagnosis of AKI did not impact on recovery of renal function or dialysis dependency at hospital discharge. This paper was innovative in that it underscored the importance of attending to appropriate volume resuscitation, and challenged clinicians to re-examine the original (and probably sound) notion of goal-directed fluid resuscitation to physiological end points. Given the practical point that total fluid volume administered to a critically ill patient may be underestimated when multiple care teams are involved over time, this paper described how the administration of large volumes of fluid does not improve and probably adversely impacts on outcomes. Well-conducted studies of restricted-volume resuscitation for AKI are now needed if we are to manage this condition better. Clearly, 'more is not better', even in those not requiring dialysis.

References

Goldstein SL, Currier H, Graf CD, Cosio CC, Brewer ED, Sachdeva R (2001). Outcome in children receiving continuous venovenous hemofiltration. *Pediatrics* **107**, 1309–1312.

Payen D, de Pont AC, Sakr Y, *et al.* (2008). A positive fluid balance is associated with a worse outcome in patients with acute renal failure. *Crit Care* **12**, R74.

Rivers E, Nguyen B, Havstad S, *et al.* (2001). Early goal-directed therapy in the treatment of severe sepsis and septic shock. *N Engl J Med* **345**, 1368–1377.

Waikar SS, Bonventre JV (2009) Creatinine kinetics and the definition of acute kidney injury. *J Am Soc Nephrol* **20**, 672–679.

10.9 Intensity of continuous renal-replacement therapy in critically ill patients

Authors

The RENAL Replacement Therapy Study Investigators: R Bellomo, A Cass, L Cole, S Finfer, M Gallagher, S Lo, C McArthur, S McGuinness, J Myburgh, R Norton, C Scheinkestel, S Su

Reference

New England Journal of Medicine 2009, **361**, 1627–1638.

Abstract

Background: The optimal intensity of continuous renal-replacement therapy remains unclear. We conducted a multicenter, randomized trial to compare the effect of this therapy, delivered at two different levels of intensity, on 90-day mortality among critically ill patients with acute kidney injury.

Methods: We randomly assigned critically ill adults with acute kidney injury to continuous renal-replacement therapy in the form of postdilution continuous venovenous hemodiafiltration with an effluent flow of either 40 ml per kilogram of body weight per hour (higher intensity) or 25 ml per kilogram per hour (lower intensity). The primary outcome measure was death within 90 days after randomization.

Results: Of the 1508 enrolled patients, 747 were randomly assigned to higher-intensity therapy, and 761 to lower-intensity therapy with continuous venovenous hemodiafiltration. Data on primary outcomes were available for 1464 patients (97.1%): 721 in the higher-intensity group and 743 in the lower-intensity group. The two study groups had similar baseline characteristics and received the study treatment for an average of 6.3 and 5.9 days, respectively (P = 0.35). At 90 days after randomization, 322 deaths had occurred in the higher-intensity group and 332 deaths in the lower-intensity group, for a mortality of 44.7% in each group (odds ratio, 1.00; 95% confidence interval [CI], 0.81 to 1.23; P = 0.99). At 90 days, 6.8% of survivors in the higher-intensity group (27 of 399), as compared with 4.4% of survivors in the lower-intensity group (18 of 411), were still receiving renal-replacement therapy (odds ratio, 1.59; 95% CI, 0.86 to 2.92; P = 0.14). Hypophosphatemia was more common in the higher-intensity group than in the lower-intensity group (65% vs. 54%, P < 0.001).

Conclusions: In critically ill patients with acute kidney injury, treatment with higher-intensity continuous renal-replacement therapy did not reduce mortality at 90 days.

Importance

Continuous renal replacement therapy (CRRT) in critically ill patients was first introduced in 1977, and the question of the optimal dose of CRRT has been asked since its inception. Whilst intuitively 'more dialysis' should be better, the question of optimal dosing of CRRT had proved challenging to answer. A number of studies had tried to address this question but all had limitations due to differences in patient selection, primary end points, and study design.

The selection of primary end point as death at 90 days in this RENAL trial was longer than in the original studies by Ronco *et al.* (2000), and was certainly sufficient to determine treatment efficacy and morbidity in a group of high-risk patients. Note is made of the fact that other trials, such as the Acute Renal Failure Trial Network (ATN) study (Palevsky *et al.*, 2008), had used similar end points and drew similar conclusions. However, this trial was sufficiently powered to identify important differences in the primary end point, and was carefully designed and executed so that fluid removal per 24 h and achieved dose as a percentage of target were similar in both groups. The trial demonstrated unequivocally that there was no additional value to increased intensity of dialysis in critically ill individuals.

These findings are applicable to current practice. The RENAL trial used post-dilution continuous venovenous haemofiltration, which is accepted as the current standard of care in many centres. A number of other studies had used pre-dilution haemofiltration, which is less commonly used in critical care settings (Saudan *et al.*, 2006; Tolwani *et al.*, 2008). Furthermore, the inclusion of over 1500 general ICU patients minimized the selection bias and improved generalizability, which had been a shortcoming of previous trials.

Lastly, the RENAL trial was a large RCT in multiple centres across Australia and New Zealand, within the context of a relatively 'universal' healthcare system. Whilst the ATN trial was also a large multicentre study, all centres were in the USA but in a variety of healthcare settings. The ATN study also used entry criteria that were relatively delayed compared with the RENAL trial (150 versus 50 h), and many had prior exposure to intermittent haemodialysis. The concordance of the results of the RENAL and ATN trials, however, is reassuring, and is simply summarized as: 'more is not necessarily better'—increasing the dose of haemofiltration is not of value in critically ill patients. From accumulating data from this and other studies, delivering more dialysis in seriously ill patients who requiring dialysis is not of value in reducing mortality.

A number of issues remain unresolved. What is not addressed in this or other studies is the question of when to initiate dialysis, how to address and achieve volume targets, and other questions that may have a greater influence on patient outcomes than how much clearance is delivered by CRRT. Lastly, it is important to note that 84% of the population achieved the prescribed dose of CRRT. Often in the critical care setting, insufficient attention is paid to achieving prescribed doses or even customizing prescriptions. These studies demonstrate that, in the context of achieving prescribed doses in CRRT, increasing the dose does not matter; this is not the same as saying that dose does not matter at all.

References

Palevsky PM, Zhang JH, O'Connor TZ, *et al.* (2008). Intensity of renal support in critically ill patients with acute kidney injury. *N Engl J Med* **359**, 7–20.

Ronco C, Bellomo R, Homel P, *et al.* (2000). Effects of different doses in continuous veno-venous haemofiltration on outcomes of acute renal failure: a prospective randomised trial. *Lancet* **356**, 26–30.

Saudan P, Niederberger M, de Seigneux S, *et al.* (2006). Adding a dialysis dose to continuous hemofiltration increases survival in patients with acute renal failure. *Kidney Int* **70**, 1312–1317.

Tolwani AJ, Campbell RC, Stofan BS, Lai KR, Oster RA, Wille KM (2008). Standard versus high-dose CVVHDF for ICU-related acute renal failure. *J Am Soc Nephrol* **19**, 1233–1238.

10.10 Glomerular filtration rate, proteinuria, and the incidence and consequences of acute kidney injury: a cohort study

Authors

MT James, BR Hemmelgarn, N Wiebe, N Pannu, BJ Manns, SW Klarenbach, M Tonelli, for the Alberta Kidney Disease Network

Reference

Lancet 2010, **376**, 2096–2103.

Abstract

Background: Low values of estimated glomerular filtration rate (eGFR) predispose to acute kidney injury, and proteinuria is a marker of kidney disease. We aimed to investigate how eGFR and proteinuria jointly modified the risks of acute kidney injury and subsequent adverse clinical outcomes.

Methods: We did a cohort study of 920 985 adults residing in Alberta, Canada, between 2002 and 2007. Participants not needing chronic dialysis at baseline and with at least one outpatient measurement of both serum creatinine concentration and proteinuria (urine dipstick or albumin-creatinine ratio) were included. We assessed hospital admission with acute kidney injury with validated administrative codes; other outcomes were all-cause mortality and a composite renal outcome of end-stage renal disease or doubling of serum creatinine concentration.

Findings: During median follow-up of 35 months (range 0–59 months), 6520 (0·7%) participants were admitted with acute kidney injury. In those with eGFR 60 mL/min per 1·73 m^2 or greater, the adjusted risk of admission with this disorder was about 4 times higher in those with heavy proteinuria measured by dipstick (rate ratio 4·4 vs no proteinuria, 95% CI 3·7–5·2). The adjusted rates of admission with acute kidney injury and kidney injury needing dialysis remained high in participants with heavy dipstick proteinuria for all values of eGFR. The adjusted rates of death and the composite renal outcome were also high in participants admitted with acute kidney injury, although the rise associated with this injury was attenuated in those with low baseline eGFR and heavy proteinuria.

Interpretation: These findings suggest that information on proteinuria and eGFR should be used together when identifying people at risk of acute kidney injury, and that an episode of acute kidney injury provides further long-term prognostic information in addition to eGFR and proteinuria.

Importance

AKI is a common occurrence in hospitalized patients and carries with it significant morbidity and mortality. Chronic kidney disease (CKD) is common in outpatient populations and is associated with equally dismal clinical outcomes. Proteinuria has been shown to be a significant risk factor for progression of CKD to end-stage renal disease (ESRD) and its presence, independent of the degree of decline in estimated glomerular filtration rate (eGFR), is also associated with higher mortality and morbidity. Data are accumulating that describe the independence of proteinuria and eGFR in predicting outcomes. Whilst most would have anticipated an impact of lower eGFR on the outcomes studied in this epidemiological analysis, many would not have anticipated the impact of proteinuria alone, irrespective of eGFR, on the risk for developing AKI. This paper elegantly demonstrated the importance of proteinuria, as a marker of pre-existing kidney disease, cardiovascular disease, or both, in predicting AKI.

This is the largest cohort study conducted and included over 900,000 patients in the province of Alberta, Canada. It demonstrated the association between eGFR and proteinuria and the risk of hospitalization for AKI. Mortality, as well as the renal-specific end points of developing ESRD and doubling of serum creatinine, were secondary end points. As in other publications, hospitalization for AKI was associated with higher mortality regardless of eGFR and the presence of proteinuria (Ricci *et al.*, 2008). However, the novel finding was that incremental reductions in eGFR and higher degrees of proteinuria were independently associated with an increased risk of hospitalization for AKI. Finally, the risk of developing ESRD and doubling of serum creatinine increased with heavier proteinuria, and an episode of hospitalization for AKI further magnified the risk for these longer-term renal outcomes.

Although the association between eGFR and proteinuria and adverse outcomes has been reported previously, the contribution of both of these to an episode of AKI and to mortality and disease progression is less appreciated by many physicians (Ruggenenti *et al.*, 1997). The importance of proteinuria in risk stratification for CKD has been reviewed recently and is consistent with these findings (Levey *et al.*, 2009). The hope is that this publication will allow risk stratification for AKI to include not only eGFR but also proteinuria. This general population cohort provides a powerful information base to clinicians and researchers with respect to risk prediction.

References

Levey AS, Cattran D, Friedman A, *et al.* (2009). Proteinuria as a surrogate outcome in CKD: report of a scientific workshop sponsored by the National Kidney Foundation and the US Food and Drug Administration. *Am J Kid Dis* **54**, 205–226.

Ricci Z, Cruz C, Ronco C (2008). The RIFLE criteria and mortality in acute kidney injury: a systematic review. *Kidney Int* **73**, 538–546.

Ruggenenti P, Perna A, Matalone M, Pisoni R, Gaspari F, Remuzzi G (1997). Proteinuria predicts end stage renal failure in non diabetic chronic nephropathies. *Kidney Int* **63**, S54–S57.

Chapter 11

Chronic kidney disease

Maarten Taal

Introduction

It is easy to forget that the term 'chronic kidney disease' (CKD) and its associated definition were proposed as recently as 2002. Such has been the success of the subsequent campaign to raise awareness of CKD as a priority for research and public health that this three-letter abbreviation has become universally accepted to the point that it now dominates the literature in nephrology and is widely recognized as an important topic for investigation and discussion in many other fields of health care. Yet the entity of progressive renal scarring resulting in loss of kidney function was recognized almost 200 years ago by Richard Bright (see papers 3.1 and 5.3). Research into the mechanisms that underpin the concept of CKD dates back several decades and was at the heart of early progress in understanding renal pathophysiology. In this chapter, we will explore landmark developments in research to understand the mechanisms that contribute to the progression of CKD as well as interventions that impact on these mechanisms to slow progression. It is this extensive body of evidence that supported arguments for defining CKD as an important clinical entity, and this in turn has led to further research that has greatly expanded our understanding of the epidemiology of CKD as well as its associated risks, which are also addressed.

The focus on CKD over the past decade has seen nephrology transformed from a specialty that focused previously on discreet renal pathologies, each of which was relatively rare, to one that has been challenged to develop strategies to identify and risk-stratify CKD that is prevalent in a substantial proportion of the general population in order to apply interventions that will attenuate progression to end-stage renal disease (ESRD) as well as the associated risk of cardiovascular disease. A thorough understanding of the concepts that contribute to the pathophysiology of CKD and comprehensive knowledge of the research evidence that supports current renal protective strategies is therefore essential for all clinicians involved in the care of patients with kidney disease and those who are at risk of CKD.

11.1 A simple method of estimating progression of chronic renal failure

Authors

WE Mitch, M Walser, GA Buffington, J Lemann Jr

Reference

Lancet 1976, **ii**, 326–328.

Abstract

In 31 of 34 patients with chronic renal insufficiency caused by various diseases, reciprocal serum-creatinine concentration declined linearly as creatinine concentration rose from a mean of 2·6 mg/dl to 14·8 mg/dl over an average of 71 months. These results indicate that in most cases reciprocal serum-creatinine declines linearly with time as chronic renal failure progresses. Analysis of this relation in individual patients gives an estimate of the progression of the disease, may help to determine the effects of therapy, and could be used to predict when dialysis will become necessary.

Importance

Viewed from the perspective of the modern era of mega-trials and molecular biology, it seems surprising that the simple observation that the reciprocal of serum creatinine [proportional to glomerular filtration rate (GFR)] declined linearly over time in a small cohort of patients with different forms of CKD should have been considered worthy of publication in a journal as prominent as *The Lancet*. Yet subsequent developments have shown that the editors quite rightly identified this as an observation with profound significance. As noted by the authors, the observation had immediate clinical relevance because it provided a simple method for predicting the need for renal replacement therapy, thereby facilitating timely preparation for dialysis and transplantation. Nevertheless, it could be argued that the insight that this observation gave to our understanding of the pathogenesis of CKD progression was of even greater significance. In the first instance, the observed linear decline in GFR was consistent with the 'intact nephron' hypothesis of Bricker *et al.* (1960), which proposed that kidney diseases progressed through the destruction of some nephrons while remaining nephrons remained functionally intact. Furthermore realization that a wide range of different forms of kidney disease all seem to progress in a linear fashion gave rise to the notion that the progression of CKD is driven by a 'common pathway' of mechanisms that is largely independent of the initiating cause. This in turn suggested that, if the common pathway could be interrupted or retarded, it might be possible to arrest or slow the rate of CKD progression. Such interventions would be expected to be effective in kidney diseases of diverse aetiology. The notion of common pathway mechanisms underpins the whole concept of 'CKD', as it provides the justification for grouping apparently diverse forms of kidney disease into a single entity. These fundamental insights spawned a field of research in nephrology that has resulted in crucial insights into CKD progression, which in turn have been translated into effective renal protective therapies that can readily be applied to the increasing numbers of patients affected by CKD.

Reference

Bricker NS, Morrin PAF, Kime SW (1960). An exposition of the 'intact nephron hypothesis'. *Am J Med* **28**, 77–97.

11.2 Hyperfiltration in remnant nephrons: a potentially adverse response to renal ablation

Authors

TH Hostetter, JL Olson, HG Rennke, MA Venkatachalam, BM Brenner

Reference

American Journal of Physiology 1981, **241**, F85–F93.

Abstract

Micropuncture studies were performed in three groups of male Munich-Wistar rats 1 wk after surgery: group I, eight control rats that underwent laparotomy and were fed a normal diet; group II, nine rats that underwent right nephrectomy and segmental infarction of five-sixths of the left kidney and were fed a normal diet; and group III, seven rats that underwent the same renal ablative procedure and were fed a low protein diet. Single nephron glomerular filtration rate (SNGFR) was higher in the remnant kidney of group II rats compared with group I rats due to higher average values for mean glomerular transcapillary hydraulic pressure difference (ΔP) and initial glomerular plasma flow rate (Q_A) in group II. Glomeruli in remnant kidneys of group II showed striking alterations in morphology, including epithelial cell protein reabsorption droplets, foot process fusion, and mesangial expansion. Group III rats demonstrated a mean SNGFR not statistically different from that of group I, but significantly less than that of group II rats. This lack of absolute hyperfiltration in remnant glomeruli of group III rats relative to group I obtained because Q_A and ΔP did not increase above values found in group I. The glomerular structural lesions seen in group II were also largely attenuated in group III. These studies demonstrate that alterations in glomerular hemodynamics associated with renal ablation are accompanied by structural lesions and suggest that sustained single nephron hyperfiltration may have maladaptive consequences by damaging remnant glomeruli.

Importance

To produce an experimental model of progressive CKD, rats were subjected to unilateral nephrectomy and infarction (or surgical ablation in some studies) of two-thirds of the remaining kidney, resulting in a '5/6 nephrectomy'. In this model, animals rapidly developed hypertension and proteinuria associated with progressive kidney damage characterized histologically by focal and segmental glomerulosclerosis. The identification of a rat strain (Munich Wistar) with glomeruli that were visible on the surface of the kidneys made possible the development of micropuncture techniques to measure directly the pressure and flow of blood in glomerular capillaries and led to the first breakthrough in our understanding the common pathway of mechanisms that drive CKD progression. These investigations found that glomerular capillary hydraulic pressure increased significantly (from 49 ± 1 to 63 ± 2 mmHg) after substantial nephron loss (actually '11/12 nephrectomy' in this experiment) and that single-nephron GFR (SNGFR) more than doubled (from 27.8 ± 3.2 to 62.5 ± 6.4 nl/min). Whereas such changes could be considered adaptive as they allowed partial compensation for the loss of nephrons, electron microscopy studies showed that they were associated with podocyte and endothelial cell damage as well as mesangial expansion as early as 7 days after 5/6 nephrectomy. Subsequent longer term studies found that these early lesions progressed to focal segmental glomerulosclerosis over time. Importantly, normalization of glomerular pressure and SNGFR by dietary protein restriction was associated with attenuation of the glomerular injury, implying that the haemodynamic adaptations to nephron loss were a key factor in the subsequent development of injury in remaining glomeruli. These observations formed the basis of the 'haemodynamic theory' of Brenner *et al.* (1982), which proposed that the haemodynamic adaptations in response to nephron loss result in progressive damage to remaining glomeruli and therefore establish a vicious circle of glomerular damage that drives CKD progression. Subsequent studies in the same model showed that treatment with an angiotensin-converting enzyme inhibitor (ACEI) resulted in normalization of glomerular pressure but did not decrease SNGFR, yet afforded renal protection similar to that observed with dietary protein restriction, implying that it was glomerular hypertension rather than hyperfiltration that was the key haemodynamic factor responsible for glomerular damage (Anderson *et al.*, 1986). Treatment with other anti-hypertensives did not attenuate glomerular hypertension and afforded no renal protection. These observations thus identified angiotensin II as a key mediator of glomerular haemodynamic adaptations and subsequent glomerular damage after nephron loss, and led to clinical trails that confirmed the renal protective effects of ACEI treatment in humans.

References

Anderson S, Rennke HG, Brenner BM (1986). Therapeutic advantage of converting enzyme inhibitors in arresting progressive renal disease associated with systemic hypertension in the rat. *J Clin Invest* **77**, 1993–2000.

Brenner BM, Meyer TW, Hostetter TH (1982). Dietary protein intake and the progressive nature of kidney disease: the role of hemodynamically mediated glomerular injury in the pathogenesis of progressive glomerular sclerosis in aging, renal ablation and intrinsic renal disease. *N Engl J Med* **307**, 652–659.

11.3 The effects of dietary protein restriction and blood-pressure control on the progression of chronic renal disease

Authors

S Klahr, AS Levey, GJ Beck, AW Caggiula, L Hunsicker, JW Kusek, G Striker, for the Modification of Diet in Renal Disease Study Group

Reference

New England Journal of Medicine 1994, **330**, 877–884.

Abstract

Background: Restricting protein intake and controlling hypertension delay the progression of renal disease in animals. We tested these interventions in 840 patients with various chronic renal diseases.

Methods: In study 1, 585 patients with glomerular filtration rates of 25 to 55 ml per minute per 1.73 m^2 of body-surface area were randomly assigned to a usual-protein diet or a low-protein diet (1.3 or 0.58 g of protein per kilogram of body weight per day) and to a usual- or a low-blood-pressure group (mean arterial pressure, 107 or 92 mm Hg). In study 2, 255 patients with glomerular filtration rates of 13 to 24 ml per minute per 1.73 m^2 were randomly assigned to the low-protein diet (0.58 g per kilogram per day) or a very-low-protein diet (0.28 g per kilogram per day) with a keto acid-amino acid supplement, and a usual- or a low-blood-pressure group (same values as those in study 1). An 18-to-45-month follow-up was planned, with monthly evaluations of the patients.

Results: The mean follow-up was 2.2 years. In study 1, the projected mean decline in the glomerular filtration rate at three years did not differ significantly between the diet groups or the blood-pressure groups. As compared with the usual-protein group and the usual-blood-pressure group, the low-protein group and the low-blood-pressure group had a more rapid decline in the glomerular filtration rate during the first four months after randomization and a slower decline thereafter. In study 2, the very-low-protein group had a marginally slower decline in the glomerular filtration rate than did the low-protein group (P = 0.07). There was no delay in the time to the occurrence of end-stage renal disease or death. In both studies, patients in the low-blood-pressure group who had more pronounced proteinuria at base line had a significantly slower rate of decline in the glomerular filtration rate.

Conclusions: Among patients with moderate renal insufficiency, the slower decline in renal function that started four months after the introduction of a low-protein diet suggests a small benefit of this dietary intervention. Among patients with more severe renal insufficiency, a very-low-protein diet, as compared with a low-protein diet, did not significantly slow the progression of renal disease.

Importance

The Modification of Diet in Renal Disease (MDRD) study was the first large randomized controlled trial to evaluate potential renal protective interventions, previously identified in animal studies, in humans with CKD. At the time of publication, it was by far the largest clinical trial conducted in nephrology and it therefore represented a major step forward in the development of clinical research. Participants were randomized in two strata, defined by GFR, in a 2 × 2 factorial manner to a 'usual' or 'low' protein diet (or 'low' and 'very low' protein diet in the case of study 2) and to 'usual' [mean arterial pressure (MAP) <107 mmHg, equivalent to <140/90 mmHg] or 'low' (MAP <92 mmHg, equivalent to <125/75 mmHg) blood pressure (BP) targets.

The primary analysis revealed no difference in the mean rate of GFR decline in 'low' versus 'usual' dietary protein groups in study 1, and only a trend towards slower decline in the 'very low' protein group in study 2. Secondary analyses showed that, in study 1, the 'low' protein diet was associated with an initial reduction in GFR, probably due to functional effects, that obscured a later reduction in the rate of GFR decline that might have proved beneficial if follow-up had been extended. Unfortunately, long-term follow-up of participants from study 2 beyond the randomization period found no renal protective benefit in the 'very low' protein diet group but did report higher mortality in this group (Menon *et al.*, 2009). Three subsequent meta-analyses have each reported that dietary protein restriction is associated with significant renal protection, but conclusive proof of efficacy in humans remains elusive.

Similarly, there was no difference in rate of change in GFR between groups randomized to different BP targets, but participants in the 'low' BP group showed an early decrease in GFR, probably due to renal haemodynamic effects, that masked a subsequent slower rate of GFR decline. Furthermore, the effect of BP control was strongly influenced by the magnitude of proteinuria. Among participants with >3 g/day of proteinuria at baseline, the 'low' BP target was associated with a significantly slower GFR decline. Follow-up of patients beyond the randomization period (mean 6.6 years) revealed a significant reduction in the risk of ESRD or a combined end point of ESRD or death among patients in the 'low' BP group, indicating that the benefits of lower BP may become evident only over a longer period (Sarnak *et al.*, 2005). Nevertheless, optimal targets for BP control in CKD remain controversial (Lewis, 2010).

References

Lewis JB (2010). Blood pressure control in chronic kidney disease: is less really more? *J Am Soc Nephrol* **21**, 1086–1092.

Menon V, Kopple JD, Wang X, *et al.* (2009). Effect of a very low-protein diet on outcomes: long-term follow-up of the Modification of Diet in Renal Disease (MDRD) Study. *Am J Kidney Dis* **53**, 208–217.

Sarnak MJ, Greene T, Wang X, *et al.* (2005). The effect of a lower target blood pressure on the progression of kidney disease: long-term follow-up of the modification of diet in renal disease study. *Ann Intern Med* **142**, 342–351.

11.4 Randomised placebo-controlled trial of effect of ramipril on decline in glomerular filtration rate and risk of terminal renal failure in proteinuric, non-diabetic nephropathy

Authors

The GISEN Group (Gruppo Italiano di Studi Epidemiologici in Nefrologia)

Reference

Lancet 1997, **349**, 1857–1863.

Abstract

Background: In diabetic nephropathy, angiotensin-converting-enzyme (ACE) inhibitors have a greater effect than other antihypertensive drugs on proteinuria and the progressive decline in glomerular filtration rate (GFR). Whether this difference applies to progression of nondiabetic proteinuric nephropathies is not clear....

Methods: In this prospective double-blind trial, 352 patients were classified according to baseline proteinuria (stratum 1: 1–3 g/24 h; stratum 2: ≥3 g/24 h), and randomly assigned ramipril or placebo plus conventional antihypertensive therapy targeted at achieving diastolic blood pressure under 90 mm Hg. The primary endpoint was the rate of GFR decline. Analysis was by intention to treat.

Findings: At the second planned interim analysis, the difference in decline in GFR between the ramipril and placebo groups in stratum 2 was highly significant (p=0·001). The Independent Adjudicating Panel therefore decided to ... do the final analysis in this stratum (stratum 1 continued in the trial).... The decline in GFR per month was significantly lower in the ramipril group than the placebo group (0·53 [0·08] *vs* 0·88 [0·13] mL/min, p=0·03). Among the ramipril-assigned patients, percentage reduction in proteinuria was inversely correlated with decline in GFR (p 0·035) and predicted the reduction in risk of doubling of baseline creatinine or endstage renal failure (18 ramipril *vs* 40 placebo, p = 0·04). The risk of progression was still significantly reduced after adjustment for changes in systolic (p = 0·04) and diastolic (p = 0·04) blood pressure, but not after adjustment for changes in proteinuria. Blood-pressure control and the overall number of cardiovascular events were similar in the two treatment groups.

Interpretation: In chronic nephropathies with proteinuria of 3 g or more per 24 h, ramipril safely reduces proteinuria and the rate of GFR decline to an extent that seems to exceed the reduction expected for the degree of blood-pressure lowering. [Extract.]

Importance

The Ramipril in Non-diabetic Renal Failure (REIN) study was the first large randomized clinical trial to show that treatment with an ACEI produced significant renal protection in addition to that attributable to lowering BP in proteinuric non-diabetic CKD. The renoprotective benefits of ACEI treatment had been established previously in patients with type 1 diabetes (see Chapter 9), but a previous randomized trial in non-diabetic CKD was confounded by significantly lower BP in the group randomized to ACEI treatment, leaving unanswered the question of whether the renal protective benefit observed was attributable to a reduction in BP or a specific effect of ACEI treatment (Maschio *et al.*, 1996). In the REIN study, participants in the placebo arm were therefore treated with other anti-hypertensive medication to ensure close matching of BP in the two arms. In stratum 2 of the study (patients with proteinuria ≥3g/day), interim analysis revealed a significant renal protective benefit in the group randomized to ACEI treatment, prompting premature termination of the study. Analysis showed a slower rate of GFR decline (primary end-point) in those treated with ACEI (0.53 versus 0.88 ml/min/month) and a lower risk of reaching the combined end point of serum creatinine doubling or ESKD. In stratum 1 (patients with proteinuria 1–3 g/day), there was no significant difference in the rate of GFR decline between randomized groups after a median follow-up of 31 months, but progression to ESRD or overt proteinuria was significantly less common in those receiving ACEI treatment, and patients with GFR <45 ml/min/1.73 m^2 as well as proteinuria >1.5 g/day showed the greatest benefit (Ruggenenti et al., 1999). A subsequent meta-analysis of 11 studies that included 1860 patients with non-diabetic CKD confirmed that ACEI treatment was associated with significantly lower risks of ESRD [relative risk 0.69, 95% confidence interval (CI) 0.51–0.94] and the combined end point of serum creatinine doubling or ESRD (relative risk 0.70; 95% CI 0.55–0.88) and that the benefits of ACEI treatment were greater in patients with higher levels of baseline proteinuria but were not significant in patients with less than 0.5 g/day of proteinuria at baseline (Jafar et al., 2001). The REIN study therefore provided the core evidence to support the use of ACEI treatment as a critical component of renoprotective strategies in proteinuric CKD and confirmed the central role of angiotensin II in the pathogenesis of CKD progression. This in turn prompted investigation into the renoprotective effects of other inhibitors of the renin–angiotensin–aldosterone system including angiotensin-receptor blockers, aldosterone antagonists, and direct renin inhibitors.

References

Jafar TH, Schmid CH, Landa M, et al. (2001). Angiotensin-converting enzyme inhibitors and progression of nondiabetic renal disease. A meta-analysis of patient-level data. *Ann Intern Med* **135**, 73–87.

Maschio G, Alberti D, Janin G, et al. (1996). Effect of the angiotensin-converting-enzyme inhibitor benazepril on the progression of chronic renal insufficiency. The Angiotensin-Converting-Enzyme Inhibition in Progressive Renal Insufficiency Study Group. *N Engl J Med* **334**, 939–945.

Ruggenenti P, Perna A, Gherardi G, et al. (1999). Renoprotective properties of ACE-inhibition in non-diabetic nephropathies with non-nephrotic proteinuria. *Lancet* **354**, 359–364.

11.5 A new dimension to the Barker hypothesis: low birthweight and susceptibility to renal disease

Authors

WE Hoy, M Rees, E Kile, JD Mathews, Z Wang

Reference

Kidney International 1999, **56**, 1072–1077.

Abstract

Background: There is an epidemic of renal failure among Aborigines in the Australia's Northern Territory. The incidence is more than 1000 per million, and is doubling every three to four years. We evaluated the relationship of birthweight to renal disease in adults in one high-risk community.

Methods: We screened more than 80% of people in the community for renal disease, using the urine albumin/creatinine ratio (ACR, g/mol) as the marker, and reviewed records for birthweights.

Results: Birthweights were available with increasing frequency for people born after 1956. In 317 adults aged 20 to 38 years at screening, the mean birthweight (SD) was 2.712 ± 0.4 kg, and 35% had been low birthweight (LBW, less than 2.5 kg). Birthweight was positively correlated with body mass index (BMI), blood pressure, and diabetes rates, but was inversely correlated with ACR. The odds ratio for overt albuminuria in LBW persons compared with those of higher birthweights was 2.82 (CI, 1.26 to 6.31) after adjusting for other factors, and LBW contributed to an estimated 27% (CI, 3 to 45%) of the population-based prevalence of overt albuminuria. Multivariate models suggest that increasing BMI and blood pressure and decreasing birthweight act in concert to amplify the increases in ACR that accompany increasing age.

Conclusions: LBW contributes to renal disease in this high-risk population. The association might be mediated through impaired nephrogenesis caused by intrauterine malnutrition. The renal disease epidemic in Aborigines may partly be the legacy of greatly improved survival of LBW babies over the last four decades. Disease rates should eventually plateau as birthweights continue to improve, if postnatal risk factors can also be contained.

Importance

Barker *et al.* (1993) proposed that low birth weight resulting from intrauterine malnutrition is associated with 'fetal programming' that results in an increased risk of type 2 diabetes, hypertension, dyslipidaemia, and cardiovascular events in later life. Further research into the potential renal consequences of low birth weight revealed that it was associated with a lower number of nephrons per kidney (nephron endowment) in both animal models and humans (Manalich *et al.*, 2000). In animal models, reduced nephron number was associated with reduced sodium excretion and increased albuminuria (Celsi *et al.*, 1998). In one post-mortem study in humans who died in accidents, ten adults with essential hypertension were found to have a significantly lower nephron number than ten matched controls without hypertension (Keller *et al.*, 2003). These observations supported Brenner's proposal that low nephron endowment would result in reduced capacity for sodium excretion and glomerular hyperfiltration that in turn would predispose people with LBW to later life hypertension and CKD, particularly if an individual was exposed to other risk factors for CKD such as diabetes or obesity (Brenner *et al.*, 1988). Observations in Pima Indians supported this hypothesis, but the majority of the CKD observed was due to diabetic nephropathy and it was therefore difficult to separate the potential effects of nephron endowment from those of diabetes. In this landmark study, the investigators screened a cohort of relatively young adult Australian Aborigines, a population previously documented to have a high prevalence of LBW, and an incidence of ESRD 20-fold higher than the non-Aboriginal population. The results revealed a high overall prevalence of overt albuminuria [urine albumin to creatinine ratio (ACR) $\geq$ 34 g/mol] that was almost twofold higher in those with a history of low birth weight (16.2 versus 8.7%; $P = 0.04$). After multivariable adjustment, the odds ratio for overt albuminuria was 2.82 (95% CI 1.26–6.31) versus normal birth weight. Multivariable analysis showed an inverse relationship between birth weight and urine ACR or risk of overt albuminuria after correction for age, sex, body mass index (BMI), and BP. Further multivariable analysis demonstrated that high BP, high BMI, and low birth weight interact to amplify the risk of overt albuminuria with increasing age. The data therefore provide clear support for Brenner's hypothesis that reduced nephron endowment is a risk factor for future CKD. These observations are relevant not just in underdeveloped countries where LBW results from maternal malnutrition but also in developed countries where fertility treatments result in increased multiple births (associated with low birth weight) and improved neonatal care has improved the survival of very low birth weight babies.

References

Barker DJ, Hales CN, Fall CH, Osmond C, Phipps K, Clark PM (1993). Type 2 (non-insulin-dependent) diabetes mellitus, hypertension and hyperlipidaemia (syndrome X): relation to reduced fetal growth. *Diabetologia* **36**, 62–67.

Brenner BM, Garcia DL, Anderson S (1988). Glomeruli and blood pressure. Less of one, more the other? *Am J Hypertens* **1**, 335–347.

Celsi G, Kistner A, Aizman R, *et al.* (1998). Prenatal dexamethasone causes oligonephronia, sodium retention, and higher blood pressure in the offspring. *Pediatr Res* **44**, 317–322.

Keller G, Zimmer G, Mall G, Ritz E, Amann K (2003). Nephron number in patients with primary hypertension. *N Engl J Med* **348**, 101–108.

Manalich R, Reyes L, Herrera M, Melendi C, Fundora I (2000). Relationship between weight at birth and the number and size of renal glomeruli in humans: a histomorphometric study. *Kidney Int* **58**, 770–773.

11.6 Effect of blood pressure lowering and antihypertensive drug class on progression of hypertensive kidney disease: results from the AASK trial

Authors

JT Wright Jr, G Bakris, T Greene, LY Agodoa, LJ Appel, J Charleston, D Cheek, JG Douglas-Baltimore, J Gassman, R Glassock, L Hebert, K Jamerson, J Lewis, RA Phillips, RD Toto, JP Middleton, SG Rostand; African American Study of Kidney Disease and Hypertension Study Group

Reference

Journal of the American Medical Association 2002, **288**, 2421–2431.

Abstract

Context: Hypertension is a leading cause of end-stage renal disease (ESRD) in the United States, with no known treatment to prevent progressive declines leading to ESRD....

Setting and participants: A total of 1094 African Americans aged 18 to 70 years with hypertensive renal disease (GFR, 20–6 mL/min per 1.73 m^2) were recruited from 21 clinical centers throughout the United States and followed up for 3 to 6.4 years.

Interventions: Participants were randomly assigned to 1 of 2 mean arterial pressure goals, 102 to 107 mm Hg (usual; n = 554) or 92 mm Hg or less (lower; n = 540), and to initial treatment with either a β-blocker (metoprolol 50–200 mg/d; n = 441), an angiotensin-converting enzyme inhibitor (ramipril 2.5–10 mg/d; n = 436) or a dihydropyridine calcium channel blocker, (amlodipine 5–10 mg/d; n = 217)....

Results: ...The mean (SE) GFR slope from baseline through 4 years did not differ significantly between the lower BP group (−2.21 [0.17] mL/min per 1.73 m^2 per year) and the usual BP group (−1.95 [0.17] mL/min per 1.73 m^2 per year; P = .24), and the lower BP goal did not significantly reduce the rate of the clinical composite outcome (risk reduction for lower BP group = 2%; 95% confidence interval [CI], −22% to 21%; P = .85). None of the drug group comparisons showed consistent significant differences in the GFR slope. However, compared with the metoprolol and amlodipine groups, the ramipril group manifested risk reductions in the clinical composite outcome of 22% (95% CI, 1%-38%; P = .04) and 38% (95% CI, 14%-56%; P = .004), respectively. There was no significant difference in the clinical composite outcome between the amlodipine and metoprolol groups.

Conclusions: No additional benefit of slowing progression of hypertensive nephrosclerosis was observed with the lower BP goal. ACEI appear to be more effective than β-blockers or dihydropyridine calcium channel blockers in slowing GFR decline. [Extract.]

Importance

Despite the publication of the REIN study, there remained uncertainty regarding the renal protective efficacy of ACEI treatment in African Americans because ACEI treatment was less effective at lowering BP in African Americans and the latter were poorly represented in previous trials. This is important because hypertensive CKD is a leading cause of ESRD in African Americans and ESRD is sixfold more common in African versus white Americans. The African American Study of Kidney Disease and Hypertension (AASK) was designed to address this uncertainty and also to investigate the benefit of lower BP targets in African Americans who were similarly under-represented in the MDRD study. Participants were randomized in a 2 × 3 factorial manner to treatment with a 'low' or 'usual' BP target (same targets as the MDRD study) and treatment with an ACEI (ramipril), dihidropyridine calcium channel blocker (amlodipine), or β-blocker (metoprolol). The amlodipine arm of the study was terminated prematurely because an interim analysis showed a slower rate of GFR decline and reduced clinical end points in the ramipril and metoprolol groups versus the amlodipine group (Agodoa *et al.*, 2001). The analysis was complicated by the observation that amlodipine treatment provoked an increase in GFR during the first 3 months of treatment (acute phase), whereas GFR tended to decrease in the ramipril and metoprolol groups. There was no consistent difference in rate of GFR decline between the drug treatment groups, but ramipril was associated with a slower rate of decline in the acute phase than metoprolol and in the chronic phase than amlodipine. Nevertheless, ramipril was associated with a significantly lower risk of the composite end point of reduction in GFR by ≥50%, ESRD, or death than metoprolol or amlodipine (22 and 38% risk reduction, respectively). Furthermore, amlodipine was associated with an initial increase in proteinuria, whereas ramipril and metoprolol provoked an initial decrease. At the end of the study, proteinuria was higher in the amlodipine group than the other two groups. There was no difference in rate of GFR decline or risk of composite end point between the two BP target groups, but the lower BP target was associated with a significantly lower magnitude of proteinuria. Taken together, the results of this complex study confirmed that ACEI treatment does afford more effective renal protection than other anti-hypertensives in African Americans, but, like the MDRD study, it failed to provide conclusive evidence in favour of lower BP targets.

Reference

Agodoa LY, Appel L, Bakris GL, *et al.* (2001). Effect of ramipril vs amlodipine on renal outcomes in hypertensive nephrosclerosis: a randomized controlled trial. *JAMA* **285**, 2719–2728.

11.7 K/DOQI Clinical Practice Guidelines on Chronic Kidney Disease. Definition and classification of stages of chronic kidney disease

Authors

National Kidney Foundation

Reference

American Journal of Kidney Disease 2002, **39**, S46–S64.

Table

Stages of chronic kidney disease

Stage	Description	GFR (ml/min/1.73 m²)
1	Kidney damage with normal or ↑GFR	> 90
2	Kidney damage with mild ↓GFR	60–89
3	Moderate ↓GFR	30–59
4	Severe ↓GFR	15–29
5	Kidney failure	< 15 (or dialysis)

Chronic kidney disease is defined as either kidney damage or GFR <60 mL/min/1.73 m2 for >3 months. Kidney damage is defined as pathologic abnormalities or markers of damage, including abnormalities in blood or urine tests or imaging studies.

Importance

Despite failing to answer conclusively its two primary research questions, the MDRD study (see paper 11.3) had a profound effect on developments in nephrology because data from the study were subsequently used to develop a simple formula for estimating GFR from serum creatinine concentration. The original MDRD formula utilized six variables including serum concentration of creatinine, urea, and albumin, as well as age, gender, and ethnicity (Levey *et al.*, 1999), but a subsequent version that utilized only four variables—creatinine, age, gender, and ethnicity—was shown to perform almost as well, especially when serum creatinine values were calibrated to isotope-dilution mass spectrometry (Manjunath *et al.*, 2001; see paper 3.5). As the MDRD formula did not require a 24 h urine collection or knowledge of the subject's weight, it afforded the opportunity for the first time for laboratories to report automatically an estimated GFR (eGFR) with every serum creatinine result.

The stage was therefore set for the remarkable impact of this landmark description of a new classification for CKD proposed by the Kidney and Dialysis Outcomes Quality Improvement (K/DOQI) of the National Kidney Foundation in the USA. The MDRD formula has made it possible to conduct large epidemiological studies showing that CKD is far more common than previously appreciated, for example affecting up to 13% of the adult population in the USA (Coresh *et al.*, 2007). Thus, the focus in nephrology has shifted from caring for those with rare and complex kidney diseases or ESRD to developing strategies for improving the detection and management of a substantial proportion of the general population with previously undiagnosed CKD. Epidemiological studies also reported an association between early-stage CKD and an increased risk of cardiovascular events that often outweighs the risk of ESRD (Coresh *et al.*, 2007) and has stimulated rapid growth in research to identify the mechanisms responsible.

The classification has not been without controversy. One weakness of the MDRD formula is that it tends to underestimate GFR above a value of 60 ml/min/1.73 m^2 leading to an overestimation of early stages of CKD, and an improved formula for estimating GFR, the CKD-EPI formula has now been proposed (Levey *et al.*, 2009). There has been criticism that the classification is based on eGFR alone, and refinements giving greater emphasis to the importance of albuminuria have recently been presented (Levey *et al.*, 2011). There is also concern that widespread use of the classification may lead to inappropriate 'disease labelling', especially in older people with moderate reductions in eGFR.

However, despite these continuing controversies, this landmark proposal for the classification of CKD has transformed clinical and epidemiological research, and clinical practice, in nephrology.

References

Coresh J, Selvin E, Stevens LA Manzi J, Kusek JW, Eggers P, van Lente F, Levey AS (2007). The prevalence of chronic kidney disease in the United States. *JAMA* **298**, 2038–2047.

Levey AS, Bosch JP, Lewis JB, Greene T, Rogers N, Roth D (1999). A more accurate method to estimate glomerular filtration rate from serum creatinine: a new prediction equation. Modification of Diet in Renal Disease Study Group. *Ann Int Med* **130**, 461–470.

Levey AS, de Jong PE, Coresh J, *et al.* (2011). The definition, classification, and prognosis of chronic kidney disease: a KDIGO Controversies Conference report. *Kidney Int* **80**, 17–28.

Levey AS, Stevens LA, Schmid CH *et al.* (2009). A new equation to estimate glomerular filtration rate. *Ann Intern Med* **150**, 604–612.

Manjunath G, Sarnak MJ, Levey AS (2001). Prediction equations to estimate glomerular filtration rate: an update. *Curr Opin Nephrol Hypertens* **10**, 785–792.

11.8 Renoprotection of Optimal Antiproteinuric Doses (ROAD) Study: a randomized controlled study of benazepril and losartan in chronic renal insufficiency

Authors

FF Hou, D Xie, X Zhang, PY Chen, WR Zhang, M Liang, ZJ Guo, JP Jiang

Reference

Journal of the American Society of Nephrology 2007, **18**, 1889–1898.

Abstract

The Renoprotection of Optimal Antiproteinuric Doses (ROAD) study was performed to determine whether titration of benazepril or losartan to optimal antiproteinuric doses would safely improve the renal outcome in chronic renal insufficiency. A total of 360 patients who did not have diabetes and had proteinuria and chronic renal insufficiency were randomly assigned to four groups. Patients received open-label treatment with a conventional dosage of benazepril (10 mg/d), individual uptitration of benazepril (median 20 mg/d; range 10 to 40), a conventional dosage of losartan (50 mg/d), or individual uptitration of losartan (median 100 mg/d; range 50 to 200). Uptitration was performed to optimal antiproteinuric and tolerated dosages, and then these dosages were maintained. Median follow-up was 3.7 yr. The primary end point was time to the composite of a doubling of the serum creatinine, ESRD, or death. Secondary end points included changes in the level of proteinuria and the rate of progression of renal disease. Compared with the conventional dosages, optimal antiproteinuric dosages of benazepril and losartan that were achieved through uptitration were associated with a 51 and 53% reduction in the risk for the primary end point ($P = 0.028$ and 0.022, respectively). Optimal antiproteinuric dosages of benazepril and losartan, at comparable BP control, achieved a greater reduction in both proteinuria and the rate of decline in renal function compared with their conventional dosages. There was no significant difference for the overall incidence of major adverse events between groups that were given conventional and optimal dosages in both arms. It is concluded that uptitration of benazepril or losartan against proteinuria conferred further benefit on renal outcome in patients who did not have diabetes and had proteinuria and renal insufficiency.

Importance

It has long been recognized that the magnitude of proteinuria is a marker of severity and prognosis in a wide range of kidney diseases. However, the observation from the REIN trial and other studies that the extent of proteinuria reduction achieved during the first 3 months of ACEI therapy correlated inversely with the subsequent rate of decline in GFR led to the notion that proteinuria may contribute to renal damage (Ruggenenti *et al.*, 2003). Subsequent studies found that when tubule cells are cultured in a medium containing high concentrations of plasma proteins they secrete increased amounts of pro-inflammatory and pro-fibrotic cytokines. Further investigations in animal models of proteinuric nephropathy found that accumulation of plasma proteins in proximal tubule cells was associated with increased inflammatory cells locally in the interstitium (Abbate *et al.*, 1998). Together, these observations supported the hypothesis that plasma proteins that appear in tubular fluid due to damage to the glomerular filtration barrier are absorbed by tubule cells and provoke a pro-inflammatory phenotype characterized by cytokine production. These cytokines are secreted into the interstitum where they provoke an inflammatory and fibrotic response that contributes to tubulo-interstitial damage. One implication of this theory is that a reduction in proteinuria should be seen as a therapeutic goal if maximum renal protection is to be achieved. The ROAD study was the first randomized clinical trial to test this hypothesis. Patients with proteinuric CKD were randomized to four arms: in two arms, patients received either ACEI or angiotensin-receptor blocker (ARB) treatment at 'standard' doses. In the remaining two arms, the ACEI or ARB dose was titrated upwards until the maximum achievable anti-proteinuric effect was achieved. BP was carefully matched in all arms with other anti-hypertensives. The study found that those arms with therapy targeted to the maximum anti-proteinuric effect did indeed achieve greater lowering of proteinuria, but, more importantly, this strategy was associated with a lower incidence of the primary end point of creatinine doubling, ESRD, or death. Thus, regardless of whether or not proteinuria does contribute directly to renal damage, the ROAD study established that proteinuria reduction should be regarded as a separate goal in renal protective strategies. Whether or not greater reduction of proteinuria through the use of supramaximal doses of ARB or ACEI and ARB combination therapy would result in improved renal protection remains controversial and cannot be recommended at present due to an excess of adverse effects reported in some trials (Mann *et al.*, 2008).

References

Abbate M, Zoja C, Corna D, Capitanio M, Bertani T, Remuzzi G (1998). In progressive nephropathies, overload of tubular cells with filtered proteins translates glomerular permeability dysfunction into cellular signals of interstitial inflammation. *J Am Soc Nephrol* **9**, 1213–1224.

Mann JF, Schmieder RE, McQueen M, *et al.* (2008). Renal outcomes with telmisartan, ramipril, or both, in people at high vascular risk (the ONTARGET study): a multicentre, randomised, double-blind, controlled trial. *Lancet* **372**, 547–553.

Ruggenenti P, Perna A, Remuzzi G (2003). Retarding progression of chronic renal disease: The neglected issue of residual proteinuria. *Kidney Int* **63**, 2254–2261.

11.9 Outcomes following diagnosis of acute renal failure in U.S. veterans: focus on acute tubular necrosis

Authors

RL Amdur, LS Chawla, S Amodeo, PL Kimmel, CE Palant

Reference

Kidney International 2009, **76**, 1089–1097.

Abstract

When patients develop acute kidney injury, a small fraction of them will develop end-stage renal disease later. The severity of renal impairment in the remaining patients is uncertain because studies have not carefully examined renal function over time or the precise timing of entry into a late stage of chronic kidney disease. To determine these factors, we used a United States Department of Veterans Affairs database to ascertain long-term renal function in 113,272 patients. Of these, 44,377 had established chronic kidney disease and were analyzed separately. A cohort of 63,491 patients was hospitalized for acute myocardial infarction or pneumonia and designated as controls. The remaining 5,404 patients had diagnostic codes indicating acute renal failure or acute tubular necrosis. Serum creatinine, estimated glomerular filtration rates, and dates of death over a 75-month period were followed. Renal function deteriorated over time in all groups, but with significantly greater severity in those who had acute renal failure and acute tubular necrosis compared to controls. Patients with acute kidney injury, especially those with acute tubular necrosis, were more likely than controls to enter stage 4 chronic kidney disease, but this entry time was similar to that of patients who initially had chronic kidney disease. The risk of death was elevated in those with acute kidney injury and chronic kidney disease compared to controls after accounting for covariates. We found that patients who had an episode of acute tubular necrosis were at high risk for the development of stage 4 disease and had a reduced survival time when compared to control patients.

Importance

For many years, it was held that patients who recovered renal function after an episode of acute kidney injury (AKI) suffered no long-term consequences. Recent studies have shown, however, that this perception was incorrect and that recovery from AKI is associated with significant risk of progressive CKD and increased mortality. In this large epidemiological study, outcomes with respect to GFR and survival were compared among three groups of patients admitted to hospital: those with CKD, those with acute myocardial infarction or pneumonia (but no AKI, designated 'controls') and those with AKI or a diagnosis of 'acute tubular necrosis' (ATN). The analysis showed a decline in GFR in all groups over time, but this was significantly greater in those admitted with AKI or ATN than in those with acute myocardial infarction or pneumonia. Furthermore, the risk of developing CKD stage 4 over time was as high in the group that had ATN (20.0%) as in the group with pre-existing CKD (24.7%). The risk of developing CKD stage 4 was lower in those with AKI (13.2%), but this was still significantly higher than in the controls (3.3%). AKI was also associated with increased mortality over time versus controls. Several other studies published at about the same time similarly reported a substantial increase in the risk of developing CKD stage 4 or 5 and increased mortality in patients who developed AKI (Ishani *et al.*, 2009; Lo *et al.*, 2009).

The interaction between AKI and CKD progression is illustrated by a study of 39,805 patients with eGFR <45 ml/min/1.73 m^2 prior to hospitalization. Those who survived an episode of AKI that required dialysis treatment had a high risk of developing ESRD within 30 days of hospital discharge that was related to pre-admission eGFR. Among patients who survived without ESRD, the incidence of ESRD and death at 6 months was 12.7 and 19.7%, respectively, versus 1.7 and 7.4% in the comparitor group with CKD but no AKI (Hsu *et al.*, 2009). Taken together, these data indicated that an episode of AKI may initiate renal damage that results in progressive CKD and that an episode of AKI may accelerate the rate of progression of pre-existing CKD (see also paper 10.10). The mechanisms for this interaction require further exploration, but given the high prevalence of CKD and the high risk of developing AKI in the elderly, AKI is increasingly being recognized as a risk factor for CKD progression, and efforts are being focused on measures to reduce the risk of developing AKI in the context of acute illness.

References

Hsu CY, Chertow GM, McCulloch CE, Fan D, Ordoñez JD, Go AS (2009). Nonrecovery of kidney function and death after acute on chronic renal failure. *Clin J Am Soc Nephrol* **4**, 891–898.

Ishani A, Xue JL, Himmelfarb J, *et al.* (2009). Acute kidney injury increases risk of ESRD among elderly. *J Am Soc Nephrol* **20**, 223–228.

Lo LJ, Go AS, Chertow GM, *et al.* (2009). Dialysis-requiring acute renal failure increases the risk of progressive chronic kidney disease. *Kidney Int* **76**, 893–899.

11.10 Lower estimated GFR and higher albuminuria are associated with adverse kidney outcomes. A collaborative meta-analysis of general and high-risk population cohorts

Authors

RT Gansevoort, K Matsushita, M van der Velde, BC Astor, M Woodward, AS Levey, PE de Jong, J Coresh; Chronic Kidney Disease Prognosis Consortium

Reference

Kidney International 2011, **80**, 93–104.

Abstract

Both a low estimated glomerular filtration rate (eGFR) and albuminuria are known risk factors for end-stage renal disease (ESRD). To determine their joint contribution to ESRD and other kidney outcomes, we performed a meta-analysis of nine general population cohorts with 845,125 participants and an additional eight cohorts with 173,892 patients, the latter selected because of their high risk for chronic kidney disease (CKD). In the general population, the risk for ESRD was unrelated to eGFR at values between 75 and 105 ml/min per 1.73 m^2 but increased exponentially at lower levels. Hazard ratios for eGFRs averaging 60, 45, and 15 were 4, 29, and 454, respectively, compared with an eGFR of 95, after adjustment for albuminuria and cardiovascular risk factors. Log albuminuria was linearly associated with log ESRD risk without thresholds. Adjusted hazard ratios at albumin-to-creatinine ratios of 30, 300, and 1000 mg/g were 5, 13, and 28, respectively, compared with an albumin-to-creatinine ratio of 5. Albuminuria and eGFR were associated with ESRD, without evidence for multiplicative interaction. Similar associations were found for acute kidney injury and progressive CKD. In high-risk cohorts, the findings were generally comparable. Thus, lower eGFR and higher albuminuria are risk factors for ESRD, acute kidney injury and progressive CKD in both general and high-risk populations, independent of each other and of cardiovascular risk factors.

Importance

The worldwide adoption of a CKD definition based on GFR together with the introduction of automated reporting of eGFR has resulted in the detection of large numbers of people with previously undiagnosed CKD. Epidemiological studies have shown that the majority are at low risk of progressing to ESRD but are at increased risk of cardiovascular events. In many people with CKD, the risk of cardiovascular events substantially outweighs the risk of progression to ESRD (Hallan *et al.*, 2006). There is therefore an urgent need for methods to predict both renal and cardiovascular risk in people with CKD. This would facilitate targeted intervention for those at high risk while sparing the majority unnecessary treatment and anxiety. Several cohort studies have attempted to develop risk-scoring equations based on a small number of clinical and biochemical variables (Taal and Brenner, 2008). From these studies, it was clear that GFR and a measure of proteinuria were the two dominant risk factors. In this collaborative study, data from a number of cohorts was combined to generate a large dataset that would allow robust assessment of eGFR and albuminuria as risk factors in patients with CKD. The analysis showed that the risk of developing ESRD increased sharply once eGFR fell below 60 ml/min/1.73 m^2, providing strong support for the use of this GFR threshold to define CKD in the absence of urinary abnormalities. Analysis of albuminuria data revealed that the risk of ESRD increased with increasing albuminuria, even in the normal range, with no threshold effect. Similar associations were found for AKI and progressive CKD. Further analyses by the same collaborative study group showed that the risk of all-cause mortality also increased when eGFR fell below 60 ml/min/1.73 m^2. Furthermore, all-cause mortality increased with albuminuria with no threshold effect. Similar associations were evident with cardiovascular mortality (Matsushita *et al.*, 2010). Thus, eGFR and albuminuria were confirmed as powerful independent risk factors for progression of CKD and all-cause as well as cardiovascular mortality. Importantly, even small increases in albuminuria within the normal range were associated with increased risk. These observations provided support for a revised classification for CKD that subdivides stage 3 into 3A (GFR 59–45 ml/min/1.73 m^2) and 3B (GFR 44–30 ml/min/1.73 m^2) and has in addition an albuminuria stage (Levey *et al.*, 2011). The benefit of this revised system is that it reflects not only the current stage of CKD but also the risk of future progression and death. Further research is still required to develop a simple and robust risk assessment tool applicable to people with CKD.

References

Hallan SI, Dahl K, Oien CM, *et al.* (2006). Screening strategies for chronic kidney disease in the general population: follow-up of cross sectional health survey. *Brit Med J* **333**, 1047.

Levey AS, de Jong PE, Coresh J, *et al.* (2011). The definition, classification and prognosis of chronic kidney disease: a KDIGO Controversies Conference report. *Kidney Int* **80**, 17–28.

Matsushita K, van der Velde M, Astor BC, *et al.* (2010). Association of estimated glomerular filtration rate and albuminuria with all-cause and cardiovascular mortality in general population cohorts: a collaborative meta-analysis. *Lancet* **375**, 2073–2081.

Taal MW, Brenner BM (2008). Renal risk scores: progress and prospects. *Kidney Int* **73**, 1216–1219.

Chapter 12

Haemodialysis

Nathan W. Levin and Thomas A. Depner

Introduction

The remarkable growth of haemodialysis since 1944 when Willem Kolff first described his rotating drum kidney wrapped with cellophane tubing has been due in part to the growing prevalence of end-stage renal disease (ESRD) and in part to a human eagerness to prolong useful life. Interest in haemodialysis as a scientific and technological discipline has also been stimulated by commercial ramifications. Our final selection of ten papers for this chapter cover 66 years, starting with Kolff's description of his pioneering work, and include the first application of dialysis to prolong life in patients with irreversible renal failure by Scribner and co-workers in 1960, who described two patients treated with continuous dialysis for days at a time. In 1965, a pioneering demonstration that overnight, unobserved dialysis could be safely done in English homes was presented by Baillod and colleagues. In 1967, Stewart, Lipps and co-workers described the first functional hollow-fibre kidney that rapidly replaced previous devices and is the only dialysis device used in any number today. In an attempt to mimic the glomerular filter, Henderson and co-workers in 1975 applied hydrostatic pressure to highly permeable Amicon filters and introduced haemodiafiltration. This convective therapy successfully removed larger retained solutes and is increasingly used internationally, althpough not in the USA. In his original work, Henderson's *in vivo* clearances of inulin, urea, and creatinine were similar to haemodialysis, but significant protein loss occurred. In 1977, reports by Platts and others of encephalopathy and spontaneous fractures caused by a toxic effect of aluminium in dialysate water led to the development of chemical and biological standards for water purity. The identification in 1985 that dialysis amyloid consists of polymerized β_2-microglobulin (Geyjo 1985) was a strong stimulus to the development of high-flux dialysers. A mechanistic analysis of the National Cooperative Dialysis Study by Gotch and Sargent in 1985 demonstrated the value of modelled urea clearance, expressed as Kt/V (where K is dialyser clearance of urea, t is dialysis time, and V is volume of distribution of urea, approximately equal to the patient's total body water) to measure the dose of dialysis. This measurement eventually received universal acceptance and has been applied in dialysis clinics throughout the world. Finally, we have selected two multi-authored papers published this century that present results and interpretation of randomized clinical trials (HEMO and FHN), which have guided prescriptions of haemodialysis dose, membrane flux, and frequency of treatments.

12.1 The artificial kidney: a dialyser with a great area

Authors

WJ Kolff, HTJ Berk, M ter Welle, AJW van der Ley, EC van Dijk, J van Noordwijk

Reference

Acta Medica Scandinavica 1944, **117**, 121–128.

Abstract

Background: When the kidneys fail, solutes normally found in the urine accumulate in the blood and tissues. At the present time, treatment consists of albumen restriction in the diet to reduce urea production, replacement of fluids lost by vomiting, administration of alkali to treat acidosis, and removal of edema fluid. Attempts to remove the accumulated toxic solutes by dialysis have failed in the past due to technical limitations in the apparatus and other complications.

Methods: We describe a new dialysis apparatus consisting of cellophane tubing 25–30 m in length, 2 m^2 in area, spirally wound on a horizontal aluminium cylinder that rotates while dipping into a 100 liter tank of rinsing solution containing 0.7% saline and 1.5% glucose, clean but not sterile, and warmed to 37–39° C. A small volume of heparin-treated venous blood was continuously or intermittently driven through the sterile tubing by the rotation of the cylinder on an axis attached to two sterile blood couplers.

Results: A 4.17% solution of urea in 500 ml water was reduced to 1.68% after 5 min and to 0.57% after 10 min of dialysis. In one patient, 24, 40, and 35 grams of urea were dialyzed out in 1.5, 4.0 and 6.0 hours respectively. Uric acid, creatinine, non-urea nitrogen, and indoxyl were also removed. The patient improved temporarily but became anuric and died after the 12th dialysis when all access sites were depleted. We believe we can keep patients suffering from uremia alive so long as blood vessels for puncture are available, while awaiting the possibility of the kidneys to regenerate.

Importance

This pioneering and revolutionary method for treating acute renal failure is the world's first artificial internal organ. The method is described in remarkable detail and includes insights by the investigator, Willem Kolff, that are increasingly recognized and emphasized in modern times. These include a distinction between convective and diffusive forces across the dialyser membrane, measuring dialysis by urea removal, and a proposed osmotic effect of glucose to extract more water from the patient. He also recognized the importance of anti-coagulation by heparin either continuously or intermittently infused, and that a reduction in blood pressure (BP) during dialysis contributed to reduced urine output. He emphasized the importance of sterility and blood cultures, and he devised a prototypical single-needle method that required only one venepuncture. The propelling of blood by rotation of the aluminium cylinder as well as the blood couplers attached to the cylinder axis were unique to the Kolff dialyser and reflected his innovative spirit and self-professed inventiveness. In later publications, he called himself a 'tinkerer.' In the present publication, Kolff first described his clinical experience with what was later to be called the 'rotating drum kidney.' To his credit, despite multiple failures treating apparently irreversible renal failure, he eventually accomplished the goal stated in this paper of allowing the native kidney to regenerate. In this sense, his artificial kidney was thought to provide a bridge of time by preventing death from uraemia and perhaps a more optimal environment for healing to take place in patients with acute kidney failure. His initial work was done during World War II when Holland was under siege and both support and materials for building his device were in short supply.

This seminal description of the first successful artificial kidney is certainly a landmark. Kolff had a remarkable vision of the future, but even he did not anticipate the impact his invention would have on the lives of millions of people throughout the world or the academic interest and extensive industry that was to develop during the next 60 years. Kidney replacement by dialysis was amazingly successful but was limited to treatment of patients with acute renal failure for the next 17 years, primarily because of the need to sacrifice a large vein and/or artery for each treatment, as noted by Kolff in this 1944 publication. Application of his method to replace kidney function in patients with ESRD had to await development of the arteriovenous shunt and fistula.

12.2 The treatment of chronic uremia by means of intermittent haemodialysis: a preliminary report

Authors

BH Scribner, R Buri, JE Caner, R Hegstrom, JM Burnell

Reference

Transactions of the American Society for Artificial Internal Organs 1960, **6**, 114–122.

Summary

Development of the technique for permanent indwelling cannulations made it possible to perform repeated dialyses in patients with kidney failure. Prolongation of life had been limited to patients with acute reversible extra renal factors that jeopardized their existing minimal renal function. Previous work had found that maintenance of nutrition and of mental function was unsuccessful. This paper provides detailed information of the course of two patients who became ambulatory and were at work part-time or working at home. They were not strong enough to work full-time. They ate 0.5 g of protein/kg of body weight. Each dialysis lasted for 24–60 h with intervals between dialyses being 4–21 days. Both patients were severely ill with severe vomiting before dialysis was initiated. At the time of writing the two patients had been treated for 10 and 8 weeks, respectively, with excellent symptomatic responses. Neither had shown the loss of weight and mental deterioration reported with previous dialytic treatments.

Importance

This was the first report of haemodialysis prolonging life in patients with ESRD. The paper is a chronological record of the progress of two patients who became famous during their transition from severe uraemia to chronic dialysis. Clyde Shields survived 11 years and Harvey Gentry, who had a urea clearance of a few millilitres per minute, received a kidney transplant 8 years later, with survival after first dialysis for 27 years. In addition to demonstrating the work of a master clinician, many issues are discussed, which have continued to be relevant over the 50 years since these events took place. Access to the circulation was now possible due to the eponymous shunt (see paper 13.1). Despite decades of experience with arteriovenous fistulae and grafts, vascular access still remained a major problem. Scribner proposed the study of the effect of variation in amount and type of dietary protein on the relationship of amino acid turnover to protein synthesis and the appearance of toxic substances. He drew attention to the importance of sodium restriction and ultrafiltration to reduce extracellular fluid volume and possibly modify the response to anti-hypertensive drugs. Fluid overload remained a major problem, despite the persistence of Scribner's advocacy (Scribner *et al.*, 1960; Dorhout Mees, 1995). Erythropoietin deficiency as a cause, and use of the hormone as therapy for anaemia, were suggested as subjects for research. Patients on dialysis were suggested as ideal for the study of non-renal actions of drugs, such as the effect of aldosterone on potassium metabolism. Scribner speculated about how long dialysis could prolong life. These two patients had received ten times as much dialysis as any previous patients, and the question asked was whether a non-dialysable toxin could accumulate with loss of weight and mental deterioration occurring. While today dialyser membranes are far more efficient and safer than the initial cellulose membranes, the problem still exists of removing uraemic toxins of molecular weight higher than those excreted even by today's high-flux dialysers. Concern about vascular disease developing with longer survival has been fully realized (see Chapter 16). As is the case today, Scribner's group treated access infection due to *Staphylococcus pyogenes* with vancomycin, and controlled skin and nares colonization with anti-bacterial ointment.

This original paper combined astute observation with the application of available technology to achieve unprecedented patient survival and to introduce important clinical and research concepts that remain relevant today.

References

Dorhout Mees EJ (1995). Volaemia and blood pressure in renal failure: have old truths been forgotten? *Nephrol Dial Transplant* **10**, 1297–1298.

Scribner B H, Caner JEZ, Buri R, Quinton W (1960). The technique of continuous haemodialysis. *Trans Am Soc Artif Intern Organs* **6**, 88–103.

12.3 Overnight haemodialysis in the home

Authors

RA Baillod, C Comty, M Ilahi, FID Kotoney-Ahula, L Sevitt, S Shaldon

Reference

Proceedings of the European Dialysis and Transplant Association 1965 **2**, 99–103.

Abstract

Background: Although haemodialysis is an effective form of treatment for chronic renal failure, the economic burden has limited its expansion. In addition, the total dependence of the patient on the hospital unit has produced many psychological problems. For this reason, we have undertaken a programme of home haemodialysis for patients with the assistance of their spouses.

Methods: Kiil dialyzers powered by the patient's blood pressure (no blood pump) were assembled and perfused with dialysate prepared by batch mode in 500 litre rigid polythene tanks. The blood path and tanks were sterilized with 1% formalin and blood access was via Scribner shunt.

Results: Six patients have been dialyzed in the home, longest for 10 months. Patient and spouse required 2–3 months of in-hospital training, and then professional support was gradually withdrawn. Dialysis time averaged 26–28 hours per week, 15 hours during sleep. Overnight unobserved dialysis was monitored with alarms for blood pressure, dialysate pressure, blood leaks, and bed weight. The latter was used to control ultrafiltration during dialysis. No emergency night calls were encountered. Five technical complications were handled by the patient/spouse with technical advice given by phone. Supplies were stocked monthly in the home. Patients and spouses expressed a preference for dialyzing in the home which also considerably reduced the cost of dialysis. [Adapted.]

Importance

Home haemodialysis was recognized early by investigators as a possible solution to the high cost of the treatment when performed in the hospital. They also found that putting the responsibility and control of treatment into the hands of the patient had psychological benefits that improved dialysis tolerance and added to its success. Although selection bias was certainly a factor that contributed to its success, committees that identified candidate patients for in-centre haemodialysis in the early days also selected independent patients with few other health problems. Methods for performing home haemodialysis in England, as described by Baillod and her colleagues in this article, were later adopted and expanded by Scribner in the USA for the original chronic haemodialysis programme in Seattle, Washington. Concern about the cost of haemodialysis led the Seattle team to place more and more emphasis on treatment in the home, eventually making eligibility for home treatment a necessary requirement for dialysis candidacy. Baillod and colleagues recognized the importance of a helper, who for the six patients in this study was the patient's spouse. Both patient and spouse were empowered by 2–3 months of intensive training that gave them a sense of satisfaction such that they favoured home treatments even though they had to do all the work, including ordering of supplies, set-up, monitoring, and take-down. When government subsidy through the US Medicare programme became a reality in 1973, home haemodialysis began to wane in popularity but more recently has undergone a resurgence for the same reasons enumerated by Baillod in this 1965 article: cost and psychological advantage. Accumulating data also suggest an improvement in outcomes, including overall survival (Culleton *et al.*, 2007; Suri *et al.*, 2007; Pierratos, 2008).

The advantages of self-haemodialysis in the home were therefore recognized by Baillod and colleagues in 1965, only 5 years after haemodialysis was first applied to manage patients with ESRD and 15 years before continuous peritoneal dialysis was beginning to appear. These investigators and those that followed successfully addressed the major potential stumbling blocks of home haemodialysis by including a helper, establishing surveillance techniques at home, and anticipating emergency procedures in the home. These efforts reassured patients and contributed to the early success of home haemodialysis. More recently, dialysis in the home, independent of frequency, has been shown to affect nutrition and cardiovascular outcomes favourably (Rocco *et al.*, 2011). Postulated reasons for these benefits include reduced exposure to infectious agents, elimination of travel and deadlines, reduced stress from interaction with patients and staff, and improved access to food.

References

Culleton BF, Walsh M, Klarenbach SW, *et al.* (2007). Effect of frequent nocturnal haemodialysis vs conventional haemodialysis on left ventricular mass and quality of life: a randomized controlled trial. *JAMA* **298**, 1291–1299.

Pierratos A (2008). Does frequent nocturnal haemodialysis result in better outcomes than conventional thrice-weekly haemodialysis? *Nat Clin Pract Nephrol* **4**, 132–133.

Rocco MV, Lockridge RS Jr, Beck GJ, *et al.* (2011). The effects of frequent nocturnal home haemodialysis: the Frequent Haemodialysis Network Nocturnal Trial. *Kidney Int* **80**, 1080–1091.

Suri RS, Garg AX, Chertow GM, *et al.* (2007). Frequent Haemodialysis Network (FHN) randomized trials: study design. *Kidney Int* **71**, 349–359.

12.4 The hollow fiber artificial kidney

Authors

BJ Lipps, RD Steward, HA Perkins, GW Holmes, McLain EA, MR Rolfs, PD Oja

Reference

Transactions of the American Society for Artificial Internal Organs 1967 **13**, 200–207.

Abstract

Background: Studies of small prototype hollow fiber artificial kidneys (HFAK) had been reported by Stewart. Urea clearances of 2 mL/min at a blood flow of 10 mL/min were observed. Two major obstacles to use as a clinical hemodialyser were a high incidence of damage to the fine fibers during cell assembly, resulting in leaky and inoperable cells, and marked coagulation severely limiting the duration of the haemodialysis.

Methods: The current HFAKs were assembled on a semi automatic fabrication process train with automatic deacetylation, plasticization, drying, and sealing. The dialyser consisted of 6000 cellulose diacetate hollow fibers with an area of 4000 cm^2 sealed at each end with DOW-Corning silastic medical grade elastomer because this potting compound was compatible with blood. In operation, blood passes through the lumen of the fibers and dialysate is pumped around the outside of the fibers, counter flowing to the blood flow.

Results: The HFAK size initially estimated for clinical use would consist of 7500–8000 fibers of 200–250 microns internal diameter, and have a urea dialysance of about 125 ml/min at a blood flow of 200–250 ml/min. Transport performance studies showed that dialysate-side transport resistance is virtually eliminated at dialysate flows of 500 ml/min and blood flows of 200–300 ml/min in vitro. In vitro permeability was similar to that of cellulose. Fiber potency was reduced over time due to platelet aggregation. Circulating an amine-containing vinyl monomer grafting solution through a full assembled HFAK followed by circulation of aqueous heparin to heparinise the cationic surfaces resulted in prolongation of PT and PTT. Dialyses with heparined dialysers in systematically heparined dogs showed no fiber occlusion. [Adapted].

Importance

Although Twardowski had designed an early capillary dialyser with an internal diameter of 1000 µm, it was patented only in Poland in 1965. Twardowski's hollow fibre concept did not address optimizing diffusive clearance with priming volume. Prior to the development of the hollow-fibre artificial kidney (HFAK) by Stewart and Lipps (Stewart *et al.*, 1964, 1968), dialysers continued to possess high blood compartment resistance and variable compliance resulting in haemodynamic instability. Providing for fluid loss by prescribing changes in transmembrane pressure was an uncertain process (Clark and Turk, 2004), and the devices were inefficient due to long diffusive paths. Parallel flow dialysers were less compliant but were also relatively inefficient asattempts to reduce blood channel widths resulted in increased resistance. On the other hand, the fibres in the hollow fibre dialyser were constant in internal diameter with short diffusive distances between blood and dialysate and blood rheology was favourable with relatively low pressure drops and low resistance.

Ben Lipps, the primary author of this paper, who is still a leader in the dialysis industry, recently wrote, 'In 1966, there were fewer than 1,000 chronic dialysis patients (with a liberal definition of "chronic") and there was no concept that approximately 1.5 million patients would be maintained by chronic dialysis 40 years later.' Lipps' thought at that time was to combine his experience with non-thrombogenic surfaces and the concept of hollow fibre membranes for creation of a unique artificial kidney or lung. Although no one in the industry or government foresaw a long-term application of this product, Lipps drove a proof-of-concept approach of which this paper is a part. William Murphy of Cordis Corporation saw the human and commercial need 3 years later and initiated a new company devoted to production of hollow fibre dialysers. Currently, the hollow-fibre kidney made by tens of companies using a wide variety of membranes is virtually the only version of an artificial kidney used for haemodialysis everywhere. The configuration is also used for devices with a variety of functions including plasmapheresis, haemodiafiltration, continuous haemofiltration in the intensive care unit, virus removal, and sorbent binding.

References

Clark WR, Turk KR Jr (2004). The NxStage system one. *Semin Dial* **17**, 167–170.

Stewart RD, Cerny JC, Mahon HI (1964). The capillary "kidney": primary report. *Med Bull (Ann Arbor)* **30**, 116–118.

Stewart RD, Lipps BJ, Baretta ED, Piering WR, Roth DA, Sargent JA (1968). Short-term haemodialysis with the capillary kidney. *Trans Am Soc Artif Intern Organs* **14**, 121–125.

12.5 Kinetics of hemodiafiltration. II. Clinical characterization of a new blood cleansing modality

Authors

LW Henderson, CK Colton, CA Ford

Reference

Journal of Laboratory and Clinical Medicine 1965, **85**, 372–391.

Abstract

Hemodiafiltration, a process in which whole blood is first diluted with a physiologic electrolyte solution and then ultrafiltered across a membrane to convectively remove solutes and excess water, has been applied clinically for the first time. Six-hour hemodiafiltration with a 1.6 m.^{2} hollow-fiber ultrafilter was applied intermittently to an anephric patient as an alternative to 6-hour haemodialysis using a 1.45 m.^{2} coil. A quantitative basis for evaluating clinical hemodiafiltration kinetics was developed, and the results were compared with data from prototype devices. With blood, diluting fluid, and ultrafiltrate flow rates of 200 ml. per minute, removal rates of urea and creatinine by both hemodiafiltration and dialysis were comparable, but for solutes of larger molecular weight (uric acid, phosphate, and inulin) removal rate was significantly greater for hemodiafiltration. The observed ultrafiltrate flux was similar to values predicted from in vitro studies. With the present membrane formulation the measured sieving coefficients for inulin, creatinine, and urea were not significantly different from one, and whole blood clearances for these solutes were 117, 108, and 101 ml. per minutes, respectively. This solute clearance pattern is very similar to the human kidney and in sharp contrast to standard coil hemodialysis.

Importance

This article describes the first successful renal replacement therapy with haemofiltration, a process likened to glomerular filtration and therefore more like native kidney function than haemodialysis. Henderson and colleagues combined haemofiltration with haemodialysis in a process they called 'haemodiafiltration', but the main pathway for solute removal was hydrostatically driven filtration rather than passive diffusion across the hollow-fibre membranes. The membranes employed were specially constructed for filtration, designed to tolerate high pressure gradients, and were poorly adept at dialysis because of their thickness and relatively long pathway for diffusion. The filter had only one filtration port, so there was no dialysate. Later use of the term 'haemodiafiltration' defined it as a combination of haemodialysis and haemofiltration where dialysate passed between two ports across the dialysate or filtrate side of the membrane. In Henderson's device, blood was diluted with replacement fluid before entering the filtration device, i.e. pre-filter replacement. Henderson showed in this patient, similar to previous bench studies, that larger molecules were removed more efficiently than by standard coil haemodialysis using cellophane-derived membranes. For example, the clearance of inulin (molecular weight 5200 Da), was not significantly different from the clearance of creatinine (molecular weight 113 Da), whereas the clearance of inulin by haemodialysis was less than 5% of the creatinine clearance. This was a major step forward because, at that time, retained solutes in the molecular weight range of 500–5000 were considered to be significant uraemic toxins that limited the success of haemodialysis.

After several years of development, membranes capable of removing larger molecules without significant removal of serum albumin were successfully applied to the treatment of uraemic patients. The clinical description and data supplied by Henderson and colleagues spurred the industry for several subsequent decades, targeting the development of membranes with larger, more uniform pore sizes. Both the improved removal of larger solutes and the improved biocompatibility of these synthetic membranes eventually lead to the abandonment of cellulose-derived membranes for haemodialysis in the USA and near elimination of dialysis-associated amyloidosis, a disease mediated by accumulation of β_2-microglobulin (molecular weight 11,800 Da). The effect of removing larger, so-called 'middle molecules' on patient outcomes remains controversial, but the improvements in membrane chemistry as developed by Henderson and subsequent investigators have almost certainly reduced morbidity and improved patient well being.

12.6 Composition of the domestic water supply and the incidence of fractures and encephalopathy in patients on home dialysis

Authors

MM Platts, GC Goode, JS Hislopp

Reference

British Medical Journal 1977, **2**, 657–660.

Abstract

Of the 202 patients undergoing home dialysis in the Trent region, 11 developed dialysis encephalopathy, 21 suffered spontaneous fractures, and 36 who had undergone dialysis for over four years had neither of these complications. Because the incidence of complications seemed to be unevenly distributed the water supplies were analysed. Water supplied to the homes of the patients with fractures or encephalopathy contained significantly less calcium and fluorine and significantly more aluminium and manganese than that piped to patients without these complications. The high aluminium concentration in the bone of patients with encephalopathy was confirmed, but aluminium concentrations in the brains from three patients with encephalopathy were not increased. Patients who undergo dialysis in areas where water contains high aluminium concentrations should be supplied with deionisers.

Importance

This was the first paper that brought to public attention the problem of significant disease resulting from toxins in dialysate, in this instance aluminium. The stimuli to this paper were Alfrey *et al.* (1976) in the USA, who proposed that ingestion of aluminium salts was the cause of dialysis encephalopathy, and Flendrig *et al.* (1976) in the Netherlands, who suggested that exposure to aluminium in the water used for dialysate was responsible. The discussion was muddied by the finding of increased aluminium tissue levels in non-dialysed patients with renal failure, presumably due to an inability to excrete the metal. In a subsequent comprehensive epidemiological study in 18 English dialysis units, the severity of both osteomalacia and encephalopathy was found to correlate with aluminium concentrations in the dialysate (Parkinson *et al.*, 1979). Noteworthy features were that several years of exposure were required before pathology was evident, and both bone and brain grey matter (but not in this initial account) contained significant quantities of aluminium. Initially overdiagnosed clinically, the dysarthria, dysphasia, and apraxia (especially affecting writing) and myoclonic jerks combined with EEG findings were diagnostic. Patients presenting with osteomalacia alone required bone biopsy with positive aluminium staining to establish the specific diagnosis. Evidence that use of aluminium-containing phosphate binders was associated with bone and brain disease is limited, and recently the question has been reopened by Mudge *et al.*, who suggests a randomized trial of alumimium-containing phosphate binders because of their efficiency and low cost. Most dialysis units use reverse osmosis or deionization to remove aluminium from water. In some communities, aluminium sulfate is added as a flocculating agent to water reservoirs, which increases concentrations acutely and adds risk unless the information is communicated to the dialysis unit. The aluminium story focused attention on the many toxic substances found in water used for dialysate. Screening for these is universally routine, with increased attention now being paid to endotoxin measurement with the objective being to achieve ultrapure water.

Platts' paper was the first epidemiological study that related aluminium in dialysate to severe bone and brain disease. Reverse osmosis and deionization systems have solved the problem. Aluminium-containing phosphate binders appear to play a minor role, with some calling for their continued use. These clinical issues provoked attention to water purity for dialysate by international standard organizations (Flendrig *et al.*, 1976).

References

Alfrey AC, LeGendre GR, Kaehny WD (1976). The dialysis encephalopathy syndrome. Possible aluminum intoxication. *N Engl J Med* **294**, 184–188.

Flendrig JA, Kruis H, Das HA (1976). Aluminium and dialysis dementia. *Lancet* **i**, 1235.

Mudge DW, Johnson DW, Hawley CM, *et al.* (2011). Do aluminium-based phosphate binders continue to have a role in contemporary nephrology practice? *BMC Nephrol* **12**, 20.

Parkinson IS, Ward MK, Feest TG, Fawcett RW, Kerr DN (1979). Fracturing dialysis osteodystrophy and dialysis encephalopathy. An epidemiological survey. *Lancet* **i**, 406–409.

12.7 β₂-microglobulin: a new form of amyloid protein associated with chronic hemodialysis

Authors

F Gejyo, S Odani, T Yamada, N Honma, H Saito, Y Suzuki, Y Nakagawa, H Kobayashi, Y Maruyama, Y Hirasawa, M Suzuki, M Arakawa

Reference

Kidney International 1986, **30**, 385–390.

Abstract

Carpal tunnel syndrome is being increasingly reported in haemodialysis patients and amyloidal tissue has been reported to be present in the perineural tissue of the median nerve and in other tissues of patients operated on for this syndrome. Amyloid tissue was homogenized and the sediments repeatedly centrifuged. The high content of amyloid in the lyophised sample was confirmed by Congo Red staining. After solubilisation in guanidine HCl, a significant amount of protein was located in a homogeneous low molecular weight fraction homogeneous fraction. The protein was found to be identical to β_2-microglobulin, with regard to its molecular weight of 11,000, amino acid composition and 16 amino-terminal amino acids: Ile-Gln-Arg-Thr-Pro-Lys-Ile-Gln-Val-Tyr-Ser-Arg-His-Pro-Ala-Glu. These results demonstrate that the amyloid associated with chronic haemodialysis contains as major component a new form of amyloid fibril protein that is homologous to β_2-microglobulin. [Adapted.]

Importance

Beginning in 1979, increased incidence of carpal tunnel syndrome had been recognized in haemodialysis patients in whom amyloid was identified in the median nerve and in other tissues including the heart, gut, and skin. The biochemical analysis in this paper determined that β_2-microglobulin (B2M) was its basic constituent. That a normal constituent of body fluid and a component of the β-chain HLA surface antigen was pathogenic, and responsible for a puzzling and significant illness, came as a surprise. Assuming a normal B2M production rate in kidney failure, neither its metabolism nor excretion was adequate to maintain normal levels, and the dialysis membranes then in use could not remove it. Whilst there was much discussion of the need to remove 'middle molecules' during dialysis, this 1986 report was a stimulus for commercial interest in increasing the permeability of dialyser membranes to larger molecules and producing what were soon called 'high-flux' dialysers. These were constructed of modified cellulose and later by extensive development of synthetic membranes that were also more biocompatible. Substances with a molecular weight of up 12,000–15,000 Da could be removed with some later dialysers engineered to remove albumin-bound uraemic toxins, which removed up to 6 g of albumin per treatment. High-flux dialysers have become the most frequently used dialysers worldwide, particularly in much of Europe and North America. Increased fluid permeability resulted in a need to control ultrafiltration, later achieved by the development of volumetric and other precise methods. In the Hemodialysis (HEMO) study, increased serum B2M concentrations were associated with an increase in all-cause mortality, and an increase in Kt/V for B2M with reduction in infectious mortality (Cheung *et al.*, 2006, 2008). Another HEMO study had also provided evidence that use of peracetic acid for dialyser reprocessing reduced subsequent B2M clearance during dialysis (Cheung *et al.*, 2999). Several randomized controlled trials (RCTs) have shown improvement in morbidity and mortality with use of high-flux membranes, particularly the HEMO and Membrane Permeability Outcome (MPO) trials, but in each case, only in subpopulations within the main study (Locatelli *et al.*, 2009). The role of B2M removal in this reduced mortality is uncertain.

Identification in this landmark paper on B2M as the proximate cause of dialysis amyloidosis not only answered an important question but was a major reason for stimulating the development and use of high-flux dialysers, which extended the molecular weight range of uraemic toxins that could be removed by dialysis. Use of high-flux dialysers has resulted in the almost complete prevention of dialysis-related amyloidosis, with other favourable effects on morbidity in patients.

References

Cheung AK, Agodoa LY, Daugirdas JT, *et al.* (1999). Effects of hemodialyzer reuse on clearances of urea and β_2-microglobulin. The Haemodialysis (HEMO) Study Group. *J Am Soc Nephrol* **10**, 117–127.

Cheung AK, Rocco MV, Yan G, *et al.* (2006). Serum β_2 microglobulin levels predict mortality in dialysis patients: results of the HEMO study. *Clin J Am Soc Nephrol* **17**, 546–555.

Cheung AK, Greene T, Leypoldt JK, *et al.* (2008). Association between serum 2-microglobulin level and infectious mortality in haemodialysis patients. *Clin J Am Soc Nephrol* **3**, 69–77.

Locatelli F, Martin-Malo A, Hannedouche T, *et al.* (2009). Effect of membrane permeability on survival of haemodialysis patients. *J Am Soc Nephrol*, **20**, 645–54

12.8 A mechanistic analysis of the National Cooperative Dialysis Study (NCDS)

Authors

FA Gotch, JA Sargent

Reference

Kidney International 1985, **28**, 525–534.

Abstract

The purpose of the NCDS was to determine the probability of clinical failure (PF) as a function of the level of dialysis and protein catabolic rate (pcr, g/kg/day). The level of dialysis prescribed in the NCDS was mechanistically defined as Kt/V (product of dialyzer urea clearance and treatment time divided by body urea volume), which exponentially determines decrease in BUN during dialysis and is also a mathematical analogue of pcr, BUN. Mechanistic analysis (MA) showed that PF was a discontinuous function of Kt/V as it was prescribed in the NCDS and that a dependence of PF on pcr could not be assessed because of the study design. The MA results were compared to those reported with statistical analysis (SA) that used BUN and pcr. The SA predicts PF is strongly dependent on pcr with nutrition-dependent high PF for pcr less than or equal to ≤0.8 and low PF with high pcr and intensive dialysis. The MA suggests that SA may not be valid because a continuous outcome function is assumed and, due to study design, Kt/V was a dependent variable of pcr and these two variables cannot be clearly separated by analysis of BUN and pcr alone.

Importance

This article was published 5 years after the results of the National Cooperative Dialysis Study (NCDS) were first revealed (Lowrie *et al.*, 1981) and were viewed sceptically at first, even by some of the investigators themselves. It constitutes a reinterpretation of the NCDS, which was designed from its inception to show the potential benefits of removing larger retention solutes. Because high-flux membranes were not available when the study was designed, treatment time was used as a surrogate for molecular size, as larger solutes were considered 'membrane restricted' as opposed to the 'flow restriction' exhibited by urea and other small solutes. As membrane exposure time is more important for removal of larger molecules, the study proposed to demonstrate the importance of larger molecules by separating both flow and treatment time in a 2 × 2 randomized protocol, using the blood urea nitrogen concentration (BUN) and treatment time as targets for intervention. After study completion, it was clear that control of BUN was far more important than treatment time, reducing subsequent emphasis on the middle-molecule hypothesis. However, as urea generation, principally from protein catabolism, measured as protein catabolic rate (pcr), also determines the patient's BUN, Gotch and Sargent focused on urea clearance, showing that this pcr-independent parameter was the strongest determinant of outcome. They expressed urea clearance as a fraction of total body water cleared per dialysis, or *Kt/V*. Body water volume was equated to the volume of urea distribution, as urea rapidly and uniformly distributes in all body water compartments. This expression of the dialysis dose, *Kt/V*, eventually became the cornerstone of dialysis prescriptions and assessment of adequacy throughout the world (National

Kidney Foundation, 2006). Its acceptance is based on ease of measurement and lack of confounding by differing rates of urea generation in the patient.

As originally constituted, Kt/V applies to a single haemodialysis when given three times weekly. A standard value of 1.2–1.4 vols per dialysis has been established in several countries, and the standard has been applied to continuous peritoneal dialysis by extrapolating to a weekly expression. In the absence of residual native kidney function, values lower than 1.0 per dialysis, as shown by Gotch and Sargent in this analysis of NCDS data, lead to increased morbidity and are associated with increased mortality (Shinzato *et al.*, 1997), but higher values have not been shown to improve outcomes (see paper 12.9).

References

Lowrie EG, Laird NM, Parker TF, Sargent JA (1981).Effect of the haemodialysis prescription on patient morbidity: report from the National Cooperative Dialysis Study. *N Engl J Med* **305**, 1176–1181.

National Kidney Foundation (2006). K/DOQI clinical practice guidelines and clinical practice recommendations for 2006 updates: haemodialysis adequacy, peritoneal dialysis adequacy, and vascular access. *Am J Kidney Dis* **48** (Suppl. 1), S1–s322.

Shinzato T, Nakai S, Akiba T, *et al.* (1997). Survival in long-term haemodialysis patients: results from the annual survey of the Japanese Society for Dialysis Therapy. *Nephrol Dial Transplant* **12**, 884–888.

12.9 Effect of dialysis dose and membrane flux in maintenance haemodialysis

Authors

G Eknoyan, GJ Beck, AK Cheung, JT Daugirdas, T Greene, JW Kusek, M Allon, J Bailey, JA Delmez, TA Depner, JT Dwyer, AS Levey, NW Levin, E Milford, DB Ornt, MV Rocco, G Schulman, SJ Schwab, BP Teehan, R Toto, for the Haemodialysis (HEMO) Study Group

Reference

New England Journal of Medicine 2002, **347**, 2010–2019.

Abstract

Background: The effects of the dose of dialysis and the level of flux of the dialyzer membrane on mortality and morbidity among patients undergoing maintenance haemodialysis are uncertain.

Methods: We undertook a randomized clinical trial in 1846 patients undergoing thrice-weekly dialysis, using a two-by-two factorial design to assign patients randomly to a standard or high dose of dialysis and to a low-flux or high-flux dialyzer.

Results: In the standard-dose group, the mean (±SD) urea-reduction ratio was 66.3 ± 2.5 percent, the single-pool Kt/V was 1.32 ± 0.09, and the equilibrated Kt/V was 1.16 ± 0.08; in the high-dose group, the values were 75.2 ± 2.5 percent, 1.71 ± 0.11, and 1.53 ± 0.09, respectively. Flux, estimated on the basis of beta$_2$-microglobulin clearance, was 3 ± 7 ml per minute in the low-flux group and 34 ± 11 ml per minute in the high-flux group. The primary outcome, death from any cause, was not significantly influenced by the dose or flux assignment: the relative risk of death in the high-dose group as compared with the standard-dose group was 0.96 (95 percent confidence interval, 0.84 to 1.10; P = 0.53), and the relative risk of death in the high-flux group as compared with the low-flux group was 0.92 (95 percent confidence interval, 0.81 to 1.05; P = 0.23). The main secondary outcomes (first hospitalization for cardiac causes or death from any cause, first hospitalization for infection or death from any cause, first 15 percent decrease in the serum albumin level or death from any cause, and all hospitalizations not related to vascular access) also did not differ significantly between either the dose groups or the flux groups. Possible benefits of the dose or flux interventions were suggested in two of seven prespecified subgroups of patients.

Conclusions: Patients undergoing haemodialysis thrice weekly appear to have no major benefit from a higher dialysis dose than that recommended by current U.S. guidelines or from the use of a high-flux membrane.

Importance

This article first revealed the results of the HEMO study, a National Institutes of Health-sponsored RCT that was designed to discover whether or not a higher dose of dialysis, measured as urea clearance and expressed as *Kt/V* given three times weekly, would improve patient outcomes. The results were not equivocal. No benefit was seen either in survival or in several other measures of patient outcome including hospitalization for cardiovascular complications or infection, hospitalizations for non-access related causes, death from cardiac or infectious causes, and serum albumin concentration. Higher doses were achieved by increasing the dialyser clearance or by increasing the treatment time, neither of which showed a benefit. The study also included a comparison of standard and high-flux dialysers, both with synthetic membranes, with intent to answer the lingering question about retained toxins in the larger molecular size range. This arm of the 2×2 study also showed no benefit with regard to the patient outcome measures. Subgroup analyses, however, showed a possible benefit of a higher dialysis dose in women compared with men, and a possible benefit of high-flux dialysis in patients who had more than 3.7 years of dialysis before randomization. Subgroup analyses, however, are prone to error and do not share the rigor of RCTs, so the latter conclusions could only be presented as speculative and in need of confirmation.

This study showed conclusively that previously established standards for dosing dialysis three times per week were sufficient, and that high-flux dialysers, although not harmful, were not as beneficial as previously imagined. These unequivocal findings opened the door to explore other aspects of kidney replacement in search of methods to reduce the current patient mortality rate that remains unacceptably high.

12.10 In-center haemodialysis six times per week versus three times per week

Authors

The FHN Trial Group: GM Chertow, NW Levin, GJ Beck, TA Depner, PW Eggers, JJ Gassman, I Gorodetskaya, T Greene, S James, B Larive, RM Lindsay, RL Mehta, B Miller, DB Ornt, S Rajagopalan, A Rastogi, MV Rocco, B Schiller, O Sergeyeva, G Schulman, GO Ting, ML Unruh, RA Star, AS Kliger

Reference

New England Journal of Medicine 2010, **363**, 2287–2300.

Abstract

Background: In this randomized clinical trial, we aimed to determine whether increasing the frequency of in-center haemodialysis would result in beneficial changes in left ventricular mass, self-reported physical health, and other intermediate outcomes among patients undergoing maintenance haemodialysis.

Methods: Patients were randomly assigned to undergo haemodialysis six times per week (frequent haemodialysis, 125 patients) or three times per week (conventional haemodialysis, 120 patients) for 12 months. The two co-primary composite outcomes were death or change (from baseline to 12 months) in left ventricular mass, as assessed by cardiac magnetic resonance imaging, and death or change in the physical-health composite score of the RAND 36-item health survey. Secondary outcomes included cognitive performance; self-reported depression; laboratory markers of nutrition, mineral metabolism, and anemia; blood pressure; and rates of hospitalization and of intervention related to vascular access.

Results: Patients in the frequent-haemodialysis group averaged 5.2 sessions per week; the weekly standard Kt/V_{urea} (the product of the urea clearance and the duration of the dialysis session normalized to the volume of distribution of urea) was significantly higher in the frequent-haemodialysis group than in the conventional-haemodialysis group (3.54 ± 0.56 vs. 2.49 ± 0.27). Frequent haemodialysis was associated with significant benefits with respect to both co-primary composite outcomes (hazard ratio for death or increase in left ventricular mass, 0.61; 95% confidence interval [CI], 0.46 to 0.82; hazard ratio for death or a decrease in the physical-health composite score, 0.70; 95% CI, 0.53 to 0.92). Patients randomly assigned to frequent haemodialysis were more likely to undergo interventions related to vascular access than were patients assigned to conventional haemodialysis (hazard ratio, 1.71; 95% CI, 1.08 to 2.73). Frequent haemodialysis was associated with improved control of hypertension and hyperphosphatemia. There were no significant effects of frequent haemodialysis on cognitive performance, self-reported depression, serum albumin concentration, or use of erythropoiesis-stimulating agents.

Importance

This was the first RCT with adequate power to examine the effect of six times per week versus three times per week dialysis on intermediate outcomes, although it was not powered to examine survival. The results confirmed previous less stringent studies (Suri *et al.*, 2006). Some 3500 patients were approached to derive the 245 studied. The favourable effects of treatment on composites of mortality and left ventricular mass change (dominated by the latter) and on self-reported physical health were impressive. Mean dialysis time was 154 min per session in the interventional group. Cognitive function did not improve. A major question was compliance in the intervention group, but 78% of patient attended more than 80% of sessions. Of the specified secondary outcomes, pre-dialysis serum phosphorus and pre-dialysis BP were both reduced. Interdialytic weight gain per treatment was also significantly reduced. While daily dialysis was clearly superior to conventional treatment number with regard to primary outcomes, it is questionable whether this therapy will be widely used for reasons of patient travel and time burdens, and of costs. However, an increase in treatment number to four or five weekly might represent favourable options for some patients, especially those able to dialyse at home. While not fully discussed, the favourable effect of the intervention might be due to fluid overload reduction in the interventional group. This approach in principle is similar to the effects of salt restriction. which also reduces interdialytic weight gain, BP, and left ventricular mass (Ozhahya *et al.*, 2002). Serum phosphorus levels were significantly reduced, which may be relevant to outcomes (Ayus *et al.*, 2005). Interventions for vascular access problems were more frequent, but overall access survival between the interventions arms did not differ. The same study group also undertook a trial of frequent nocturnal home haemodialysis, which did not show significant differences between the treatment arms (Rocco *et al.*, 2011). However the inclusion criteria in that study had permitted patients with significant urine volumes, which reduced differences in interdialytic weight gain between treatment groups (Rocco *et al.*, 2011).

The primary results of this landmark RCT were that frequent dialysis provided over a year reduced left ventricular mass and improved a self-reported physical health measure. Interdialytic weight gain, pre-dialysis BP, and serum phosphorus levels were all reduced. These may be variably related to outcomes. Widespread application of this increase in frequency of treatment may lead to an increase in home dialysis.

References

Ayus JC, Mizani MR, Achinger SG, Thadhani R, Go AS, Lee S (2005). Effects of short daily versus conventional haemodialysis on left ventricular hypertrophy and inflammatory markers: a prospective, controlled study. *J Am Soc Nephrol* **16**, 2778–2788.

Ozhahya M, Toz H, Qzerkan F, *et al.* (2002). Impact of volume control on left ventricular hypertrophy in dialysis patients. *J Nephrol* **15**, 655–660.

Rocco MV, Lockridge RS, Beck GJ, *et al.* (2011). The effects of frequent nocturnal home haemodialysis: the Frequent Haemodialysis Network Nocturnal Trial. *Kidney Int* **80**, 1080–1091.

Suri RS, Nesrallah GE, Mainra R, *et al.* (2006). Daily haemodialysis: a systematic review. *Clin J Am Soc Nephrol* **1**, 33–42.

Chapter 13

Vascular access for haemodialysis

Jan H. M. Tordoir

Introduction

For maintenance haemodialysis repeated access to the blood vessels is mandatory, and this was and remains the Achilles heel of successful haemodialysis.

Initially glass cannulae were used for vessel cannulation and the arteries as well as veins were sacrificed after every single dialysis. Repeated vascular access was not possible until a double cannula system fabricated from a new PTFE material with heparin lock between dialysis sessions was introduced by Paul Teschan . In Canada Graham Murray performed the first dialysis in 1946 with the use of a vein-to-vein blood circuit with a special pulsatile blood pump which produced minimum breakdown of red blood cells, to move blood from the vena cava to a peripheral vein. Nils Alwall from Sweden had tried to connect the venous and arterial glass cannulae together with rubber tubing in between dialyses sessions to form a continuously flowing shunt, but they clotted after a few uses. Nevertheless, with the use of a coil kidney and glass cannulae for access, patients were kept alive for weeks to some months, before there was simply no more access.

Femoral vein catheters for acute dialysis were introduced in 1964 by Stanley Shaldon from UK; and later the subclavian (Uldall catheter) and jugular veins with single and double lumen catheters were employed.

The great breakthrough in chronic haemodialysis treatment came from Belding Scribner, Wayne Quinton and David Dillard. Unaware of the experiments of Nils Alwall 12 years before, they developed an external shunt. The first two patients were dialysed in March 1960 and survived for 11 years on dialysis, the other for 8 years before transplantation. The shunt was a combination of PTFE and silicon rubber and the PTFE was quickly relegated to the arterial and venous tips, and to a bridge connector, the bulk of the shunt being silicon rubber. However, the arterial and venous connections tended to need revision frequently and typically the patency of these shunts was no more than several months.

A more durable solution for long-term vascular access was proposed in 1966 by nephrologists Michael Brescia and James Cimino, surgeon Keith Appel and resident Baruch Hurwich. They attempted veno-venous dialysis using a simple occlusion cuff and wide bore needles, but because not all patients had veins of sufficient calibre for cannulation, they developed the idea of enlarging the veins using a surgically created arterio-venous anastomosis. The advantages for the patient were immediately obvious. In subsequent decades, variations in surgical technique and location for arteriovenous fistula formation were developed and fistulae are nowadays still successfully used in most patients.

Alternatives for failed fistulae came from the development of prosthetic materials like PTFE and polyurethane as implants for vascular access. Lately, the need for access surveillance and prophylactic balloon angioplasty of stenoses to prolong the effective life of AV fistulae were recognised.

13.1 Cannulation of blood vessels for prolonged hemodialysis

Authors

W Quinton, D Dillard, BH Scribner

Reference

Transactions of the American Society for Artificial Internal Organs 1960, **6**, 104–113.

Abstract

An external shunt connecting the radial artery and cephalic vein has been developed and used in 6 patients. The cannulas are placed in the vessels through a subcutaneous space so that they emerge from the skin some distance from the site of vessel cannulation. A fitting connects the arterial to the venous cannula thereby creating an arteriovenous shunt. Dialysis can be performed at any time by replacing the shunt and connect [sic] it to the tubes of the dialysis machine. No anticoagulation is required when the shunt is in place and the risk of infection is minimized by the subcutaneous tunnel.

Importance

The first dialysis treatments were performed by means of repeated cannulation of an artery and vein using glass tubes. The main disadvantages were that the vessels could be used only for one dialysis session and that heparin was needed to keep these tubes open. This resulted frequently in bleeding complications. Quinton, Dillard, and Scribner substantially improved the possibility of external vascular access and made one of the most important contributions to the field of haemodialysis vascular access. In their initial publication, an extensive technical description of the external arteriovenous shunt was given, pointing out the importance of the use of Teflon tubes to insert into the vessels. In the six patients they treated with the external shunt, no clotting or infection occurred. One patient had eight dialysis treatments over a period of 8 weeks. Tissue reaction was absent and the vessels showed no inflammation adjacent to the tips of the cannulae. Over three decades, the Quinton–Scribner shunt was used successfully in millions of patients with acute and chronic renal failure (Clark and Parsons, 1966). Its use was largely abandoned after the introduction of the double-lumen central venous catheter, and today the necessary materials for the Scribner shunt are no longer commercially available. A number of modifications of the external shunt were developed in the years after its introduction, including the Buselmeier shunt and the Allen–Brown shunt (Adams *et al.*, 1991) connecting the vessels in the groin with tubes mounted on vascular grafts. In addition, conversion from the temporary external shunt to permanent internal arteriovenous fistula the description of the Brescia–Cimino fistula (Simonian *et al.*, 1977).

The invention and subsequent application of the external arteriovenous shunt by Quinton, Dillard, and Scribner described in this landmark paper made chronic intermittent haemodialysis treatment possible over prolonged periods of time (Blagg, 2011). Its publication was an important step forward in the treatment of patients with renal failure.

References

Adams WJ, Thompson JF, Liounis B, Ekberg H, Rotenko I (1991). The Allen Brown shunt: a useful option for vascular access. *Am J Surg* **162**, 24–30.

Blagg CR (2011). The 50th anniversary of long-term hemodialysis: University of Washington Hospital, March 9th, 1960. *J Nephrol* **24** (Suppl. 17), S84–S88.

Clark PB, Parsons FM (1966). Routine use of the Scribner shunt for haemodialysis. *Br Med J* **1**, 1200–1202.

Simonian SJ, Stuart FP, Hill JL, Mahajan SK (1977). Conversion of a Scribner shunt to an arteriovenous fistula for chronic dialysis. *Surgery* **82**, 448–451.

13.2 Chronic hemodialysis using venipuncture and a surgically created arteriovenous fistula

Authors

MJ Brescia, JE Cimino, K Appel, BJ Hurwich

Reference

New England Journal of Medicine 1966, **275**, 1089–1092.

Abstract

In our experience complications involving external Scribner shunts have been the greatest cause of morbidity. Moreover, cannula revisions along with treatment of infections and clotting were responsible for most hospital days. Therefore we considered the possibility of creating an internal arteriovenous fistula.

An arteriovenous fistula between the radial artery and available vein was surgically created in 16 patients undergoing chronic dialysis. A successfully combination of a radiocephalic fistula and venipuncture using 14 gauge, thin walled needles for over 800 dialysis in 13 patients was accomplished.

Importance

This publication by Brescia and colleagues is probably the most important paper in the field of dialysis vascular access. Even today, the arteriovenous fistula at the wrist is still named after its inventors: the Brescia–Cimino or Cimino–Brescia fistula. It is peculiar that the surgeon (Kenneth Appel) who actually performed the operations is never named. This surgical technique, used 45 years ago, is still valid with slight modifications in anastomosis length and type (end-to-side versus side-to-side vein to artery). Their perfect results with only two early failures from the 16 fistulae (12%) and no long-term complications reflect the composition of the dialysis population at that time. The mean age of their patients was 38 years (range 28–54) and all were suffering from chronic glomerulonephritis. Today, the dialysis population is much older and the cause for renal failure is mostly vascular disease or diabetes mellitus. The creation of a fistula between an often sclerotic, obstructed radial artery and cephalic vein in such patients is a much more difficult operation with a less good outcome. The authors mentioned as a major disadvantage of any arteriovenous fistula an increase in cardiac output, although heart failure was not a problem in their patients and cardiac function remained stable. This observation is of great importance and is even more relevant to the present dialysis patient population in whom cardiac dysfunction is much more common, yet high-output heart failure due to an arteriovenous fistula is uncommon (Basile *et al.*, 2008). Although a distal radiocephalic fistula is still recommended as the primary access option, even in elderly patients, high failure rates necessitate the creation of more proximal fistulae with their inherent high flow rates and the associated risk of cardiac failure and distal ischaemia. To overcome these potential complications, efforts continue to make successful distal fistulae, employing radiological and surgical interventions, aimed at increasing arterial inflow (Turmel-Rodrigues *et al.*, 2009).

The invention of the Brescia–Cimino or radiocephalic arteriovenous fistula was therefore a major step forward in the treatment of patients with intermittent haemodialysis. Nowadays, the dialysis population is different from that 45 years ago, making the creation of a radiocephalic fistula a difficult operation. It remains the 'gold standard' for vascular access, although sustained efforts are needed to maintain the function of these distal fistulae.

References

Basile C, Lomonte C, Vernaglione L, Casucci F, Antonelli M, Losurdo N (2008). The relationship between the flow of arteriovenous fistula and cardiac output in haemodialysis patients. *Nephrol Dial Transplant* **23**, 282–287.

Turmel-Rodrigues L, Boutin JM, Camiade C, Brillet G, Fodil-Chérif M, Mouton A (2009). Percutaneous dilation of the radial artery in nonmaturing autogenous radial-cephalic fistulas for haemodialysis. *Nephrol Dial Transplant* **24**, 3782–3788.

13.3. Clinical experience with the expanded polytetrafluoroethylene vascular prosthesis. The arteriovenous graft

Author

M Haimov

Reference

Angiology 1978, **29**, 1–6.

Abstract

Expanded polytetrafluoroethylene grafts were used in 44 patients in the last 18 months. In 13 patients the graft was used for various types of peripheral vascular reconstructive procedures, as a substitute of the autogenous saphenous veins. In 31 patients the prosthesis was used for the construction of vascular access for hemodialysis. Results of the use of this new vascular prosthesis are comparable to those achieved with the autogenous saphenous vein when used for the same purposes. A much longer period of observation is necessary before a definitive verdict can be reached on the safety and clinical applicability of any new vascular prosthetic material. But preliminary clinical results with the PTFE vascular prosthesis are encouraging and seem to justify continued cautious application of this vascular substitute.

Importance

Haimov was the first to report on the clinical use of PTFE prosthesis for both peripheral bypass and arteriovenous access. From that time, PTFE has been used as the most common graft for vascular access purpose (Munda *et al.*, 1983; Palder *et al.*, 1985). In this first report, the graft was implanted in the forearm, arm, or leg position with patencies ranging from 50 to 100% over 6–18 months of follow-up. The PTFE prosthesis was thought to cause less infection and aneurysm formation compared with bovine heterografts. These properties are still the main advantages of PTFE grafts, although the patency rates are comparable to those of bovine grafts (Hurlbert *et al.*, 1998). At the time of Haimov's publication, it was believed that a new intima formed throughout the inner surface of the graft and across the suture lines. The bloodstream lining was thought to be of stratified, elongated cells resembling true endothelium. This is a misunderstanding, and current knowledge has shown that a fibrin layer lines the graft surface with only a limited ingrowth of endothelial cells from the anastomotic sites into the graft (Delorme *et al.*, 1992).

We now know that the main disadvantage of PTFE grafts is progressive intimal hyperplasia at the venous anastomosis, causing stenosis formation resulting in thrombotic occlusion. This feature accounts for the poor patency rates achieved with this type of graft. This report was the starting point of the implantation of PTFE grafts on a large scale. PTFE remains the most important prosthesis available as a substitute for autogenous fistulae.

References

Delorme JM, Guidoin R, Canizales S, *et al.* (1992). Vascular access for hemodialysis: pathologic features of surgically excised ePTFE grafts. *Ann Vasc Surg* **6**, 517–524.

Hurlbert SN, Mattos MA, Henretta JP, *et al.* (1998). Long-term patency rates, complications and cost-effectiveness of polytetrafluoroethylene (PTFE) grafts for hemodialysis access: a prospective study that compares Impra versus Gore-tex grafts. *Cardiovasc Surg* **6**, 652–656.

Munda R, First MR, Alexander JW, Linnemann CC Jr, Fidler JP, Kittur D (1983).Polytetrafluoroethylene graft survival in hemodialysis. *JAMA* **249**, 219–222.

Palder SB, Kirkman RL, Whittemore AD, Hakim RM, Lazarus JM, Tilney NL (1985). Vascular access for hemodialysis. Patency rates and results of revision. *Ann Surg* **202**, 235–239.

13.4 Experience using central venous access for long-term hemodialysis. A new concept

Authors

DJ McGonigle, LG Schrock, RO Hickman

Reference

American Journal of Surgery 1983, **145**, 571–573.

Abstract

Central venous access for acute renal failure has been used for a number of years. The femoral vein and, more recently, the subclavian vein have been the routes of access. This technique has many advantages, however, it also has some significant limitations. We have recently been using a catheter for long- as well as short-term hemodialysis. The catheter is placed by means of a short incision through an opening in the internal jugular vein, and maneuvered so that the tip lies in the superior portion of the right atrium. After dialysis, the catheter is filled with heparin. The catheter then requires no additional care between between [sic] hemodialysis sessions. We have reported an experience of 50 patients in whom this catheter has been used. The complications have been remarkably few, and none were serious or fatal. At present, the patient using the catheter for the longest period of time has had it in position for approximately 19 months. We believe this technique provides a significant new choice among the ways in which hemodialysis can be achieved for short- or long-term needs.

Importance

This article was the first report on the experience of tunnelled central venous catheters for long-term use in haemodialysis vascular access. The novelty of this single-lumen Silastic catheter was the incorporation of a Dacron cuff at the external end to provide anchorage of the catheter in the percutaneous tunnel (Weijmer *et al.*, 2004). The authors were ahead of the times in using a jugular- rather than a subclavian-vein approach. Catheters were placed with an open surgical technique with venotomy, whereas nowadays a percutaneous insertion technique using a guide wire is employed.

In 38 out of 50 patients with central venous access, the catheter was used for long-term dialysis, with three patients having the catheter for more than 1 year. Technical catheter-related problems resulted in catheter removal in eight patients for outflow obstruction and Dacron cuff erosion in four patients. The catheter lock solution at that time was heparin and might have contributed to the high rate of septicaemia, which occurred in five patients without any deaths.

The major advantages of the technique were long-term use with minimal care, the lack of a need for systemic anti-coagulation, reduced length of hospitalization, minimal surgical intervention, and its role in providing bridging access while waiting for fistula maturation or while complications temporarily prevented fistula use. The major disadvantages remained the high rates of intervention for cuff erosion, catheter thrombosis, and infection (Oliver *et al.*, 2000). Cuff erosion is related to surgical technique and can be relatively simply solved by technical modifications. In contrast, thrombosis and infection may be due to catheter design and the locking solution used, which at that time were the major drawbacks of using central-vein catheters for long-term use.

Nevertheless, the concept of using central-vein catheters for long-term chronic haemodialysis treatment was a major step forward in the management of the dialysis population. Since that time, developments in catheter design and use of locking solutions have improved the outcome of catheter dialysis and lowered the incidence of infection and septicaemia. Although fistulae are to be preferred for long-term dialysis (Rayner *et al.*, 2004), central-vein catheters remain indispensable in daily dialysis practice.

References

Oliver MJ, Callery SM, Thorpe KE, Schwab SJ, Churchill DN (2000). Risk of bacteremia from temporary hemodialysis catheters by site of insertion and duration of use: a prospective study. *Kidney Int* **58**, 2543–2545.

Rayner HC, Besarab A, Brown WW, Disney A, Saito A, Pisoni RL (2004). Vascular access results from the Dialysis Outcomes and Practice Patterns Study (DOPPS): performance against Kidney Disease Outcomes Quality Initiative (K/DOQI) Clinical Practice Guidelines. *Am J Kidney Dis* **44**, 22–26.

Weijmer MC, Vervloet MG, ter Wee PM (2004). Compared to tunnelled cuffed haemodialysis catheters, temporary untunnelled catheters are associated with more complications already within 2 weeks of use. *Nephrol Dial Transplant* **19**, 670–677.

13.5 Insufficient dialysis shunts: improved long-term patency rates with close hemodynamic monitoring, repeated percutaneous balloon angioplasty, and stent placement

Authors

L Turmel-Rodrigues, J Pengloan, D Blanchier, M Abaza, B Birmelé, O Haillot, D Blanchard

Reference

Radiology 1993, **187**, 273–278.

Abstract

Over 54 months, 70 short stenoses of 63 shunts (32 Brescia–Cimino fistulas, 31 grafts) in 59 patients necessitated a first percutaneous transluminal angioplasty (PTA). Restenosis led to 63 redilations in 38 lesions. Nine stents were inserted in seven grafts and two proximal veins in seven patients, the indication being that stenosis had recurred twice in 6 months. In three of these stenoses, five delayed intrastent redilations were necessary. Three previously dilated occluded grafts were recovered with local thrombolysis. Morbidity was 4.08%, with one immediate rupture, four delayed pseudoaneurysms (1–28 months), and two periprocedural bacteremias. Half (15 of 29) of graft stenoses and only 14% (four of 27) of Brescia-Cimino fistula stenoses had a mean restenosis interval of less than 6 months. The mean restenosis interval increased from 3.6 months +/− 0.5 (standard deviation) before stent placement to 15.2 months +/− 0.4 after stent placement (P < .001). Insertion of a stent can be advised when stenoses of graft venous anastomoses have recurred twice in less than 6 months. The combination of all interventional radiologic procedures allowed a significant improvement in secondary patency rates after PTA, with 82% at 1 year, 79% at 2 years, and 71% at 3 years.

Importance

The concept of access monitoring by venous pressure measurement was adapted in the late 1980s, and application of pre-emptive intervention by percutaneous transluminal angioplasty (PTA) with or without stent placement was relatively a new procedure. Turmel-Rodrigues and colleagues were one of the first to publish a large endovascular intervention series in both autogenous fistulae and prosthetic grafts, in which suspicion of stenoses was based on poor arterial inflow or poor outflow indicated by high venous pressures. They reported on a total of 147 interventions, including 70 primary dilations, 68 re-interventions, and nine stent placements for significant stenoses. Thrombosed accesses were not included. Good angiographic and haemodynamic result was achieved in 65 (93%) out of the 70 primary procedures. Restenosis necessitated repeated PTA in 38 patients, which was a primary patency of 44%. Fistulae did better than grafts, with a patency of 62 versus 25%. If only PTA was employed, the secondary patency was significantly worse compared with all radiological procedures (71 versus 82%). Stenoses in grafts did recur earlier than fistulae, and for recurrent stenoses, stent implantation was advised.

Multiple publications have since addressed the use of pre-emptive endovascular treatment for fistulae and grafts and the outcomes are usually good (Tessitore *et al.*, 2004; Casey *et al.*, 2008; Tonelli *et al.*, 2008), although there is still discussion about the usefulness of this strategy for prolongation of access survival, particularly for arteriovenous grafts. Nevertheless, its application continues to be recommended in most clinical practice guidelines for vascular access.

References

Casey ET, Murad MH, Rizvi AZ, *et al.* (2008). Surveillance of arteriovenous hemodialysis access: a systematic review and meta-analysis. *J Vasc Surg* **48**, S48–S54.

Tessitore N, Lipari G, Poli A, *et al.* (2004). Can blood flow surveillance and pre-emptive repair of subclinical stenosis prolong the useful life of arteriovenous fistulae? A randomized controlled study. *Nephrol Dial Transplant* **19**, 2325–2333.

Tonelli M, James M, Wiebe N, Jindal K, Hemmelgarn B; Alberta Kidney Disease Network (2008). Ultrasound monitoring to detect access stenosis in hemodialysis patients: a systematic review. *Am J Kidney Dis* **51**, 630–640.

13.6 The relationship of recirculation to access blood flow

Authors

A Besarab, R Sherman

Reference

American Journal of Kidney Diseases 1997, **29**, 223–229.

Abstract

The relationship between vascular access recirculation and access blood flow has been obscured by measurement techniques that overestimate recirculation. We measured brachial artery blood flow (a surrogate for access blood flow) using Doppler ultrasound and access recirculation using a two-needle slow/stop flow method and the standard peripheral vein method in 77 chronic hemodialysis patients. These patients had 25 native arteriovenous fistulae and 52 polytetrafluoroethylene grafts. Access recirculation by the slow/stop flow method was uniformly absent in these patients unless their access blood flow rate was less than the dialyzer blood flow rate. The peripheral vein method averaged 10.7% in these patients; many values were considerably higher. We conclude that access recirculation is a function of access blood flow and does not occur (in the absence of or reversed needle cannulation) unless access blood flow is markedly impaired.

Importance

This report by Besarab and Sherman was the first of numerous publications on access monitoring and surveillance. The rationale of this research was the high incidence of thrombosis due to neointimal stenosis formation in prosthetic graft vascular access, which at that time compromised over 80% of vascular accesses in the USA. In a cohort of 77 patients with 52 PTFE grafts and 25 native fistulae, brachial-artery flow as a measure of access flow by Doppler method was correlated to the percentage of recirculation (Paulson *et al.*, 1998). They showed with an elegant study design that recirculation measurement with the two-needle slow/stop flow was more accurate compared with the peripheral vein method. In addition, they showed that recirculation can occur only when access flow is lower than dialysis flow. In other words, there must be flow reversal in the access during dialysis if recirculation is noticed. This was an important observation and has led to a better understanding of the flow haemodynamics in vascular access during dialysis. This observation is more important for arteriovenous grafts than for native fistulae, which will remain functional even with very low flow rates. In this study, it was shown that recirculation is a very late sign of impeding access failure that is better used for monitoring of native fistulae than for grafts.

Subsequent studies have focused mainly on flow measurement for access monitoring (Moist *et al.*, 2003; Lopot *et al.*, 2004) with the knowledge that recirculation is a very late sign of impeding access failure and therefore of little value. However, this was the first report showing the relative importance of recirculation measurement for surveillance, particularly in arteriovenous grafts. It nicely showed the relationship of recirculation to access flow and gave insight into access haemodynamics during dialysis treatment.

References

Lopot F, Nejedlý B, Sulková S, Bláha J (2004). Comparison of different techniques of hemodialysis vascular access flow evaluation. *J Vasc Acces* **5**, 25–32.

Moist LM, Churchill DN, House AA, *et al.* (2003). Regular monitoring of access flow compared with monitoring of venous pressure fails to improve graft survival. *J Am Soc Nephrol* **14**, 2645–2653.

Paulson WD, Gadallah MF, Bieber BJ, Altman SD, Birk CG, Work J (1998). Accuracy and reproducibility of urea recirculation in detecting haemodialysis access stenosis. *Nephrol Dial Transplant* **13**, 118–124.

13.7 Tailoring the initial vascular access for dialysis patients

Authors

K Konner, TE Hulbert-Shearon, EC Roys, FK Port

Reference

Kidney International 2002, **62**, 329–338.

Abstract

Background: Creating a functioning initial arteriovenous (AV) access for aging and diabetic end-stage renal disease (ESRD) hemodialysis patients has been a challenge.

Methods: This study describes 748 consecutive primary AV access creations and their primary (unassisted) and secondary (assisted) access survival at a single center. Twenty-four percent of the patients had diabetes as their cause of ESRD and the average age was 59.6 years. No patient receiving an initial AV access required synthetic graft material. All received an AV fistula. Three types of fistulae were created and their distribution varied significantly for diabetic and non-diabetic patients (respective percentages): forearm AV fistula (24%, 62%), perforating vein fistula (PVF) at the elbow (48%, 21%) and non-PVF at the elbow (29%, 17%).

Results: Results of access survival for age groups <65 and 65+ years, male and female, diabetic and non-diabetic subgroups ranged from 51 to 75% for unassisted and from 75 to 96% for assisted two year access survival. PVF appeared to be advantageous over non-PVF access at the elbow. First intervention for peripheral steal syndrome was required at a rate of 7 and 0.6 per 100 patient-years at risk for diabetic and non-diabetic patients, respectively. The thrombosis rates per patient year of 0.03 for non-diabetics and 0.07 for diabetics are superior to previously published results for AV fistulae or for a combined AV fistula-AV graft approach.

Conclusions: Potential explanations for these excellent results among elderly and diabetic patients include preoperative evaluation, exclusive use of native vessels, a variable surgical approach including PVF, and the experience of a single operator.

Importance

This experience with a large cohort of native arteriovenous fistulae in a single centre, performed by a single operator, was of great importance at a time when successful vascular access creation was increasingly reported to be difficult, particularly in diabetic and elderly patients. As a counterpoint to the great number of prosthetic graft implantations in these patient groups, in particular in the USA, Klaus Konner and his colleagues showed excellent results of primary fistula creation in a consecutive series of 748 patients. It was remarkable that there was no need to implant grafts as a primary access, given that 24% of patients had diabetes and 40% were over 65 years of age, indicating a high risk of peripheral arterial disease with the likelihood of unsuitable vessels for native fistula creation. With only three types of fistulae in the forearm and elbow (using the perforating vein, cephalic, or basilic vein), it was possible to create access in all patients. Most of the non-diabetic patients (62%) received forearm fistulae, whilst among the diabetics only 24% had forearm fistulae. This clearly indicates peripheral vessel disease in diabetic patients. Early fistula thrombosis occurred in only one out of 181 diabetic patients and 18 out of 567 non-diabetic patients. In addition, no differences in primary and secondary patencies at 1 and 2 years were found between patients with and without diabetes and over 65 years of age. Thrombosis rates were very low, only 0.03 and 0.07 events per patient-year for diabetic and non-diabetic patients respectively. Only peripheral ischaemia was significantly more frequently in diabetics (0.07 versus 0.006 events per patient-year). These results are superior to almost all publications reporting the outcome of native fistulae (Ravani *et al.*, 2002; Basile *et al.*, 2004; Jennings, 2006). The reasons for these excellent results lie in the fact that a tailored selection of type and location of the initial vascular access was performed by a single very experienced operator. Pre-operative clinical evaluation combined with ultrasonography was considered mandatory and indicative of which type and location of fistula should be chosen.

This publication reported on the largest series of native fistulae in the literature. It showed that a strategy of creating fistulae in all patient groups, in spite of the presence of diabetes or high age, resulted in excellent outcome with a low rate of complications. To achieve these goals, adequate pre-operative vessel assessment and patient-specific tailoring of access location is mandatory. However, probably the most important factor for good access outcome is the experience of the person who performs the surgery.

References

Basile C, Ruggieri G, Vernaglione L, Montanaro A, Giordano R (2004). The natural history of autogenous radio-cephalic wrist arteriovenous fistulas of haemodialysis patients: a prospective observational study. *Nephrol Dial Transplant* **19**, 1231–1236.

Jennings WC (2006). Creating arteriovenous fistulas in 132 consecutive patients: exploiting the proximal radial artery arteriovenous fistula: reliable, safe, and simple forearm and upper arm hemodialysis access. *Arch Surg* **141**, 27–32.

Ravani P, Marcelli D, Malberti F (2002). Vascular access surgery managed by renal physicians: the choice of native arteriovenous fistulas for hemodialysis. *Am J Kidney Dis* **40**, 1264–1276.

13.8 Salvage of the nonfunctioning arteriovenous fistula

Authors

GA Beathard, SM Settle, MW Shields

Reference

American Journal of Kidney Diseases 1999, **33**, 910–916.

Abstract

Two factors are necessary for an arteriovenous fistula (AVF) to be usable as dialysis access. It must have adequate blood flow, and it must have a size that will allow for cannulation. An AVF can remain patent in the face of relatively low blood flow. For effective dialysis, the AVF only has to deliver a blood flow that is marginally greater than the pump rate. Unfortunately, dialysis may not be technically possible in those cases with lower flow because the AVF does not mature sufficiently to a size adequate for cannulation. In this prospective observational series of 63 patients, failure of AVF development was the result of venous stenosis and/or the presence of accessory veins (venous side branches). The presence of these anomalies could be diagnosed by physical examination. After documentation by angiography, the patients were treated with angioplasty, venous ligation, or a combination of both. Three levels of venous ligation were performed depending on individual requirements: ligation of accessory veins (AVL), ligation of the median cubital vein, and temporary banding of the main fistula itself. The determining factor was the appearance of the fistula after each of the procedures was accomplished relative to potential for cannulation. Of these 63 patients with nonfunctional fistulae that ranged in age from 33 to 418 days, access was salvaged in 52 patients (82.5%). This included 9 of 12 patients who required repeat procedures. The results of this study validate angioplasty and AVL as therapy for the salvage of AVFs that fail to develop.

Importance

During the 1990s, particularly in the USA, the attitude towards access creation needed to change in view of the high complication rate and the cost of the use of prosthetic graft fistulae. Clinical practice guidelines from the Kidney Disease Outcomes Quality Initiative (KDOQI) in the USA stressed the preferential use of native fistulae for dialysis; however, this strategy resulted in a high percentage of non-functioning accesses due to poor maturation. In this landmark paper, Beathard and colleagues highlighted the possibility of salvaging these non-functioning fistulae. Their hypothesis was that non-maturation was due to stenosis development, accessory vein flow diversion, or low intraluminal vein pressure. They made a diagnosis of non-maturation solely by clinical examination, whereas nowadays access flow measurement by ultrasound examination is believed to be the 'gold standard' for such assessment.

A group of 63 patients with non-matured radiocephalic (56 patients) and brachiocephalic (seven patients) fistulae had angiography and subsequently intervention. It is remarkable that all patients showed one or more abnormalities, which could all be treated. Some of the patients had multiple interventions, with angioplasty for venous stenosis followed by either accessory vein ligation or narrowing of the main draining vein to increase intraluminal pressure. The total success rate for the 63 patients was 82.5% with a 1-year fistula patency of 75%.

Although the strategy of salvaging poorly maturing fistulae is widely accepted, the rationale to occlude accessory veins, ligate the medial cubital vein, or band the mainstream vein continues to be debated. This is because current theory of the aetiology of non-maturation is different from that postulated in this paper. Adequate arterial inflow increases wall shear stress, initiating outward vein remodelling. Augmentation of blood flow will further influence vessel adaptation. In this respect, the presence of accessory veins is probably of less importance. High vein resistance due to venous stenosis does not advantageously influence maturation but usually will induce non-maturation. Nowadays, the objectives for treatment of non-maturing fistulae are focused on enhancement of blood flow by arterial inflow and venous outflow improvement by either endovascular or surgical means (Turmel-Rodrigues *et al.*, 2001, 2009; Dammers *et al.*, 2002; Tordoir *et al.*, 2003; Planken *et al.*, 2007).

This publication showed that salvage of non-functioning native fistulae, due to non-maturation, is worthwhile and leads to increasing numbers of fistulae. However, although the interventions for fistula salvation led to a high success rate, the rationale behind the methods used is debatable.

References

Dammers R, Tordoir JH, Welten RJ, Kitslaar PJ, Hoeks AP (2002). The effect of chronic flow changes on brachial artery diameter and shear stress in arteriovenous fistulas for hemodialysis. *Int J Artif Organs* **25**, 124–128.

Planken RN, Duijm LE, Kessels AG, *et al.* (2007). Accessory veins and radial-cephalic arteriovenous fistula non-maturation: a prospective analysis using contrast-enhanced magnetic resonance angiography. *J Vasc Access* **8**, 281–286.

Tordoir JH, Rooyens P, Dammers R, van der Sande FM, de Haan M, Yo TI (2003). Prospective evaluation of failure modes in autogenous radiocephalic wrist access for haemodialysis. *Nephrol Dial Transplant* **18**, 378–383.

Turmel-Rodrigues L, Mouton A, Birmelé B, *et al.* (2001). Salvage of immature forearm fistulas for haemodialysis by interventional radiology. *Nephrol Dial Transplant* **16**, 2365–2371.

Turmel-Rodrigues L, Boutin JM, Camiade C, Brillet G, Fodil-Chérif M, Mouton A (2009). Percutaneous dilation of the radial artery in nonmaturing autogenous radial-cephalic fistulas for haemodialysis. *Nephrol Dial Transplant* **24**, 3782–3788.

13.9 Vascular access use and outcomes: an international perspective from the Dialysis Outcomes and Practice Patterns Study

Authors

J Ethier, DC Mendelssohn, SJ Elder, T Hasegawa, T Akizawa, T Akiba, BJ Canaud, RL Pisoni

Reference

Nephrology Dialysis Transplantation 2008, **23**, 3219–3226. [Erratum: **23**, 4088.]

Abstract

Background:…DOPPS is a prospective, observational study of haemodialysis (HD) practices and patient outcomes at >300 HD units from 12 countries and has collected data thus far from >35,000 randomly selected patients.

Methods: VA [vascular access] data were collected for each patient at study entry (1996–2007). Practice pattern data from the facility medical director, nurse manager and VA surgeon were also analysed.

Results: Since 2005, a native arteriovenous fistula (AVF) was used by 67–91% of prevalent patients in Japan, Italy, Germany, France, Spain, the UK, Australia and New Zealand, and 50–59% in Belgium, Sweden and Canada. From 1996 to 2007, AVF use rose from 24% to 47% in the USA but declined in Italy, Germany and Spain. Moreover, graft use fell by 50% in the USA from 58% use in 1996 to 28% by 2007. Across three phases of data collection, patients consistently were less likely to use an AVF versus other VA types if female, of older age, having greater body mass index, diabetes, peripheral vascular disease or recurrent cellulitis/gangrene. In addition, countries with a greater prevalence of diabetes in HD patients had a significantly lower percentage of patients using an AVF. Despite poorer outcomes for central vein catheters, catheter use rose 1.5- to 3-fold among prevalent patients in many countries from 1996 to 2007, even among non-diabetic patients 18–70 years old.…Patients were significantly ($P < 0.05$) less likely to start dialysis with a permanent VA if treated in a facility that (1) had a longer time from referral to access surgery evaluation or from evaluation to access creation and (2) had longer time from access creation until first AVF cannulation.…

Conclusions: Most countries meet the contemporary National Kidney Foundation's Kidney Disease Outcomes Quality Initiative goal for AVF use; however, there is still a wide variation in VA preference.…[Extract.]

Importance

The Dialysis Outcome Practice Pattern Study (DOPPS) is one of the largest databases collecting information on several aspects of dialysis treatment. In DOPPS, patients from a selection of dialysis facilities in Europe, Japan, Australia, New Zealand, Canada, and the USA have been followed sequentially during three different time periods (DOPPS I–III). This allows determination of trends in dialysis practices. The importance of the current study was assessment of the influence on vascular access practice of clinical practice guidelines such as KDOQI in the USA, European Best Practice Guidelines, and 'Fistula First' (a US-based promotion of the preferential use of arteriovenous fistulae). Although the number of native fistulae has risen from DOPPS I to III, there are a number of countries with persistently low fistula use. Most European countries and Japan have more than 75% of prevalent patients with fistulae, but for instance Belgium, the USA, and Canada have around 50%. One of the most important features of this study was the steep rise in the use of central-vein catheters for dialysis in prevalent patients. This was not only the case in countries with previously high catheter use but also in countries such as Japan and Italy, which historically had low catheter use. The presumed reason for this development lies in the fact that more co-morbid patients, with diabetes, hypertension, and peripheral arterial disease, are now being established on dialysis treatment (Xi *et al.*, 2010). Fistula creation in these patients might be cumbersome due to sclerotic and damaged vessels, resulting in delayed or non-maturation. In addition, late referral to the nephrologist and late planning of vascular access surgery are strongly related to the chance of catheter use (Hasegawa *et al.*, 2009; Rayner and Pisoni, 2010; Ocak *et al.*, 2011). The recommendation from the guidelines to create only native fistulae may be too strong. In particular, recommendations should possibly be more liberal in difficult patient groups, allowing the option of graft implantation. Recent literature supports this view and shows acceptable outcome of both grafts and arteriovenous fistulae in defined patient groups (Lazarides *et al.*, 2007).

Nevertheless, this report from the DOPPS study serves as an important instrument to monitor implementation of guidelines recommendations in the vascular access practice. The data presented are pivotal in the planning and organization of dialysis facilities. In addition, it shows convincingly that knowledge and training of healthcare workers and physicians are of utmost importance to achieve the desired target goals.

References

Hasegawa T, Bragg-Gresham JL, Yamazaki S, *et al.* (2009). Greater first-year survival on hemodialysis in facilities in which patients are provided earlier and more frequent pre-nephrology visits. *Clin J Am Soc Nephrol* **4**, 595–602.

Lazarides MK, Georgiadis GS, Antoniou GA, Staramos DN (2007). A meta-analysis of dialysis access outcome in elderly patients. *J Vasc Surg* **45**, 420–426.

Ocak G, Halbesma N, le Cessie S, *et al.* (2011). Haemodialysis catheters increase mortality as compared to arteriovenous accesses especially in elderly patients. *Nephrol Dial Transplant* **26**, 2611–2617.

Rayner HC, Pisoni RL (2010). The increasing use of hemodialysis catheters: evidence from the DOPPS on its significance and ways to reverse it. *Semin Dial* **23**, 6–10.

Xi W, MacNab J, Lok CE, *et al.* (2010). Who should be referred for a fistula? A survey of nephrologists. *Nephrol Dial Transplant*, **25**, 2644–2651.

13.10 Effect of clopidogrel on early failure of arteriovenous fistulas for hemodialysis. A randomized controlled trial

Authors

LM Dember, GJ Beck, M Allon, JA Delmez, BS Dixon, A Greenberg, J Himmelfarb, MA Vazquez, JJ Gassman, T Greene, MK Radeva, GL Braden, TA Ikizler, MV Rocco, IJ Davidson, JS Kaufman, CM Meyers, JW Kusek, HI Feldman; Dialysis Access Consortium Study Group

Reference

Journal of the American Medical Association 2008, **299**, 2164–2171.

Abstract

Context: The arteriovenous fistula is the preferred type of vascular access for hemodialysis because of lower thrombosis and infection rates and lower health care expenditures compared with synthetic grafts or central venous catheters. Early failure of fistulas due to thrombosis or inadequate maturation is a barrier to increasing the prevalence of fistulas among patients treated with hemodialysis. Small, inconclusive trials have suggested that antiplatelet agents may reduce thrombosis of new fistulas....

Design, Setting, and Participants Randomized, double-blind, placebo-controlled trial conducted at 9 US centers composed of academic and community nephrology practices in 2003–2007. Eight hundred seventy-seven participants with end-stage renal disease or advanced chronic kidney disease were followed up until 150 to 180 days after fistula creation or 30 days after initiation of dialysis, whichever occurred later.

Intervention: Participants were randomly assigned to receive clopidogrel (300-mg loading dose followed by daily dose of 75 mg; n = 441) or placebo (n = 436) for 6 weeks starting within 1 day after fistula creation.

Main Outcome Measures: The primary outcome was fistula thrombosis, determined by physical examination at 6 weeks. The secondary outcome was failure of the fistula to become suitable for dialysis. Suitability was defined as use of the fistula at a dialysis machine blood pump rate of 300 mL/min or more during 8 of 12 dialysis sessions.

Results:...Fistula thrombosis occurred in 53 (12.2%) participants assigned to clopidogrel compared with 84 (19.5%) participants assigned to placebo (relative risk, 0.63; 95% confidence interval, 0.46–0.97; P = .018). Failure to attain suitability for dialysis did not differ between the clopidogrel and placebo groups (61.8% vs 59.5%, respectively; relative risk, 1.05; 95% confidence interval, 0.94–1.17; P = .40).

Conclusion: Clopidogrel reduces the frequency of early thrombosis of new arteriovenous fistulas but does not increase the proportion of fistulas that become suitable for dialysis. [Extract.]

Importance

Before this randomized controlled trial (RCT) was published, multiple studies had been undertaken of the effect of anti-platelet and anti-coagulant medication on the performance of native and graft arteriovenous fistulae (Saran *et al.*, 2002; Hasegawa *et al.*, 2008). Most of these studies had low power or were not randomized, so the evidence remained limited. Because of the problem of the widespread use of grafts and more recently early failure and non-maturation of native fistulae, the Dialysis Access Consortium (DAC) was established in the USA. The purpose of this consortium is to perform interventional studies in haemodialysis vascular access. In this RCT, the effect of an anti-platelet drug, clopidogrel, on early fistula outcome was measured in 877 incident patients with primary native fistulae. The primary endpoint was fistula thrombosis and secondary endpoint unsuitability of the fistula for dialysis treatment. This well-conducted study showed a significant reduction in post-operative fistula thrombosis in patients treated with clopidogrel (12.2 versus 19.5%). However, this did not result in more functional fistulae for dialysis treatment. A very high non-maturation rate of about 60% was found in both groups. The interpretation of the findings was that thrombosis risk had been reduced by clopidogrel but that vessel adaptation necessary for maturation had not been stimulated. This is an important message, especially given that this is a well-powered study.

However, some issues of study design may have influenced the outcome. The 877 patients were recruited in 27 hospitals over a 4-year period and dialysis was performed in 125 facilities. Fistula surgeries were performed by 71 surgeons, meaning an average number of only three operations per surgeon per year. One may wonder whether such limited experience is enough for the surgeons to achieve acceptable results (Gundevia *et al.*, 2008; Bourquelot *et al.*, 2011; see also paper 13.7).

In addition, although inclusion criteria for this study were well defined, it is not clear whether pre-operative vessel ultrasound evaluation to determine the strategy for access surgery was undertaken in all patients.

Compared with European studies, the non-maturation and early failure rates of both radio- and brachiocephalic fistulae were rather high and compared with the goals in most clinical practice guidelines are unacceptable. Nevertheless, this is probably the first RCT with enough power to prove any benefit of anti-platelet drugs on fistula outcome. Although fistula suitability for dialysis was not improved with clopidogrel use, one may question the design of this study, in particular taking into consideration the quality of the surgery.

References

Bourquelot P, Van-Laere O, Baaklini G, *et al.* (2011). Placement of wrist ulnar-basilic autogenous arteriovenous access for hemodialysis in adults and children using microsurgery. *J Vasc Surg* **53**, 1298–1302.

Gundevia Z, Whalley H, Ferring M, Claridge M, Smith S, Wilmink T (2008). Effect of operating surgeon on outcome of arteriovenous fistula formation. *Eur J Vasc Endovasc Surg* **35**, 614–618.

Hasegawa T, Elder SJ, Bragg-Gresham JL, *et al.* (2008). Consistent aspirin use associated with improved arteriovenous fistula survival among incident hemodialysis patients in the Dialysis Outcomes and Practice Patterns Study. *Clin J Am Soc Nephrol* **3**, 1373–1378.

Saran R, Dykstra DM, Wolfe RA, Gillespie B, Held PJ, Young EW; Dialysis Outcomes and Practice Patterns Study (2002). Association between vascular access failure and the use of specific drugs: the Dialysis Outcomes and Practice Patterns Study (DOPPS). *Am J Kidney Dis* **40**, 1255–1263.

Chapter 14

Peritoneal dialysis

Martin Wilkie and Sarah Jenkins

Introduction

The first tentative attempts at peritoneal dialysis (PD) in humans were in the 1920s, but its clinical value began to be appreciated in the 1950s when it was used in the field in the Korean War and helped save the lives of US soldiers with traumatic acute kidney injury (AKI). However, PD remained a treatment only deliverable in a hospital setting, and therefore only suitable for AKI, or as a stop-gap treatment until more definitive renal replacement therapy for end-stage renal disease (ESRD), by haemodialysis or transplantation, was established. Even for AKI, the use of PD lessened as haemodialysis became more widely available, except in small children.

However, in the late 1970s, the potential of PD as an acceptable long-term self-care therapy for ESRD began to be realized, and the ten landmark papers we have selected for this chapter all relate to the development of chronic PD and our growing understanding of its strengths and limitations.

In chronological order, we have started with the 1978 paper reporting the first experience with continuous ambulatory PD (CAPD). Then we have selected the 1989 description of the peritoneal equilibration test (PET), which has stood the test of time as a technique for evaluation of peritoneal membrane function, followed by the 1991 computer simulations of intraperitoneal volume curves based on the three-pore model of the peritoneal membrane.

From the early years of CAPD, the disadvantages of glucose as the osmotic agent in PD fluid were apparent, and we include the 1994 MIDAS Study, a description of the safety and efficacy of icodextrin, the one alternative to glucose that has stood the test of time. The long-term effect of PD fluid on peritoneal membrane structure and function is a challenge for the longevity of the technique of, so we have selected a 2001 study of long-term survivors on PD assessing the relationship between dialysate glucose exposure and changes to peritoneal membrane function, and a 2002 report of the long-term structural changes seen in the peritoneum from the Cardiff biopsy registry.

In the 1990s, the necessary dose of PD to achieve adequate dialysis was widely discussed, and to highlight this debate, we have selected the first report of ADEMEX, a randomized controlled trial (RCT) that helped establish a minimum dose of dialysis to be delivered, and also the EAPOS Study, which tested the adequacy of PD in patients with no residual renal function.

The importance of encapsulating peritoneal sclerosis as a rare but late life-threatening complication of PD is recognized in selecting the 2009 Scottish cohort study, which effectively described its epidemiology.

Finally, the remarkable variability in the use of PD across the developed world should not be ignored. Among many factors influencing these variations, we have selected a 2010 paper from Canada that explores with great care the complex barriers to self-care that need to be considered during shared decision-making about preferred dialysis modality.

14.1 Continuous ambulatory peritoneal dialysis

Authors

RP Popovich, JW Moncrief, KD Nolph, AJ Ghods, ZJ Twardowski, WK Pyle

Reference

Annals of Internal Medicine 1978, **88**, 449–456.

Abstract

The technique of continuous ambulatory peritoneal dialysis was evaluated in nine patients during 136 patient weeks. The major objectives were to see if continuous ambulatory peritoneal dialysis would provide [1] acceptable control of serum chemistries by usual criteria, [2] adequate removal of sodium and water, [3] tolerable protein losses, and [4] a low prevalence of peritonitis with episodes responsive to therapy with continuing continuous ambulatory peritoneal dialysis. Preliminary findings suggest continuous ambulatory peritoneal dialysis represents an effective ambulatory, portable, internal dialysis technique. Larger-solute clearances per week may approach values six times greater than with most hemodialysis techniques. Small-solute clearances approach dialysate flow rate (8.3 ml/min) and are comparable to other dialysis techniques on a weekly basis. Edema is readily controlled and protein losses should be tolerable with adequate protein intake. Peritonitis occurs on the average every 10 weeks but responds to therapy promptly with continuing continuous ambulatory peritoneal dialysis. If the prevalence of peritonitis can be reduced, continuous ambulatory peritoneal dialysis appears to represent a very attractive dialysis technique.

Importance

In the 1960s and 1970s, PD was recognized as a valuable addition to the range of renal replacement therapies available and was performed in hospital as an intermittent therapy. There had been case series of patients in which the mean exposure was 13.8 months, and the longest use of the technique was over 4 years (Palmer, 1971).

Against this background, Popovich had published in 1976 an abstract describing a 'novel portable/wearable equilibrium peritoneal dialysis technique' (Popovich *et al.*, 1976). Popovich's 1978 paper records a study of nine patients, selected because of problems with haemodialysis and trained to perform the dialysis themselves at home, in the new CAPD programme at the University of Missouri Medical Centre in cooperation with the University of Texas. Those patients under the care of the Texas unit disconnected from their PD system and used new tubing at every exchange, whereas the Missouri patients disconnected once a day. This paper recorded the beginnings of the home-based PD programmes that we recognize today.

The results reassured these pioneers of PD that their proposed system offered a real alternative to haemodialysis. Clearance of urea was lower than that seen with haemodialysis, but for vitamin B12 and inulin it was greater (Nolph, 1977). The dietary results and positive subjective patient reports suggested that PD enabled the patients to achieve an anabolic state. There was better blood pressure control attributed to improved salt and water balance, with the patients experiencing little oedema. However, the peritonitis rates were concerning, with 13 episodes occurring during 136 weeks of treatment and one patient requiring catheter replacement. The suggestion that improved connection and disconnection systems could influence the peritonitis rate was astute.

This paper heralded the beginning of PD as a home therapy, and it is remarkable for the foresight that the authors showed. Beyond the careful documentation of the indices of safety and efficacy, the discussion outlines most of the areas that continue to cause concern for nephrologists, including peritonitis rates, the need for improved connection technology, the effect of exposure to PD on the peritoneal membrane, and the search for biocompatible fluids. The authors suggested that chronic irritation of the membrane, due either to the dialysate itself or to contaminants including endotoxin and production materials, was of concern and 'deserved attention'. This has been amply borne out in studies of the impact of time on PD, as well as potential membrane irritants on progressive changes to the structure of the peritoneal membrane (Davies *et al.*, 1998; see also paper 14.6).

These preliminary results suggested that CAPD provided an effective and cost-efficient alternative to the time-consuming processes of haemodialysis or inpatient intermittent PD that was available at the time.

References

Davies S, Phillips L, Griffiths AM, Russell LH, Naish PF, Russell GI (1998). What really happens to people on long-term peritoneal dialysis? *Kidney Int* **54**, 2207–2217.

Nolph KD (1977). Short dialysis, middle molecules, and uremia. *Ann Intern Med* **86**, 93–97.

Palmer RA (1971). Peritoneal dialysis by indwelling catheter for chronic renal failure 1963–1968. *Can Med Assoc J* **105**, 376–379.

Popovich RP, Moncrief JW, Decherd JB, Bomar JB, Pyle WK (1976). The definition of a novel portable/ wearable equilibrium peritoneal dialysis technique. *Abstr Am Soc Artif Intern Organs* **5**, 64.

14.2 Clinical value of standardized equilibration tests in CAPD patients

Author

ZJ Twardowski

Reference

Blood Purification 1989, **7**, 95–108.

Abstract

Peritoneal transport rates, a critical determinant of peritoneal dialysis efficiency, vary widely among patients and may be easily categorized by standardized peritoneal equilibration test. Measurements of creatinine and glucose transfer are particularly useful in selecting optimal dialysis prescription. Patients with high-average peritoneal solute transport do well on standard CAPD even after losing residual renal function. Patients with high peritoneal solute transfer rates are likely to have inadequate ultrafiltration on standard CAPD. These patients do much better on dialysis regimens with short-dwell exchanges, such as nightly peritoneal dialysis or daytime ambulatory peritoneal dialysis. Patients with low-average and particularly with low peritoneal transport rates are likely to develop symptoms and signs of inadequate dialysis on standard CAPD as residual renal function becomes negligible, and may require high-dose peritoneal dialysis prescriptions.

Importance

In this landmark paper, Twardowski describes the PET, which to this day remains the routine clinical test giving a standardized evaluation of the movement of solute and water across the peritoneal membrane This deceptively simple test allows evaluation of ultrafiltration, transperitoneal movement of solute, rate of catheter flow, and estimation of the residual peritoneal volume. The standard test describes the equilibration of glucose and creatinine during a 4 h exchange of 2.27% glucose dialysate. This allows classification of patients into high, high average, low average, and low 'transporters' based on 4 h dialysate:plasma creatinine ratios A similar approach is applied to glucose reabsorption. The PET greatly simplified previous attempts to classify peritoneal membrane function using the measurement of the mass transfer coefficient for a range of solutes.

The utility of this deceptively simple test has been enormous. Twardowski has been proven correct in suggesting that it could be used to assess concordance with treatment and assess the loss of residual renal function. It also has a role in planning patient prescriptions, deciding on the most appropriate dialysis solutions for patient management, and monitoring long-term changes to the peritoneal membrane to understand mechanisms of peritoneal injury. It became clear that higher transporters had poorer outcomes on PD (Brimble *et al.*, 2006), leading to interventions to improve the outcome for these patients through the use of icodextrin and automated PD (to perform shorter cycles over night).

Variations of the PET have been developed including a version that can be conducted in the community where the patient infuses the dialysate at home so that the 4 h drain is scheduled to coincide with a nurse visit when the required samples are obtained. A 2 h version has been developed for use in children (Warady and Jennings, 2007). The Standard Permeability Assessment uses dextran 70 as a volume marker in a 3.86% glucose dialysate bag giving a larger ultrafiltration allowing for a more accurate assessment (Pannekeet *et al.*, 1995). The 'personal dialysis capacity', collects five dialysate samples over 24 h and allows a more accurate description of the parameters of the three-pore model (van Biesen *et al.*, 2003). A further approach evaluated the dialysate:plasma sodium concentration ratio ($D:P_{Na}$) as an indirect index of transcellular water transport by aquaporin channels (La Milia *et al.*, 2004).

The PET is robust, but there are possible causes of inaccuracy. The creatinine measurement should be corrected for the glucose concentration, as there is interference with the Jaffe analytical method. Secondly, the presence of an approximate 5% excess in the dialysis bags as well as the 'flush before fill' component of the twin-bag dialysis systems lead to a potential error and therefore the diaysate bags should be weighed to assess fluid volumes accurately. Thirdly, a large residual peritoneal volume can theoretically create inaccuracy by diluting the solute of the fresh bag to such an extent as to impact on the ultrafiltration volumes.

Despite developments over the last 20 years, the basic PET has not been superseded it in its utility, simplicity, and reproducibility.

References

Brimble KS, Walker M, Magetts PJ, Kundhal KK, Rabbat CG (2006). Meta-analysis: peritoneal membrane transport, mortality, and technique failure in peritoneal dialysis. *J Am Soc Nephrol* **17**, 2591–2598.

La Milia V, Di Filippo S, Crepaldi M, *et al.* (2004). Sodium removal and sodium concentration during peritoneal dialysis: effects of three methods of sodium measurement. *Nephrol Dial Transplant* **19**, 1849–1855.

Pannekeet MM, Imholz AL, Struijk DG, *et al.* (1995). The standard peritoneal permeability analysis: a tool for the assessment of peritoneal permeability characteristics in CAPD patients. *Kidney Int* **48**, 866–875.

van Biesen W, Carlsson O, Bergia R, *et al.* (2003). Personal dialysis capacity (PDC™) test: a multicentre clinical study. *Nephrol Dial Transplant* **18**, 788–796.

Warady BA, Jennings J (2007). The short PET in pediatrics. *Perit Dial Int* **27**, 441–445.

14.3 Computer simulations of peritoneal fluid transport in CAPD

Authors

B Rippe, G Stelin, B Haraldsson

Reference

Kidney International 1991, **40**, 315–325.

Abstract

To model the changes in intraperitoneal dialysate volume (IPV) occurring over dwell time under various conditions in continuous ambulatory peritoneal dialysis (CAPD), we have, using a personal computer, numerically integrated the phenomenological equations that describe the net ultrafiltration (UF) flow existing across the peritoneal membrane in every moment of a dwell. Computer modelling was performed according to a three-pore model of membrane selectivity as based on current concepts in capillary physiology. This model comprises small 'paracellular' pores (radius approximately 47 A) and 'large' pores (radius approximately 250 A), together accounting for approximately 98% of the total UF-coefficient (LpS), and also 'transcellular' pores (pore radius approximately 4 to 5 A) accounting for 1.5% of LpS. Simulated curves made a good fit to IPV versus time data obtained experimentally in adult patients, using either 1.36 or 3.86% glucose dialysis solutions, under control conditions; when the peritoneal UF-coefficient was set to 0.082 ml/min/mm Hg, the glucose reflection coefficient was 0.043 and the peritoneal lymph flow was set to 0.3 ml/min. Also, theoretical predictions regarding the IPV versus time curves agreed well with the computer simulated results for perturbed values of effective peritoneal surface area, LpS, glucose permeability-surface area product (PS or "MTAC"), intraperitoneal dialysate volume and dialysate glucose concentration. Thus, increasing the peritoneal surface area caused the IPV versus time curves to peak earlier than during control, while the maximal volume ultrafiltered was not markedly affected. However, increasing the glucose PS caused both a reduction in the IPV versus time curve "peak time" and in the "peak height" of the curves. The latter pattern was also seen when the dialysate volume was reduced. It is suggested that computer modelling based on a three-pore model of membrane selectivity may be a useful tool for describing the IPV versus time relationships under various conditions in CAPD.

Importance

This landmark paper by Rippe and colleagues described simulations of fluid movement based on the three-pore model of the capillary endothelium. They introduced the concept of the reflection coefficient, which describes the permeability of a membrane to a solute—which is equivalent to 1 when the membrane is completely impermeable and 0 when it is completely permeable. As the reflection coefficient for glucose at the level of the interendothelial small pores was as low as 0.03, they deduced that glucose could not be effective as an osmotic agent unless there was also a transcellular pore at which the reflection coefficient was 1. The presence of the transcellular pore was therefore hypothesized before it was subsequently identified as the 28 kDa water channel aquaporin (AQP), and it was shown that upregulation of AQP1 in peritoneal capillaries results in increased water permeability and ultrafiltration, without affecting the osmotic gradient or small solute permeability (Stoenoui *et al.*, 2003). Changes in AQP1 may also be a cause of ultrafiltration failure.

The three-pore model described in this simulation has now been confirmed by studies of intraperitoneal sodium mass to determine small-pore versus transcellular fluid transport, and studies using radio-iodinated serum albumin as an intraperitoneal volume marker (Asghar and Davies, 2008). These simulations also explain the phenomenon of sodium sieving with hypertonic glucose exchanges, making sodium removal less effective with ambulatory PD (APD) than with longer dwells on CAPD, possibly explaining why blood pressure may be less well controlled on APD than on CAPD. There is therefore now the possibility of modelling a range of clinical scenarios in PD patients and adjusting the PD prescription to account for individual variation, for example, to assess the effect of increasing the effective peritoneal surface area on the characteristics of the intraperitoneal volume curve with a range of solutions that increase small solute transport. Rippe and colleagues went on to model the effects of polyglucose as an osmotic agent as well as variations in glucose concentration (Rippe and Levin, 2000), and these effects have also been confirmed in the clinic (Jenkins and Wilkie, 2003). There have since been modifications of the three-pore model that take account of the role of the interstitium (the 'distributed model'), which becomes more important with time on PD, as well as the role of glycocalyx, an additional functional barrier in the interendothelial cleft.

References

Asghar RB, Davies SJ (2008). Pathways of fluid transport and reabsorption across the peritoneal membrane. *Kidney Int* **73**, 1048–1053.

Jenkins SB, Wilkie ME (2003). An exploratory study of a novel peritoneal combination dialysate (1.36% glucose/7.5% icodextrin), demonstrating improved ultrafiltration compared to either component studied alone. *Perit Dial Int* **23**, 475–480.

Rippe B, Levin L (2000). Computer simulations of ultrafiltration profiles for an icodextrin-based peritoneal fluid in CAPD. *Kidney Int* **57**, 2546–2556.

Stoenoui MS, Ni J, Verkaeren C, *et al.* (2003). Corticosteroids induce expression of aquaporin-1 and increase transcellular water transport in rat peritoneum. *J Am Soc Nephrol* **14**, 555–565.

14.4 A randomized multicenter clinical trial comparing isosmolar icodextrin with hyperosmolar glucose solutions in CAPD

Authors

CD Mistry, R Gokal, E Peers, and the MIDAS Study Group

Reference

Kidney International 1994, **46**, 496–503.

Abstract

…A randomized, controlled multicenter investigation of Icodextrin in ambulatory peritoneal dialysis (MIDAS) was undertaken to evaluate the long-term safety and efficacy by comparing daily overnight (8 to 12 hr dwell) use of isosmolar Icodextrin (282 mOsm/kg) with conventional 1.36% (346 mOsm/ kg) and 3.86% (484 mOsm/kg) glucose exchanges over six months. Two hundred and nine patients were randomized from 11 centers, with 106 allocated to receive Icodextrin (D) and 103 to remain on glucose (control group; C); 138 patients completed the six month study (71 C, 67 D). All patients were divided into weak (1.36%) or strong (3.86%) subgroups based on their use of glucose solutions overnight during the pretreatment baseline period. The mean ($\pm$ SEM) overnight ultrafiltration (UF) with D was 3.5 times greater than 1.36% glucose at eight hours [527 ± 36 vs. 150 ± 47 ml; 95% confidence interval (CI) for the difference $+ 257$ to $+497$ ml; $P < 0.0001$] and 5.5 times greater at 12 hours (561 ± 44 vs. 101 ± 48 ml, 95% CI for the difference $+329$ to $+590$; $P < 0.0001$) and no different from that of 3.86% glucose at eight hours (510 ± 48 vs. 448 ± 60 ml, 95% CI for the difference -102 to $+226$ ml; $P = 0.44$) and at 12 hours (552 ± 44 vs. 414 ± 78 ml, 95% CI for the difference -47 to $+325$ ml; $P = 0.06$). The biochemical profiles were no different in the two groups except for a small fall in serum sodium (140 to 136 mmol/liter) and chloride (103 to 99 mmol/liter) concentrations in the Icodextrin group. …This study demonstrates that the daily overnight use of an isosmolar icodextrin solution was safe and effective up to six months and could replace the overnight use of hyperosmolar glucose solutions. [Extract.]

Importance

Icodextrin (molecular weight 16,800 Da) is a starch-derived glucose polymer that was developed from a food supplement. Early work (Mistry *et al.*, 1987) showed that, despite being isosmotic with uraemic serum, icodextrin produced sustained ultrafiltration. Once the optimal concentration of 7.5% icodextrin had been determined, this 6-month study in 11 UK centres evaluated its safety and efficacy in clinical practice. Patients were randomized either to icodextrin 7.5% or to continue the pre-study glucose usage for the overnight dwell. Overnight ultrafiltration volume using icodextrin was 3.5 times greater than 1.36% glucose at 8 h and 5.5 times greater at 12 h, whereas it was equivalent to 3.86% glucose at 8 and 12 h. Icodextrin is metabolized to oligosaccharides, and the mean serum maltose in the icodextrin group increased from 0.04 g/l to a steady-state level of 1.20 g/l within 2 weeks, which was not associated with any adverse clinical effects. They went on to show that peritonitis rates did not differ with icodextrin (Gokal *et al.*, 1995).

Since this landmark paper, icodextrin has had a major impact on the long-term use of PD, especially in improving volume management, particularly in high transporters. More detailed studies of extracellular fluid volume and total body water measured using bioelectrical impedance and deuterium dilution have confirmed the benefits of icodextrin (Davies *et al.*, 2003). A more recent study in diabetic high transporters on CAPD showed that icodextrin improved volume status and also metabolic factors including glycated haemoglobin and lipid measurements (Paniagua *et al.*, 2009).

Safety concerns since the widespread introduction of icodextrin have been few, although there was an outbreak of sterile peritonitis associated with contamination by a product of bacterial cell wall (peptidoglycan), which has not recurred (Povlsen *et al.*, 2003). There are interactions between metabolites of icodextrin and certain glucose testing methods, and use of icodextrin renders serum amylase undetectable making the diagnosis of pancreatitis more difficult. Since this study, icodextrin has become incorporated as part of routine PD and has contributed to improved volume management high and high average transporters.

References

Davies S J, Woodrow G, Donovan K, *et al.* (2003). Icodextrin improves the fluid status of peritoneal dialysis patients: results of a double-blind randomized controlled trial. *J Am Soc Nephrol* **14**, 2338–2344.

Gokal R, Mistry CD, Peers EM (1995). Peritonitis occurrence in a multicenter study of icodextrin and glucose in CAPD. MIDAS Study Group. Multicenter Investigation of Icodextrin in Ambulatory Dialysis. *Perit Dial Int* **15**, 226–230.

Mistry CD, Mallick NP, Gokal R (1987). Ultrafiltration with an isosmotic solution during long peritoneal dialysis exchanges. *Lancet* **ii**, 178–182.

Paniagua R, Ventura MD, Avila-Diaz M, *et al.* (2009). Icodextrin improves metabolic and fluid management in high and high-average transport diabetic patients. *Perit Dial Int* **29**, 422–432.

Povlsen JV, Ivarsen P, Jorgensen KA, Madsen S (2003). Exposure to the peptidoglycan contaminant in icodextrin may cause sensitization of the patient maintained on peritoneal dialysis. *Perit Dial Int* **23**, 509–510.

14.5 Peritoneal glucose exposure and changes in membrane solute transport with time on peritoneal dialysis

Authors

SJ Davies, L Phillips, PF Naish, GI Russell

Reference

Journal of the American Society of Nephrology 2001, **12**, 1046–1051.

Abstract

Peritoneal solute transport increases with time on treatment in a proportion of peritoneal dialysis (PD) patients, contributing to ultrafiltration failure. Continuous exposure of the peritoneum to hypertonic glucose solutions results in morphologic damage that may have a causative role in changes in peritoneal function. The purpose of this analysis was to establish whether increased exposure to glucose preceded changes in solute transport in a selected group of long-term PD patients. Peritoneal solute transport, residual renal function, peritonitis rate, and peritoneal exposure to glucose were recorded prospectively in a cohort of 303 patients at a single dialysis center. A subgroup of individuals, treated continuously for 5 yr, were identified and defined retrospectively as having either stable or increasing transport status. Of the 22 patients who were treated continuously for 5 yr, 13 had stable solute transport (solute transport at start, 0.67 [±0.1]; at 5 yr, 0.67 [±0.1]), whereas 9 had a sustained increase (solute transport at start, 0.56 [±0.08]; at 5 yr, 0.77 [±0.09]). Compared with the stable patients, those with increasing transport had earlier loss in residual renal function and were exposed to significantly more hypertonic glucose during the first 2 yr of treatment that preceded the increase in solute transport. This was associated with greater achieved ultrafiltration compensating for the reduced urinary volumes in these patients. Further increases in glucose exposure were observed as solute transport continued to rise. Peritonitis, including severity of infection and causative organism, was similar in both groups. In this selected group of long-term survivors on PD, an increase in solute transport with time was preceded by increased peritoneal exposure to hypertonic glucose. This is supportive evidence that hypertonic glucose may play a causative role in alterations in peritoneal membrane function.

Importance

In this landmark paper, Davies and colleagues studied a group of patients who had received CAPD for a minimum of 5 years without interruption. The study was designed to answer the 'chicken and egg' question of which comes first: the use of hypertonic glucose exchanges in PD or changes to the peritoneal membrane transport characteristics. Previous studies had suggested that exposure to glucose dialysate solutions and the glucose degradation products that form advanced glycation end products is a factor in the structural changes that occur to the membrane (Krediet *et al.*, 2003).

Twenty-two patients had completed 5 years of uninterrupted PD, of whom 13 (group 1) had stable membrane solute transport over the study period (4 h PET dialysate:plasma creatinine ratio <0.1 difference from baseline) and the remaining nine patients (group 2) had a change of more than 0.1 from baseline. There were several differences between the groups. Group 2 patients had lower residual renal function at the start of the study and lost this residual function at an earlier stage. This was compensated for by an increase in ultrafiltration through the use of significantly more hypertonic exchanges. The study successfully answered the question it posed—the increased exposure to glucose seen in group 2 preceded the rise in solute transport and then continued to increase as the dialysate:plasma creatinine ratio increased.

As all patients had survived an uninterrupted 5 years on PD, they had necessarily avoided major episodes of peritonitis, making it unlikely that peritonitis was a prominent cause for the differences in membrane characteristics. The long duration of PD therapy also suggested that, even though group 2 had less residual renal function at the start of the study and lost it earlier than group 1, some other factor enabled them to be long-term technique survivors, perhaps defined by their low solute transport during the first 2 years of therapy.

This study was important because the prospective data demonstrated long-term evidence of a negative association between the higher concentration glucose dialysate use and peritoneal membrane functional status. Of equal importance was the observation that membrane function was stable in the patients who used the lower glucose dialysate concentrations. The observation that functional membrane change was associated with increased glucose exposure altered practice by emphasizing the need to use hypertonic glucose exchanges sparingly and, by implication, confirming that volume management should include fluid restriction and optimization of urine flow where possible.

Reference

Krediet RT, Zweers MM, Van Westrhenen R, Ho-dac-Pannekeet MM, Struijk DG (2003). What can we do to preserve the peritoneum? *Perit Dial Int* **23** (Suppl. 2), S14–S19.

14.6 Morphologic changes in the peritoneal membrane of patients with renal disease

Authors

JD Williams, KJ Craig, N Topley, C von Ruhland, M Fallon, GR Newman, RK Mackenzie, GT Williams, and on behalf of the Peritoneal Biopsy Study Group

Reference

Journal of the American Society of Nephrology 2002, **13**, 470–479.

Abstract

This study examined the morphologic features of the parietal peritoneal membranes of 130 patients undergoing peritoneal dialysis (PD) and compared them with the features of the peritoneal membranes of normal individuals, uremic predialysis patients, and patients undergoing hemodialysis. The median thickness of the submesothelial compact collagenous zone was 50 μm for normal subjects, 140 μm for uremic patients, 150 μm for patients undergoing hemodialysis, and 270 μm for patients undergoing PD ($P < 0.001$ for all versus normal subjects). Compact zone thickness increased significantly with the duration of PD therapy [0 to 24 mo, 180 μm ($n = 58$); 25 to 48 mo, 240 μm ($n = 24$); 49 to 72 mo, 300 μm ($n = 13$); 73 to 96 mo, 750 μm ($n = 16$); >97 mo, 700 microm ($n = 19$)]. Vascular changes included progressive subendothelial hyalinization, with luminal narrowing or obliteration. These changes were absent in samples from normal subjects but were present in 28% of samples from uremic patients and 56% of biopsies from patients undergoing PD. In the PD group, the prevalence of vasculopathy increased significantly with therapy duration ($P = 0.0001$). The density of blood vessels per unit length of peritoneum was significantly higher for patients with membrane failure and was correlated with the degree of fibrosis ($P = 0.01$). For the first time, a comprehensive cross-sectional analysis of the morphologic changes in the peritoneal membranes of patients undergoing PD is provided. The infrequency of fibrosis in the absence of vasculopathy suggests that vasculopathy may predispose patients to the development of fibrosis. This study provides a sufficiently large cohort of samples to allow structure–function relationships to be established, as well as providing a repository of tissue for further studies.

Importance

In response to the emerging evidence that PD impaired the long-term integrity of the peritoneal membrane, a peritoneal biopsy registry was established in Cardiff, UK, to examine the morphological features of the parietal peritoneal membrane in patients undergoing PD and compare them with normal individuals, uraemic but non-dialysed patients, and patients undergoing haemodialysis. A reproducible process was developed for sample collection in order to avoid artefacts due to collection or fixation.

This landmark study reported on peritoneal biopsies from 212 individuals, including nine normal patients, 25 uraemic patients, 48 patients undergoing haemodialysis, and 130 patients undergoing PD at 20 centres in Europe and Japan. Following informed consent, biopsies were collected at the time of abdominal surgery, for example from kidney-transplant donors, patients undergoing the placement of PD catheters, at the time of renal transplantation, or when the catheter was removed for intercurrent problems, excluding peritonitis.

The most prominent finding was an increase in the thickness of the submesothelial compact collagenous zone, which was associated with the duration of PD. Vascular abnormalities affecting predominantly venules, small veins, and arterioles were also noted with vessel wall thickening and capillary dilation associated with subendothelial hyaline material, luminal distortion, or obliteration. The prevalence of vasculopathy was not different after 2 years but thereafter increased in prevalence and severity with the duration of PD. The degree of fibrosis of the submesothelial compact zone was also related to the severity of the vasculopathy. Loss of mesothelium was related to both thickening of the submesothelial compact zone and the presence of vasculopathy.

This was the first systematic study of peritoneal morphology in PD, and demonstrated that the thickness of the submesothelial compact zone of the parietal peritoneum tends to increase with time on PD, although it was notable that uraemic patients who were not treated with PD also exhibited a degree of submesothelial fibrosis. The findings suggest a causal relationship between the vasculopathy and membrane thickening, raising the possibility that the vasculopathy results in a degree of ischaemia, which exacerbates the fibrosis. It seems likely that these morphological changes are a response to components of the dialysis process, and possible candidates include glucose exposure, acidic pH, the lactate buffer, and the presence of glucose degradation products. It is also likely that these structural changes underlie the changes to membrane function that can occur with time on PD, including the loss of ultrafiltration capacity and increases in small solute transport.

14.7 Effects of increased peritoneal clearances on mortality rates in peritoneal dialysis: ADEMEX, a prospective, randomized, controlled trial

Authors

R Paniagua, D Amato, E Vonesh, R Correa-Rotter, A Ramos, J Moran, S Mujais, and for the Mexican Nephrology Collaborative Study Group

Reference

Journal of the American Society of Nephrology 2002, **13**, 1307–1320.

Abstract

…A prospective, randomized, controlled, clinical trial was performed to study the effects of increased peritoneal small-solute clearances on clinical outcomes among patients with end-stage renal disease who were being treated with PD. A total of 965 subjects were randomly assigned to the intervention or control group (in a 1:1 ratio). Subjects in the control group continued to receive their preexisting PD prescriptions, which consisted of four daily exchanges with 2 L of standard PD solution. The subjects in the intervention group were treated with a modified prescription, to achieve a peritoneal creatinine clearance (pCrCl) of 60 L/wk per 1.73 m². The primary endpoint was death. The minimal follow-up period was 2 yr. …Patient survival was similar for the control and intervention groups in an intent-to-treat analysis, with a relative risk of death (intervention/control) of 1.00 [95% confidence interval (CI), 0.80 to 1.24]. Overall, the control group exhibited a 1-yr survival of 85.5% (CI, 82.2 to 88.7%) and a 2-yr survival of 68.3% (CI, 64.2 to 72.9%). Similarly, the intervention group exhibited a 1-yr survival of 83.9% (CI, 80.6 to 87.2%) and a 2-yr survival of 69.3% (CI, 65.1 to 73.6%). An as-treated analysis revealed similar results (overall relative risk = 0.93; CI, 0.71 to 1.22; P = 0.6121). Mortality rates for the two groups remained similar even after adjustment for factors known to be associated with survival for patients undergoing PD (e.g., age, diabetes mellitus, serum albumin levels, normalized protein equivalent of total nitrogen appearance, and anuria).…No clear survival advantage was obtained with increases in peritoneal small-solute clearances within the range achieved in this study. [Extract.]

Importance

The Adequacy of PD in Mexico (ADEMEX) study had the objective of determining whether an increment in small solute clearance improved patient survival. The preceding Canada and USA (CANUSA) cohort study had reported an association between small solute clearance and outcome, although subsequent reanalysis of the CANUSA study shows that patient outcome was unrelated to the PD prescription but rather to residual urine volume (Bargman *et al.*, 2001).

The ADEMEX protocol randomized patients into two different PD prescriptions, which resulted in a significant separation between the groups in both total Kt/V (see Chapter 12) and total creatinine clearance.

Survival in the two groups was identical. However, further analysis showed that discomfort and peritonitis were more common causes of study drop out in those randomized to achieve a higher Kt/V, whereas uraemia, hyperkalaemia, or congestive cardiac failure were more common causes of death in the control group. There was also a relationship of mortality risk with urine volume and peritoneal ultrafiltration consistent with the findings of other studies, including the European APD Outcome Study (Brown *et al.*, 2003; paper 14.8), that volume status is an important determinant for outcome in PD patients.

A subsequent study from Hong Kong also showed no impact on mortality when patients were randomized to three groups according to achieved *Kt/V* (Lo *et al.*, 2003), although there were more problems in those with the lowest *Kt/V*, leading the authors to recommend that the minimum *Kt/V* target should be 1.7. The importance of renal clearance and the absence of an effect of peritoneal clearance in the range of values common in current practice was confirmed in the Netherlands Cooperative Study on the Adequacy of Dialysis (Termorshuizen *et al.*, 2003).

The ADEMEX study challenged existing dogma that 'more is better' and made clear that there is no gain from uniform attempts to increase *Kt/V* above 1.7. Nevertheless, evidence from the Hong Kong study that patients start to deteriorate below a *Kt/V* of 1.7 means that this should be regarded as a minimum level of adequacy. It remains important to individualize patient care as suggested by the causes of study discontinuation and mortality in ADEMEX. Recommendations to consider combined urinary and peritoneal clearances to monitor dialysis adequacy with minimum treatment doses of Kt/V_{urea} of ≥1.7 per week or creatinine clearances of ≥50 l per week per 1.73 m² have been incorporated into current clinical practice guidelines (Woodrow and Davies, 2011).

References

Bargman JM, Thorpe KE, Churchill DN (2001). Relative contribution of residual renal function and peritoneal clearance to adequacy of dialysis: a reanalysis of the CANUSA study. *J Am Soc Nephrol* **12**, 2158–2162.

Brown EA, Davies SJ, Rutherford P, *et al.* (2003). Survival of functionally anuric patients on automated peritoneal dialysis: the European APD Outcome Study. *J Am Soc Nephrol* **14**, 2948–2957.

Lo WK, Ho YW, Li CS, *et al.* (2003). Effect of Kt/V on survival and clinical outcome in CAPD patients in a randomized prospective study. *Kidney Int* **64**, 649–656.

Termorshuizen F, Korevaar JC, Dekker FW, Van Manen JG, Boeschoten EW, Krediet RT (2003). The relative importance of residual renal function compared with peritoneal clearance for patient survival and quality of life: an analysis of the Netherlands Cooperative Study on the Adequacy of Dialysis (NECOSAD)-2. *Am J Kidney Dis* **41**, 1293–1302.

Woodrow G, Davies SJ (2011). Renal Association Clinical Practice Guideline on peritoneal dialysis. *Nephron Clin Pract* **118** (Suppl. 1), c287–c310.

14.8 Survival of functionally anuric patients on automated peritoneal dialysis: the European APD Outcome Study

Authors

EA Brown, SJ Davies, P Rutherford, F Meeus, M Borras, W Riegel, JC Divino Filho, E Vonesh, M van Bree and on behalf of the EAPOS Group

Reference

Journal of the American Society of Nephrology 2003, **14**, 2948–2957.

Abstract

The European APD Outcome Study (EAPOS) is a 2-yr, prospective, multicenter study of the feasibility and clinical outcomes of automated peritoneal dialysis (APD) in anuric patients. A total of 177 patients were enrolled with a median age of 54 yr (range, 21 to 91 yr). Previous median total time on dialysis was 38 mo (range, 1.6 to 259 mo), and 36% of patients had previously been on hemodialysis for >90 d. Diabetes and cardiovascular disease were present in 17% and 46% of patients, respectively. The APD prescription was adjusted at physician discretion to aim for creatinine clearance (Ccrea) $\geq$60 L/wk per 1.73 m^2 and ultrafiltration (UF) $\geq$750 ml/24 h during the first 6 mo. Baseline solute transport status (D/P) was determined by peritoneal equilibration test. At 1 yr, 78% and 74% achieved Ccrea and UF targets, respectively; median drained dialysate volume was 16.2 L/24 h with 50% of patients using icodextrin. Baseline D/P was not related to UF achieved at 1 yr. At 2 yr, patient survival was 78% and technique survival was 62%. Baseline predictors of poor survival were age (>65 yr; $P = 0.006$), nutritional status (Subjective Global Assessment grade C; $P = 0.009$), diabetic status ($P = 0.008$), and UF (<750 ml/24 h; $P = 0.047$). Time-averaged analyses showed that age, Subjective Global Assessment grade C and diabetic status predicted patient survival with UF the next most significant variable (risk ratio, 0.5/L per d; $P = 0.097$). Baseline Ccrea, time-averaged Ccrea, and baseline D/P had no effect on patient or technique survival. This study shows that anuric patients can successfully use APD. Baseline UF, not Ccrea or membrane permeability, is associated with patient survival.

Importance

This study examined the effect of APD in anuric patients from 13 European countries Throughout the study, the dialysis prescription was adjusted in order to achieve a creatinine clearance target of more than 60 l per week per 1.73 m^2 and an ultrafiltration target of more than 750 ml over 24 h.

The prescription algorithm for anuric PD patients was based on corrected body surface area and transport status. At baseline, the median overnight treatment time was 9.0 h (range, 7–12) with a median volume of 11.0 l (range, 6–28.75). The majority of patients also used a daytime dwell, with a median daytime dialysate volume of 4.0 l (range, 0–9.0), and many used an extra daytime exchange. The proportion of patients prescribed icodextrin for the long dwell increased throughout the study to 50% at 12 months and 60% at 24 months. A hundred and twenty patients did not complete the 2-year study and 31 (26.3%) died. The predominant cause of death was cardiovascular disease, with infection being second most common.

The 2-year actuarial patient survival was 78%, technique survival 62%, and combined patient and technique survival 49%. Parameters associated with significantly worse patient survival on univariate analysis included increasing age, worse subjective global assessment, increased comorbidity, diabetes, and reduced ultrafiltration at baseline. It is interesting to note that baseline ultrafiltration of more or less than 750 ml per day predicted outcome whereas creatinine clearance did not (Davies *et al.*, 2006).

The group that received icodextrin rather than glucose during the daytime exchange had more stable membrane function as evidenced by the 4 h dialysate:plasma creatinine ratios, which can be taken as supportive evidence that a reduction in glucose exposure is important for membrane stability

This study demonstrated that it is possible to conduct APD in anuric patients with outcomes that are similar to those from other studies of patients on PD. However, this was a selected group of patients (low transporters were under-represented) and the dialysis volumes in some patients were large. The study reinforced the importance of adequate volume management in patients on PD, which has been supported by subsequent studies and has led to an interest in exploring more closely the mechanisms of managing fluid in patients on PD.

Reference

Davies SJ, Brown EA, Reigel W, *et al.* (2006). What is the link between poor ultrafiltration and increased mortality in anuric patients on automated peritoneal dialysis? Analysis of data from EAPOS. *Perit Dial Int* **26**, 458–465.

14.9 Encapsulating peritoneal sclerosis in the new millennium: a national cohort study

Authors

MC Brown, K Simpson, J J Kerssens, RA Mactier on behalf of the Scottish Renal Registry

Reference

Clinical Journal of the American Society of Nephrology 2009, **4**, 1222–1229.

Abstract

Background and objectives: The study aim was to establish the incidence and characterize all encapsulating peritoneal sclerosis (EPS) cases in patients treated by peritoneal dialysis (PD).

Design, setting, participants, and measurements: The patient cohort, which started PD from January 1, 2000, to December 31, 2007, was identified from the Scottish Renal Registry (n = 1238). Possible EPS cases were identified by the ten adult Scottish renal units. Patient records were examined to ensure cases met diagnostic criteria.

Results: Forty-six cases were identified; 19 had their first PD exposure after January 1, 2000. The rate was 1.5%, an incidence of 4.9 per 1000 person-years. The incidence increased with PD duration, with rates of 0, 0.6, 2.0, 3.5, 8.1, 8.8 and 5% at <1, 1 to 2, >2 to 3, >3 to 4, >4 to 5, >5 to 6 and >6 yr PD exposure, respectively. The median PD duration of EPS cases was 5.1 yr (interquartile range [IQR] 3.4 to 6.1 yr). At diagnosis, 12 (26%) were on PD and 33 (72%) were diagnosed <2 yr after PD stopped. The cases had a median of 3.3 episodes of peritonitis (range 0 to 20, IQR 1 to 4.5). Thirty (65%) had used 3.86% dextrose dialysate and 45 (98%) had used Extraneal. The mortality was 42% at 1 yr postdiagnosis with a median survival of 149 d (IQR 61 to 408 d).

Conclusions: The incidence reported in this study may be used to inform patients of the minimum risk of developing EPS on PD.

Importance

Encapsulating peritoneal sclerosis (EPS) has become a feared complication of PD. Although uncommon it can have devastating consequences beyond merely PD technique failure. This landmark study was the first to report its epidemiology in a well-defined population. The Scottish Renal Registry reviewed all cases of EPS identified in Scotland, UK, from 2000 to 2007 using a cohort study of all adult patients who started PD in Scotland during that period. Using established diagnostic criteria, which rely on both clinical features and histological confirmation (Kawaguchi *et al.*, 2000), they identified an incidence of 8.7 per 1000 person-years of PD. However, the incidence was demonstrated to increase with time on PD, reaching 8.1% for those with 4–5 years exposure to the therapy. The prevalence of EPS in this and other studies in the same decade appeared to be higher than in earlier reports.

Overall, 91% of cases had undergone diagnostic imaging and 3% had undergone laparotomy or laparoscopy. At diagnosis, 26% were still on PD and the remainder were diagnosed within 2 years of stopping PD; 65% of cases had used fluids with high-concentration glucose and 98% had used icodextrin. Compared with the remainder of that PD population, a significantly larger proportion of EPS cases had stopped PD because of ultrafiltration failure or inadequate dialysis. Although the risk of EPS was near zero after 1 year of PD, the minimum risk after 4 years of PD was 1 in 12. However, the cumulative risk was modest at 2.6% by 5 years, reflecting the reality that few patients continue PD beyond 4 years so that EPS is a condition of technique survivors. The outlook, however, was poor; the mortality rate was 42% within 1 year of diagnosis, with the median survival from diagnosis being 180 days (range 1–1075 days).

Other subsequent cohort studies (Lambie *et al.*, 2010; Korte *et al.*, 2011) also seem to suggest an increased frequency or at least an improved rate of diagnosis of PD-associated EPS in recent years. Although care is needed in distinguishing association from causality, factors increasing the incidence of EPS in these reports include time on PD, dialysate glucose concentrations, and possibly the use of icodextrin. There is also an association with discontinuing PD, and perhaps with renal transplantation.

This Scottish Registry cohort provides a valuable description of EPS in a well-defined patient population. The epidemiology of EPS is complex and, given its rarity, the difficulties with delayed diagnosis, and its association with ultrafiltration failure, it remains difficult to disentangle the true risk factors. Regrettably, to date, the optimal treatment remains poorly defined. Nutritional optimization, the use of immunosuppressive agents and tamoxifen, and the role surgery at specialist centres all require further evaluation in prospective studies. (Celicout *et al.*, 1998; Augustine *et al.*, 2009).

References

Augustine T, Brown PW, Davies SD, Summers AM, Wilkie ME (2009). Encapsulating peritoneal sclerosis: clinical significance and implications. *Nephron Clin Pract* **111**, c149–c154.

Celicout B, Levard H, Hay J, Msika S, Fingerhut A, Pelissier E (1998). Sclerosing encapsulating peritonitis: early and late results of surgical management in 32 cases. French Associations for Surgical Research. *Dig Surg* **15**, 697–702.

Kawaguchi Y, Kawanishi H, Mujais S, Topley N, Oreopoulos DG, for the International Society for Peritoneal Dialysis Ad Hoc Committee on Ultrafiltration Management in Peritoneal Dialysis (2000). Encapsulating peritoneal sclerosis: definition, etiology, diagnosis, and treatment. *Perit Dial Int* **20** (Suppl. 4), S43–S55.

Korte MR, Sampimon DE, Lingsma HF, *et al.* (2011). Risk factors associated with encapsulating peritoneal sclerosis in Dutch EPS study. *Perit Dial Int* **31**, 269–278.

Lambie ML, John B, Mushahar L, Huckvale C, Davies SJ (2010). The peritoneal osmotic conductance is low well before the diagnosis of encapsulating peritoneal sclerosis is made. *Kidney Int* **78**, 611–618.

14.10 Impact of contraindications, barriers to self-care and support on incident peritoneal dialysis utilization

Authors

MJ Oliver, AX Garg, PG Blake, JF Johnson, M Verrelli, JM Zacharias, S Pandeya, RR Quinn

Reference

Nephrology Dialysis Transplantation 2010, **25**, 2737–2744.

Abstract

Background: Targets for peritoneal dialysis (PD) utilization may be difficult to achieve because many older patients have contraindications to PD or barriers to self-care. The objectives of this study were to determine the impact that contraindications and barriers to self-care have on incident PD use, and to determine whether family support increased PD utilization when home care support is available.

Methods: Consecutive incident dialysis patients were assessed for PD eligibility, offered PD if eligible and followed up for PD use. All patients lived in regions where home care assistance was available.

Results: The average patient age was 66 years. One hundred and ten (22%) of the 497 patients had absolute medical or social contraindications to PD. Of the remaining 387 patients who were potentially eligible for PD, 245 (63%) had at least one physical or cognitive barrier to self-care PD. Patients with barriers were older, weighed less and were more likely to be female, start dialysis as an inpatient and have a history of vascular disease, cardiac disease and cancer. Family support was associated with an increase in PD eligibility from 63% to 80% (P = 0.003) and PD choice from 40% to 57% (P = 0.03) in patients with barriers to self-care. Family support increased incidence PD utilization from 23% to 39% among patients with barriers to self-care (P = 0.009). When family support was available, 34% received family-assisted PD, 47% received home care-assisted PD, 12% received both family- and home care-assisted PD, and 7% performed only self-care PD. Incident PD use in an incident end-stage renal disease (ESRD) population was 30% (147 of the 497 patients).

Conclusions: Contraindications, barriers to self-care and the availability of family support are important drivers of PD utilization in the incident ESRD population even when home assistance is available. These factors should be considered when setting targets for PD.

Importance

In the developed world where the majority of dialysis patients are elderly with significant co-morbidities, barriers to self-care are one of the factors that may be responsible for the decline in PD usage. This study explored the impact on PD usage of contraindications and barriers to self-care in four Canadian dialysis centres where homecare assistance is available. Central to the study design was a 2-weekly multidisciplinary team meeting, including a nephrologist, specialist nurses, and a social worker who reviewed patients starting dialysis for contraindications to PD, barriers to self-care, and availability of support in the home.

Twenty-two per cent of the patients were judged by the multidisciplinary team to have absolute contraindications to PD. Of the remainder who were potentially eligible for PD, 63 had at least one physical or cognitive barrier to self-care PD, and in these patients the presence of a family member was associated with significant increases in PD eligibility, PD choice, and eventual PD utilization. When family support was available, 34% received family-assisted PD, 47% received homecare-assisted PD, 12% received both family- and homecare-assisted PD, and 7% performed self-care PD. Homecare assistance can increase the number of patients who can be safely offered PD (Oliver *et al.*, 2007), but the disadvantages of assisted PD should be considered. There is mixed evidence about the risk of peritonitis in patients receiving nurse or family assistance compared with autonomous patients (Verger *et al.*, 2007; Povlsen and Ivarsen, 2008; Castrale *et al.*, 2010). Nevertheless, the Broadening Options for Long-term Dialysis in the Elderly (BOLDE) study (patients aged 80 years or older) reported that dialysis modality was an independent predictor of illness intrusion, with greater intrusion felt in those on haemodialysis whilst quality of life was similar, if not better, in those on PD (Brown *et al.*, 2010).

This study demonstrated that, even when homecare assistance for PD is available, family support was an important driver of PD eligibility, choice, and use. However, despite the complex interventions described, the incident PD usage in this ESRD population was only 30%. This limitation needs to be recognized by healthcare planners who are increasingly placing emphasis on self-care modalities for renal replacement therapy.

References

Brown EA, Johansson L, Farrington K, *et al.* (2010). Broadening Options for Long-term Dialysis in the Elderly (BOLDE): differences in quality of life on peritoneal dialysis compared to haemodialysis for older patients. *Nephrol Dial Transplant* **25**, 3755–3763.

Castrale C, Evans D, Verger C, *et al.* (2010). Peritoneal dialysis in elderly patients: report from the French Peritoneal Dialysis Registry (RDPLF). *Nephrol Dial Transplant* **25**, 255–262.

Oliver MJ, Quinn RR, Richardson EP, Kiss AJ, Lamping DL, Manns BJ (2007). Home care assistance and the utilization of peritoneal dialysis. *Kidney Int* **71**, 673–678.

Povlsen JV, Ivarsen P (2008). Assisted peritoneal dialysis: also for the late referred elderly patient. *Perit Dial Int* **28**, 461–467.

Verger C, Duman M, Durand PY, Veniez G, Fabre E, Ryckelynck JP (2007). Influence of autonomy and type of home assistance on the prevention of peritonitis in assisted automated peritoneal dialysis patients. An analysis of data from the French Language Peritoneal Dialysis Registry. *Nephrol Dial Transplant* **22**, 1218–1223.

Chapter 15

Transplantation

Aisling Courtenay

Introduction

The earliest recorded attempt at renal transplantation was in 1902 in dogs and further experimental models were reported in the next decades. However sporadic efforts in humans were persistently disappointing with limited if any useful function from the engrafted organ.

The era of clinical organ transplantation really began after World War II. The surgical techniques were refined in Paris and Boston where some deceased donor transplants in the 1950s functioned for several weeks. The landmark case between identical twins in 1954 revealed the enormous potential of renal transplantation if the issue of rejection could be solved.

The immunological basis of rejection had been demonstrated by work on skin grafts in the 1940s and the concept of tissue antigens and donor antibodies was established in the late 1950s. By the mid-1960s the potential importance of HLA antigens in the outcome of renal transplantation was recognised, and humoral antibodies that resulted in hyperacute rejection were first demonstrated.

The incomplete understanding of the rejection process however did not halt further attempts at clinical renal transplantation. Initially in 1959 total body irradiation of the recipient offered some hope, with graft and patient survival exceeding 20 years in the first Boston case. However, the survival of irradiated patients overall, as a consequence of sepsis, was very discouraging. At the same time the use of 6-mercaptopurine showed promise in canine transplantation. From the early 1960s its derivative azathioprine, along with corticosteroids, became the established immunosuppressive regimen and long-term survival for patients with end-stage renal disease became a realistic option. The rate of graft loss generally however was in the region of 40% at 1-year. In the 1980s the introduction of ciclosporin improved outcomes further. There are now many alternative immunosuppressive medications with differing efficacy and safety. Graft loss due to irreversible rejection is now rare but the unwanted side-effects of long-term treatment remain concerning.

The insufficient number of donor organs available is one of the greatest challenges in transplantation. Live donor programmes have expanded and minimal invasive surgery makes this a more attractive prospect for many potential donors. The prerequisite for compatibility at ABO blood group and HLA tissue typing levels can also be overcome in selected cases with comparable long-term outcomes reported particularly for ABO incompatible transplants. Legislative changes have also allowed for sharing or exchanging organs in certain countries and provide opportunity for non-directed altruistic donation. The exploitation of live donors in so called 'transplant tourism' is an important international moral and ethical issue for the transplant community.

Many challenges remain in renal transplantation. Future developments may lead to a greater understanding and clinical application of tolerance, the ability to refine the immunological risk and immunosuppressive load for a given individual, and the use of stem cell technology to provide organs.

15.1 'Actively acquired tolerance' of foreign cells

Authors

RE Billingham, L Brent, PB Medawar

Reference

Nature 1953, **172**, 603–606.

Abstract

There is a fundamental problem with tissue homografts since the host immunological response results in destruction of the transplanted tissue. However experimental studies provide evidence that embryos are fully tolerant of grafts of foreign tissues, and in dizygotic cattle twins there is persistent of red blood cells from the zygote lineage of the twin. For long after birth the majority of cattle twins are tolerant of grafts of each other's skin.

We carried out a series of experiments in mice of different genetic strains. The natural course of skin grafts from A-line strain mice to CBA strain mice recipients was determined. Foetal CBA strain mice were then inoculated with tiny tissue clumps and cells of an adult A-line mouse, and subsequently received a skin graft from an A-line mouse at 21 days old.

In 3 out of 5 mice there was prolonged survival of the grafts which resembled autografts in every respect except their donor-specific albinism. One mouse subsequently received a second graft from an A-line donor and similarly there was no evidence of an immune response. The grafts in the remaining 2 mice were destroyed within days following the injection of lymph nodes fragments from an adult CBA mouse that had been immunised to A-line skin.

This work was extended with inoculation at birth, inoculation with different cell types, grafting of skin from a third strain, transplanting of previously tolerated grafts into CBA mice with unaltered immunity; and preliminary experiments were also conducted in chickens.

Our conclusions are: (1) mice and chicken never develop, or develop to only a limited degree, the power to react immunologically against foreign homologous tissue cells to which they have been inoculated in foetal life; (2) acquired tolerance is immunologically specific; (3) acquired tolerance is due to a specific failure of the host's immunological response. [Adapted.]

Importance

The disintegration of engrafted tissues and organs after varying time intervals was, in the first half of the last century, an insurmountable barrier to transplantation. Great urgency in elucidating the biological reasons for such failure arose during World War II with the high demand for skin engraftment following burns injuries. Peter Medawar's work on skin grafts in rabbits was pioneering and suggested that there was an immunological basis for the failure of transplantation (Medawar, 1944).

The significance of the earlier work by the immunologist Peter Gorer was unrecognized for some time. As early as 1936, he obtained antisera from rabbits inoculated with erythrocytes from three mouse strains that could identify three different blood group antigens in mice (Gorer, 1936). Tumours, containing antigen II, when engrafted into mice lacking this antigen, did not grow and the serum of such animals contained antibody to antigen II. Gorer then joined George Snell, a geneticist and future Nobel Laureate, who was studying tumour resistance genes (designated histocompatibility or H genes) in mice. Gorer's antiserum to antigen II was first to detect an allele at the H locus that was termed histocompatibility locus 2 or H-2 in 1948 (Gorer *et al.*, 1948). Other loci involved in histocompatibility were subsequently discovered; those associated with H-2, however, consistently produced a strong reaction and induced early rejection. The H-2 complex became known as the major histocompatibility complex in the mouse.

Gorer's work complemented that of Medawar and colleagues, and the series of experiments reported here involved some of the same mice strains as Gorer's original experiments, although it would be some time before the link between their discoveries was recognized. This paper is a landmark as it offered the first evidence that the immune response could be modified so as to avoid rejection. In essence, the inoculation of fetuses *in utero* with foreign donor cells, before the immunological system was sufficiently developed to distinguish between 'self' and 'non-self', produced chimaeric mice that subsequently did not react immunologically to donor tissue. The extension of this work provided important new insights into the immune system and tolerance. Medawar was awarded the Nobel Prize in 1960.

A model for the development of true tolerance in clinical transplantation remains elusive. The discovery of microchimaerism in long-standing renal and hepatic transplant recipients (Starzl *et al.*, 1992) has renewed interest in the chimaeric paradigm first raised in this paper, which retains its importance as a seminal work in the field of transplant immunobiology.

References

Gorer PA (1936). The detection of antigenic differences in mouse erythrocytes by the employment of immune sera. *Br J Exp Pathol* **17**, 42–50.

Gorer PA, Lyman S, Snell GD (1948). Studies on the genetic and antigenic basis of tumour transplantation. Linkage between a histocompatibility gene and "fused" in mice. *Proc Roy Soc Lond Biol Sci* **135**, 499–505.

Medawar PB (1944). The behaviour and fate of skin autografts and skin homografts in rabbits: a report to the War Wounds Committee of the Medical Research Council. *J Anat* **78**, 176–199.

Starzl TE, Demetris AJ, Murase N, Ildstad S, Ricordi C, Trucco M (1992). Cell migration, chimerism, and graft acceptance. *Lancet* **339**, 1579–1582.

15.2 Successful homotransplantation of the human kidney between identical twins

Authors

JP Merrill, JE Murray, JH Harrison, WR Guild

Reference

Journal of the American Medical Association 1956, **160**, 277–282.

Abstract

A patient whose illness had begun with edema and hypertension was found to have suffered extreme atrophy of both kidneys. Because of the steady worsening of the condition and the appearance of uremia with other unfavourable prognostic signs, transplantation of one kidney from the patient's healthy identical twin brother was undertaken.

Preparations included collection of evidence of monozygosity and experimental transplantation of a skin graft from the twin. During the transfer of the healthy kidney it was totally ischemic for 82 minutes. Evidence of functional activity in the transplanted kidney was obtained.

The hypertension persisted until the patient's diseased kidneys were both removed. The homograft has survived for 11 months, and the marked clinical improvement in the patient has included disappearance of the signs of malignant hypertension.

Importance

The transplantation of a kidney from Ron Herrick into his identical twin brother, Richard, 2 days before Christmas in 1954, is universally considered the world's first successful organ transplant. The recipient survived with self-supporting renal function for 8 years, and the donor for 56 years.

The ground work for renal transplantation began in the early 1900s when several investigators performed auto- and homotransplantations in animals. The most influential of these was Alexis Carrel, considered the father of transplant and vascular surgery, who established the techniques of vascular anastomoses that remain in use today. He noted a substantial difference between the function of autotransplants (transplanting a kidney from the renal fossa to the neck) and homotransplants (engrafting a kidney from another individual of the same species). The former would last indefinitely after the other kidney had been removed, but if there was function in the latter it was for a few days only.

Transplantation in humans was attempted occasionally thereafter as a bridge for anuric acute kidney injury, the first reported case being by Yu Yu Voronoy in 1936, but with limited success. In 1950, two different groups in France performed several transplants, with Rene Küss being the first to place the graft retroperitoneally in the pelvis with anastomoses to the iliac vessels (Küss *et al.*, 1951). Jean Hamburger reported 'useful' function for 23 days in a live donation from a mother to son in 1953 (Michon *et al.*, 1953), but in general there was little function beyond the few days observed in animal models.

In Boston, David Hume reported measurable graft function with urine production from 37 to 180 days (average 97 days) in four out of nine cases of renal transplants in the early 1950s (Hume *et al.*, 1955). Grafts were placed in the upper thigh and all ultimately failed.

Thus, the technical feasibility of renal transplantation was established, but with limited understanding of the rejection process, or how to modify it, the outcomes remained poor.

By chance, at the time Hume was submitting his case series for publication, a young man with advanced renal failure presented to the Boston Public Health Hospital. He had a twin brother. One of his physicians suggested renal transplantation as a possible, or indeed the only, option. It was already established that skin transplantation between identical twins was successful, and experimental observations suggested that a kidney might behave similarly if transplanted. After determining 'beyond a reasonable doubt' that the twins were monozygotic, the surgery went ahead. The kidney was placed in the pelvis, copying the work of the French, which has since been the established standard technique for renal transplantation.

There was early graft function with clinical and biochemical improvement. The recipient was sufficiently well to fall in love with one of the nurses who had volunteered to work that Christmas and who looked after him in his recovery—they later married!

This transplant procedure was remarkable neither for the technical aspect of engraftment nor for its advance of immunobiology or pharmacology. Not alluded to in the paper, but for which it is fundamentally important, was the change in public perception of kidney transplantation as a potentially viable and curative procedure. There was considerable ethical debate about the morality of removing a kidney from a healthy individual, and early transplant advocates faced overt criticism from within and without medical circles. The fact that a successful outcome was possible and life-saving, coupled with the extensive media coverage this case generated, revolutionized attitudes to renal transplantation. The landmark nature of this case is a testament to the courage as well as skill of the authors.

References

Hume DM, Merrill JP, Miller BF, Thorn GW (1955). Experiences with renal homotransplantation in the human: report of nine cases. *J Clin Invest* **34**, 327–382.

Küss R, Teinturier J, Milliez P (1951). Quelques essais de greffe de rein chez l'homme [Some attempts at kidney transplantation in man]. *Mem Acad Chir (Paris)* **77**, 755–764.

Michon L, Hamburger J, Oeconomos N, *et al.* (1953). Une tentative de transplantation rénale chez l'homme: aspects médicaux et biologiques [An attempted kidney transplantation in man: medical and biological aspects]. *Presse Med* **61**, 1419–1423.

15.3 Prolonged survival of human-kidney homografts by immunosuppressive drug therapy

Authors

JE Murray, JP Merrill, JH Harrison, RE Wilson, GJ Dammin

Reference

New England Journal of Medicine 1963, **268**, 1315–1323.

Summary

To be successful, homotransplantation requires conditioning of the recipients to suppress the immune response. Empirical approaches to this issue involve irradiation, total body or focal, with or without additional chemical suppression. However, in canine renal transplantation, drug therapy alone has successfully prolonged graft survival, and this may be a feasible option for human transplantation.

We used drugs as the sole modality for the suppression of immunity in a series of 13 patients who received a kidney homograft. The initial cases have been previously described; five recent cases are reported in detail here. Imuran and azaserine were used in combination for 21 days, at which point the latter was replaced by actinomycin C. Prednisolone was used as rescue therapy if there was rejection that was not reversed with actinomycin C.

One patient received a cadaveric kidney that is still functioning after 1 year; one had good function for 5 months after transplantation from an unrelated infant but then died of a cerebral haemorrhage; the other three all received kidneys from adult live donors, between 4 weeks and 3 months ago, which continue to function well.

Reliance solely on drug therapy without the use of irradiation is a feasible approach in the conditioning of recipients for homotransplantation. The advantages of such an approach include the ability to alter drug dosage according to clinical response, the therapy does not need to be initiated before the transplant, the extreme environmental precautions necessitated by total body irradiation are not required, and there is absence of complete inhibition of the host immune system.

Importance

The rejection of transplanted organs was an insurmountable barrier to clinical transplantation in the 1950s, which was all the more frustrating given the success of renal transplantation between monozygotic twins.

The initial attempt to overcome this immunological barrier was to pre-condition the recipient by total body irradiation. Whilst this had the desired effect in terms of preventing the rejection of the graft, and the first two recipients from 1959 lived over 20 years (Merrill *et al.*, 1960; Hamburger *et al.*, 1962), the majority of patients succumbed to infection, despite extreme environmental precautions.

Meanwhile, a young English surgeon called Roy Calne began using 6-mercaptopurine, which had been developed in the 1950s for the treatment of leukaemia, with some success in experimental transplant models (Calne, 1960). He continued his work in Boston with Joseph Murray and another future Nobel Laureate, George Hitchings, and the modified molecule azathioprine was produced. The effectiveness of this drug in canine transplantation prompted its use, as an alternative to irradiation, in human renal transplantation. The first two patients received this drug in 1961, but unfortunately the dose of azathioprine used in dogs, 12 mg/kg, was lethal in man.

The dose was titrated down and by the eighth and subsequent recipients in Boston, a tolerable dose of 3 mg/kg was used.

This landmark paper reported in detail the course of five Boston recipients and was the first to demonstrate that graft survival between genetically distinct individuals was possible in the absence of irradiation.

Such a development was highly significant for a number of reasons. Importantly, there was now an option for deceased-donor transplantation, as pre-conditioning of the recipient was not required. Unlike the consequences of radiation treatment, there was now the possibility of titrating the degree of immunosuppression with the patient's response as determined both clinically and by laboratory markers. Also, importantly, the 'drug-treated host [was] not an immunological cripple', as demonstrated by the ability of some recipients to survive sepsis successfully while on immuno-suppressive therapy. This was a significant advance.

The authors acknowledged many unknowns at that time including: the duration of time for which these drugs would be necessary, whether the possibility of rejection diminishes with the passage of time, and the uncertainty over the role of prednisolone: 'the place of corticosteroid therapy in the reversion of rejection is still unsettled'. They also did not know that the 'cautious optimism' they concluded with was indeed more than justified, with azathioprine becoming a mainstay of immunosuppressive therapy for renal transplantation.

References

Calne RY (1960). The rejection of renal homografts. Inhibition in dogs by 6-mercaptopurine. *Lancet* i, 417–418.

Hamburger J, Vaysse J, Crosnier J, Auvert J, Lalanne CM, Hopper J Jr (1962). Renal homotransplantation in man after radiation of the recipient. Experience with six patients since 1959. *Am J Med* **32**, 854–871.

Merrill JP, Murray JE, Harrison JH, Friedman EA, Dealy JB, Dammin GJ (1960). Successful homotransplantations of the kidney between non-identical twins. *N Engl J Med* **262**, 1251–1260.

15.4 The reversal of rejection in human renal homografts with subsequent development of homograft tolerance

Authors

TE Starzl, TL Marchioro, WR Waddell

Reference

Surgery, Gynecology and Obstetrics 1963, **117**, 385–395.

Summary

Long-term survival of renal homotransplants is consistently threatened by rejection, and with little prospect of successful reversal of the immunological process the outlook has been pessimistic. Our experience suggests that is possible to manage rejection successfully in the majority of cases.

The first ten recipients of renal homografts from live donors from November 1962 to May 1963 were studied. The first patient had total body irradiation, and all subsequent recipients received azathioprine pre- and post-transplantation. Splenectomy was performed in all ten patients and thymectomy in seven. Rejection crises were diagnosed clinically by a systemic febrile response, severe hypertension, oliguria or anuria, and acute renal failure.

Seven of the nine patients that survived the immediate post-operative period unequivocally suffered a severe rejection crisis. One of the others had been given 100 mg of prednisone daily from the time of transplantation, but died at 113 days from surgery from an unrecognized intra-abdominal abscess. The time to and rapidity of development of rejection varied. Prednisone and actinomycin C were used as secondary anti-rejection agents. The dose of azathioprine was increased temporarily in most cases, and to a level that induced leukopenia deliberately in two cases where second-line therapy had been ineffective. There was successful reversal of rejection, in terms of improvement in renal function, in all cases with minimal or undetectable permanent functional damage. In just one case was there recurrence of rejection.

The rejection process in humans receiving renal homografts can seldom be entirely prevented but its effects can be reversed with a high degree of regularity and completeness by the addition of actinomycin C and massive doses of prednisone to pre-existing azathioprine therapy. A state of host-graft non-reactivity seems to follow the successful treatment of a rejection crisis.

Importance

In the early 1960s, successful renal transplantation between genetically non-identical individuals was becoming a possibility. The development of azathioprine as an immunosuppressant agent meant that irradiation, with its obvious disadvantages, was no longer essential. However, despite the optimism engendered by this new agent, rejection still occurred frequently, with limited scope for its reversal.

In this landmark paper, Thomas Starzl claimed that 'the rejection process...can be reversed with a high degree of regularity and completeness'.

The report detailed with precision the clinical course, management, and outcomes of ten live-donor transplant procedures, none of which were between identical twins, over a 6-month period to May 1963. The use of live-donor organs with a very minimal ischaemic time resulted in immediate graft function in all but one transplant (which was complicated by an intra-operative cardiac arrest). This ensured that 'the onset of acute rejection [could] be diagnosed with great accuracy'. The diagnosis was based on clinical features, as there was a reluctance to biopsy transplanted kidneys at that time.

The second-line agents used to manage the rejection crises were prednisone and actinomycin C. The rationale for the latter was cytocidal action that was relatively selective for lymphocytes and which had been used in animal models. Starzl and colleagues were successful in reversing the rejection process in all of their patients in this series, with minimal sequelae. Thus, the concept that acute rejection is a reversible phenomenon in human renal transplantation was developed.

The authors in this paper also raised the question of tolerance in transplantation. They noted what they termed 'a state of relative immunological non-reactivity', as a return to previous maintenance levels of immunosuppression was sufficient to suppress the immune response following the rejection episode. In only one case was there a second episode of rejection. Further work with this cohort and subsequent recipients in Colorado led to the realization that a time-related reduction in immunosuppression was possible.

The subsequent refinement of anti-rejection therapy included the realization that splenectomy and thymectomy were not necessary, the use of prednisone as a maintenance therapy alongside azathioprine reduced rejection incidence, and the refinement of drug dosing allowing effective immunological suppression without life-threatening consequences. Successful prolonged survival without early infectious deaths became a reality from the mid-1960s onward (McGeown *et al.*, 1977).

Reference

McGeown MG, Kennedy JA, Loughridge WG, *et al.* (1977). One hundred kidney transplants in the Belfast City Hospital. *Lancet* **ii**, 648–651.

15.5 Hyperacute rejection of kidney allografts, associated with pre-existing humoral antibodies against donor cells

Authors

F Kissmeyer-Nielsen, S Olsen, VP Petersen, O Fjeldborg

Reference

Lancet 1966, **ii**, 662–665.

Summary

Transplant immunity is predominantly cellular, and circulating antibodies to donor cells after kidney transplantation have not been reported. However, very rapid rejection of grafts has been described in cases of major ABO incompatibility, presumably due to the presence of ABO antibodies in the recipient and ABO antigens in the graft. It is possible that humoral antibodies have a role in homograft rejection, but the importance of such antibodies is uncertain.

We analysed the clinical features, serology, and pathology of two cases of hyperacute rejection in our series of 21 consecutive human kidney allotransplantations.

Both cases were females in their 30s, both had several weeks of peritoneal dialysis prior to receiving a cadaveric kidney transplant, and both had had several pregnancies and blood transfusions. There was immediate function with urine production after opening the anastomoses, but quickly the grafts became soft, flabby, and cyanotic with no urine production. Graft nephrectomy was performed at 3 and 14 days after transplantation. Both patients subsequently died of sepsis.

Serological investigations demonstrated that both patients were heavily isoimmunized with extremely strong leukocyte agglutinins and complement-fixing thrombocyte antibodies. The circulating antibodies were active against antigens from the cadaver donors used. Pathology revealed widespread necrosis with extensive microthrombi in most glomeruli and juxtaglomerular arterioles but with no interstitial cell infiltrate.

It is believed that the identified humoral antibodies played a decisive part in the hyperacute rejections, which happened within 1 h of the re-establishment of renal circulation and initial urine flow.

Importance

This is a landmark paper, as it was the first time that there had been demonstrable donor-specific antibodies in the serum of renal transplant recipients, resulting in graft destruction. The presence of such antibodies had been postulated for some time but never previously identified.

W. J. Dempster, a London surgeon, made important contributions in the early days of transplantation. He worked extensively with canine models, and in 1951 concluded that the destruction of transplanted graft was due to an 'actively acquired immunity reaction' (Dempster, 1951). However, there were many unknowns, including the number and nature of genes involved in tissue incompatibility, and the troubling absence of demonstrable antibodies in the serum of transplant recipients. This report by Kissmeyer-Nielsen came 15 years after Dempster had prophesied that 'it may be that, with proper techniques, antibodies to tissue antigens will be demonstrated in the serum of the host'.

By this stage, there had been considerable advances in the understanding of immunobiology, much of which had come from the study of multiparous women and those who had received multiple blood transfusions (both characteristics of the two patients with hyperacute rejection in this paper). In 1958, the French immunologist Jean Dausset reported that the sera of seven patients, who had previously received multiple blood transfusions, reacted in a similar manner causing leukocyte agglutination in 11 out of 19 volunteers (Dausset, 1958). Dausset concluded that the antisera detected an alloantigen on human leukocytes. Dausset is thus credited with the first discovery of an HLA antigen, which was termed MAC, the first initials of three of his important volunteers. He concluded that 'in a more long time perspective, the study of leucocyte antigens might become of great importance in tissue transplantation' (translated).

Other investigators, such as Jan van Rood and Rose Payne, used sera from multiparous women to identify other leucocyte antigens, termed LA1, LA2, and so on. By the second International Histocompatibility Workshop in 1965, it was apparent that several specifities were common across different groups, including for example MAC and LA2, which became known as HLA-A2 (Bruning *et al.*, 1965). In the late 1960s came the first indication from Paul Terasaki and others that HLA matching may be important in the outcomes of kidney transplantation (Kissmeyer-Nielsen and Thorsby, 1970). This paper in 1966 added to the rapid development and clinical application of transplant immunobiology in this era.

From these early observations, there has evolved an increasingly sophisticated understanding of HLA alleles, and the development of laboratory techniques to identify donor-specific antibodies with increasing sensitivity. This field continues to evolve, with the hope that this will be of increasing benefit to clinical transplantation.

References

Bruning JW, van Leeuwen A, van Rood JJ (1965). Leukocyte antigens. In: *Histocompatibility Testing*, pp. 275–284. Edited by DB Amos and JJ van Rood. Munksgaard, Copenhagen.

Dausset J (1958). Iso-leuco-anticorps. *Acta Haematol* **20**, 156–166.

Dempster WJ (1951). Problems involved in the homotransplantation of tissues, with particular reference to skin. *Brit Med J* **2**, 1041–1049.

Kissmeyer-Nielsen F, Thorsby E (1970). Human transplantation antigens. *Transplant Rev* **4**, 1–176.

15.6 Successful seventeen-hour preservation and transplantation of human-cadaver kidney

Authors

FO Belzer, BS Ashby, PF Gulyassy, M Powell

Reference

New England Journal of Medicine 1968, **278**, 608–610.

Summary

Transplantation of cadaveric organs remains limited by the inability to store such grafts. Long-term organ preservation and the development of a true organ bank will probably not be possible until the problems of freezing and thawing have been solved, but even short-term preservation for less than 72 h would be of great benefit. Potentially the patient could remain at home rather than in a hospital on a constant standby status, and there would be time to allow tissue-typing work. On the basis of our results in canine transplantation, we attempted to preserve a human cadaver kidney.

The donor was a 44-year-old man with a fatal head injury. The right kidney was removed after a total warm ischaemia time of 25 min, and transported at 4 °C to the laboratory. It was connected to extracorporeal perfusion apparatus after a total ischaemia time of 55 min. The total anoxia time was 17 h before the kidney was transplanted in the normal fashion into a 47-year-old man with terminal uraemia.

Urine production occurred 20 min after re-establishment of the vascular supply. Despite good quantities of urine for the first 10 days, the creatinine clearance remained low. There was gradual improvement in renal function with a creatinine clearance of 31 ml/min by time of discharge from hospital 7 weeks after transplantation.

Encouraging results in laboratory experiments suggest that short-term organ preservation should be possible in transplantation. We report the successful implantation and function of a human cadaver kidney 17 h after donor death, with the use of an extracorporeal perfusion circuit for 15.5 h. We hope to convert this apparatus to be fully portable so it can be taken to the donor's hospital and thereby minimize anoxia in future cases.

Importance

Early clinical success in renal transplantation was in live donation, but clearly if transplantation was to be a useful therapeutic option, extension beyond live donation was essential. In the absence of a means of preserving organs, however, grafts from deceased donors were available only to those essentially living in the hospital awaiting a suitable organ. In addition to the obvious practical limitations with this approach, the short time frame also prohibited the possibility of tissue-typing work. By 1965, Paul Terasaki had suggested that HLA matching was an important determinant of graft outcome.

Alexis Carrel had experimented with the perfusion of organs using small pumps in the early part of the last century. Folkert Belzer, however, was the pioneer of organ preservation in clinical transplantation. He developed a perfusion device that consisted of a pump, perfusion chamber, membrane oxygenator, filter, and heat exchanger that functioned satisfactorily in animal models.

This paper was the first report of successful implantation of a deceased-donor kidney after a prolonged ischaemic time. Although the post-transplant course was complicated by a hypotensive episode due to retroperitoneal haemorrhage, the kidney ultimately functioned satisfactorily.

Belzer's plan for a 'portable' device was realized, although it was so sizeable he had to rent a truck to transport his invention whenever he went to harvest organs!

The alternative to machine perfusion in organ preservation is perfusion by gravity and subsequent cold storage. One of the first solutions was Collins' solution (Collins *et al.*, 1969), which was adapted by the Eurotransplant Organization, with the subsequent solution being termed Eurocollins. Comparative analysis suggested that this was a viable alternative to machine perfusion (Clark *et al.*, 1973), and it was certainly more practical. Belzer then worked systematically to optimize the chemistry of the preservation fluid and produced the University of Wisconsin (UW) solution, which is still considered the gold standard solution in renal transplantation, allowing successful engraftment after many hours of cold ischaemia (Ploeg *et al.*, 1992).

More recently, there has been a renaissance of interest in machine perfusion in an effort to minimize additional insults to extended criteria kidneys and organs donated after circulatory death. There is registry evidence now supported by a randomized controlled trial that pulsatile perfusion reduces the risk of delayed graft function and improves transplant outcomes (Moers *et al.*, 2009). Current devices, however, are considerably more portable than Belzer's original prototype!

Belzer's vision of an 'organ bank' has never been realized, but his work in organ preservation was fundamental in establishing deceased-donor transplantation as a viable option for multitudes requiring a renal transplant but without a living donor.

References

Clark EA, Opelz G, Mickey MR, Terasaki PI (1973). Evaluation of Belzer and Collins kidney-preservation methods. *Lancet* **i**, 361–364.

Collins GM, Bravo-Shugarman M, Terasaki PI (1969). Kidney preservation for transportation: initial perfusion and 30 hours' ice storage. *Lancet* **ii**, 1219–1222.

Moers C, Smits JM, Maathuis MH, *et al.* (2009). Machine perfusion or cold storage in deceased-donor kidney transplantation. *N Engl J Med* **360**, 7–19.

Ploeg RJ, van Bockel JH, Langendijk PT, *et al.* (1992). Effect of preservation solution on results of cadaveric kidney transplantation. The European Multicentre Study Group. *Lancet* **340**, 129–137.

15.7 Cyclosporin A in patients receiving renal allografts from cadaver donors

Authors

RY Calne, DJ White, S Thiru, DB Evans, P McMaster, DC Dunn, GN Craddock, BD Pentlow, K Rolles

Reference

Lancet 1978, **ii**, 1323–1327.

Abstract

Seven patients on dialysis with renal failure received transplants from mismatched cadaver donors and were treated with cyclosporin A (CyA), initially as the sole immunosuppressive agent. CyA was effective in inhibiting rejection but there was clear evidence of both nephrotoxicity and hepatotoxicity. A cyclophosphamide analogue was added to the CyA treatment in six of the patients. Five patients are out of hospital with functioning allografts, and two of these have received no steroids. One patient required an allograft nephrectomy because of pyelonephritis in the graft. Another died of systemic aspergillus and candida infection. Further careful study of this potentially valuable drug will be required before it can be recommended in clinical practice.

Importance

The combination of steroids and azathioprine was the standard immunosuppression therapy for renal transplantation from the mid-1960s. This therapy was revolutionary, avoiding irradiation and permitting transplantation between genetically distinct individuals and from deceased donors. Alternative immunosuppressive agents were sought, however, because severe rejection episodes did still occur, and the side-effects of both steroids and bone-marrow toxicity were marked in some individuals.

Cyclosporin A (CyA) was first isolated from a fungal extract in 1971 and was noted to have immunosuppressive qualities without cytotoxicity. Pre-clinical work was reported in 1976 at a meeting of the British Society for Immunology; attending the presentation was a member of Roy Calne's transplant research group. They were immediately interested and subsequently used CyA in transplant models in dogs, pigs, and monkeys, finding that it improved survival and function in comparison with azathioprine (Calne *et al.*, 1978, 1979).

This landmark paper was the first report of the use of CyA in human transplant recipients, and detailed the course of seven patients receiving their first deceased-donor kidney. Importantly, there was a profound immunosuppressive effect, and none of the rejection that did occur was characterized by the 'typical rejection crises' with which early transplant clinicians were so familiar.

Of the three adverse effects documented in these first cases, it was considered that nephrotoxicity was 'particular worrying'. Despite the effectiveness of this drug, which became the backbone of modern immunosuppressive therapy, this has remained the major disadvantage associated with its use. The authors considered that the direct toxic effect was probably dose dependent, but that patients varied in their susceptibility to this side-effect. Both observations have subsequently been verified.

One of the challenges with the discrepancy in pharmacokinetics between patients in relation to CyA is the assessment of drug absorption. At the time of this report, there was no means of measuring the blood concentration levels. As assays became available, the trough level has been generally the preferred timing of the sample, although there is evidence to suggest that the peak (2 h post-dose) sample has better correlation with drug exposure.

Similar to azathioprine, the dose of CyA used initially in patients was the same mg/kg dose that was effective in animal models. These first patients therefore started with 25 mg/kg/day, which was not a lethal dose but undoubtedly contributed to the severity of the hepatic and renal toxicity encountered.

At the time of this paper, the authors were uncertain about the mechanism of action of CyA, how long it would be required to be given, and the optimum dose. All of these questions now have answers, and, despite the proliferation of new classes of immunosuppressants in the past 10–15 years, the calcineurin inhibitors (CyA and tacrolimus) remain fundamental to the majority of immunosuppressive regimens still in use. One may consider this a success or failure: the impact of this work by Roy Calne and others is to be applauded, but the continued use of an agent in renal transplant medicine that is nephrotoxic might indeed be baffling to the uninformed observer.

References

Calne RY, White DJ, Rolles K, Smith DP, Herbertson BM (1978). Prolonged survival of pig orthotopic heart grafts treated with cyclosporin A. *Lancet* **i**, 1183–1185.

Calne RY, White DJ, Pentlow BD, *et al.* (1979). Cyclosporin A: preliminary observations in dogs with pancreatic duodenal allografts and patients with cadaveric renal transplants. *Transplant Proc* **11**, 860–864.

15.8 Vascular deposition of complement-split products in kidney allografts with cell-mediated rejection

Authors

HE Feucht, E Felber, MJ Gokel, G Hillebrand, U Nattermann, C Brockmeyer, E Held, G Riethmüller, W Land, E Albert

Reference

Clinical & Experimental Immunology 1991, **86**, 464–470.

Abstract

Complement activation in 73 renal transplant biopsies was investigated by indirect immunoperoxidase staining using MoAbs reactive with complement-split products. Intense deposition of complement fragments C4d and C3d in peritubular capillaries, indicating activation of the classical pathway, could be detected in the majority of transplanted kidneys with cell-mediated rejections. Abundant deposition of complement-split products was observed in 22 early biopsies from patients with high 'immunological risk' (i.e. previous rejected transplants and/or circulating antibodies against HLA-antigens). Despite negative results in the crossmatch before transplantation and paucity of immunoglobulins in transplant biopsies, antibodies directed against endothelial cell antigens should be considered as a possible cause of classic complement activation.

Importance

In the early 1950s, renal transplantation was technically feasible but the rejection of grafts in all but those between monozygotic twins seemed an insurmountable barrier to successful clinical transplantation. The discovery and description of HLA antigens, elucidation of the immune system, and development of immunosuppressant therapy followed. The rejection of allografts was subsequently categorized temporally into hyperacute, acute, and chronic rejection. In the hyperacute response, clearly the injury was antibody mediated. However, in acute rejection, as immunoglobulins were not detected by immunofluorescence in biopsy specimens, the humoral response was largely ignored. It was assumed that this was a cellular process. The pathogenic processes in chronic rejection were even less certain.

In the late 1980s, the use of monoclonal antibodies directed against split products of the complement cascade suggested that the classical complement pathway was activated in certain forms of glomerulonephritis. The C3d and C4d fragments produced by cleavage of C3 and C4 remained bound in tissue but were not detectable by conventional immunofluorescence techniques available at the time.

Helmut Feucht and colleagues used the new immunoperoxidase stain to investigate complement activation in renal transplantation. The deposition of C4d was noted in peritubular capillaries in grafts with acute rejection, being particularly 'abundant' in patients deemed at high immunological risk.

This was of interest, as it was already recognized that activation of the classical complement pathway, which the presence of C4d reflects, was generally precipitated by immunoglobulins or immune complexes (Ziccardi, 1981).

This was the first indication that the humoral immune system might also be involved in acute rejection of kidney transplants, although at that time the precipitant or target antigen of such a response was speculative.

Subsequent work following this landmark paper established that the detection of C4d in allograft biopsies is an important tool in the evaluation of graft dysfunction. C4d staining was also instrumental in the realization a decade later of the importance of antibody-mediated injury in late graft loss (Mauiyyedi *et al.*, 2001).

C4d staining is now an established marker of antibody-mediated rejection in organ transplantation (Sis *et al.*, 2010). In turn, there is now the opportunity for directed therapeutic strategies to reverse such rejection. Recently, and in completion of the complement circle, an antibody to C5, which blocks the next step in the complement cascade formation of terminal complex C5–9, appears to add effectively to the armamentarium of anti-rejection therapies.

References

Mauiyyedi S, Pelle PD, Saidman S, *et al.* (2001). Chronic humoral rejection: identification of antibody-mediated chronic renal allograft rejection by C4d deposits in peritubular capillaries. *J Am Soc Nephrol* **12**, 574–582.

Sis B, Mengel M, Haas M, *et al.* (2010). Banff '09 meeting report: antibody mediated graft deterioration and implementation of Banff working groups. *Am J Transplant* **10**, 464–471.

Ziccardi RJ (1981). Activation of the early components of the classical complement pathway under physiologic conditions. *J Immunol* **126**, 1769–1773.

15.9 Laparoscopic live donor nephrectomy

Authors

LE Ratner, LJ Ciseck, RG Moore, FG Cigarroa, HS Kaufman, LR Kavoussi

Reference

Transplantation 1995, **60**, 1047–1049.

Abstract

A laparoscopic live-donor nephrectomy was performed on a 40-year-old man. The kidney was removed intact via a 9-cm infraumbilical midline incision. Warm ischaemia was limited to less than 5 min. Immediately upon revascularization, the allograft produced urine. By the second postoperative day, the recipient's serum creatinine had decreased to 0.7 mg/dl. The donor's post-operative course was uneventful. He experienced minimal discomfort and was discharged home on the first postoperative day. We conclude that laparoscopic donor nephrectomy is feasible. It can be performed without apparent deleterious effects to either the donor or the recipient. The limited discomfort and rapid convalescence enjoyed by our patient indicate that this technique may prove to be advantageous.

Importance

The very early successes in renal transplantation were with live donors. However, with the introduction of immunosuppressive therapy and then preservation methods, deceased donation became feasible and quickly became the commonest form of transplantation in most countries. Initially, the criteria for acceptance onto a maintenance dialysis programme and transplantation were restricted, and the waiting time for transplantation was relatively short (Courtney *et al.*, 2008). However, there has been a substantial increase in waiting time for transplantation over the past three decades as there is an increasing disparity between the number of people waiting for a solid-organ transplant and the relatively static deceased-donor pool.

Kidneys donated from living persons provide an alternative source of organs, and in general grafts from living donors have better outcomes. Nephrectomy, however, with the open lumbotomy approach resulted in prolonged convalescence with high analgesic requirements. This procedure was considered to be a deterrent to potential donors.

With the advent of minimally invasive surgery, the option of laparoscopic nephrectomy became a clinical reality first in 1990 (Clayman *et al.*, 1991). However, there were legitimate concerns regarding this option for retrieval of a kidney that would then be implanted into someone else, rather than discarded. It would be essential to minimize warm ischaemic time and preserve adequate vessel length to avoid any potential detrimental effect on transplant outcomes.

This landmark paper describes the first experience of laparoscopic live-donor nephrectomy. The outcome for the donor was successful, with discharge the day after surgery, substantially reduced analgesic requirements compared with open nephrectomy, and a successful return to work after 2 weeks. The results for the recipient were similarly good, with primary graft function and an uncomplicated course.

The first donor was selected carefully: straightforward vascular anatomy, thin, and with no previous abdominal surgery. Clearly, this caution was appropriate given what was at stake; however, the authors concluded, 'we believe that the potential benefits of the minimally invasive procedure justifies its continued careful application and assessment', and so it proved.

Laparoscopic donation is now established as the preferred form of nephrectomy for kidney donors and is used for right-sided kidneys, those with multiple vessels, and for donors that are obese. In many countries, the number of live kidney donors now exceeds the deceased-donor total, and this technique has facilitated this important increase.

References

Clayman RV, Kavoussi LR, Soper NJ, *et al.* (1991). Laparoscopic nephrectomy: initial case report. *J Urol* **146**, 278–282.

Courtney AE, McNamee PT, Maxwell AP (2008). The evolution of renal transplantation in clinical practice: for better, for worse? *Quart J Med* **101**, 967–978.

15.10 Long-term results of ABO-incompatible living kidney transplantation: a single-center experience

Authors

K Tanabe, K Takahashi, K Sonda, T Tokumoto, N Ishikawa, T Kawai, S Fuchinoue, T Oshima, T Yagisawa, H Nakazawa, N Goya, S Koga, H Kawaguchi, K Ito, H Toma, T Agishi, K Ota

Reference

Transplantation 1998, **65**, 224–228.

Abstract

Background:…in Japan…a serious shortage of cadaveric organs exists.…For this purpose, ABO-incompatible living kidney transplantations (LKTs) have been performed.…we have already reported the short-term results of ABO-incompatible LKT…In this study, we have reviewed the long-term results of ABO-incompatible LKT…

Methods: Sixty-seven patients…underwent ABO-incompatible living kidney transplantation at our institute between January, 1989, and December, 1995. The mean age was 34.9 years (range, 8–58 years), with 38 males and 29 females. Incompatibility in ABO blood group antigens was as follows: A1→O, 23 patients; B→O, 19 patients; A1B→A1, 7 patients; B→A1, 8 patients; A1→B; 4 patients; A1B→B, 4 patients; A1B→O, 2 patients.…Plasmapheresis and immunoadsorption were carried out to remove the anti-AB antibodies…In the induction phase, methylprednisolone, cyclosporine, azathioprine, antilymphocyte globulin, and deoxyspergualin were used for immunosuppression. Local irradiation of the graft was performed at a dose of 150 rad, on the first, third, and fifth days after transplantation. Splenectomy was done at the time of kidney transplantation in all cases.

Results: Patient survival was 93% at 1 year and 91% at 8 years. Graft survival was 79% at 1, 2, 3, and 4 years, 75% at 5 and 6 years, and 73% at 7 and 8 years. Patient survival was not significantly different from that of ABO-compatible patients. However, graft survival was significantly different between ABO-incompatible grafts and ABO-compatible grafts. Specifically, ABO-incompatible transplant recipients experienced a significantly higher rate of early graft loss up to 3 years but showed an equivalent graft loss by year 4. Among 67 patients, 16 grafts were lost during the observation period. Loss was due to acute rejection in 5 patients…Of 16 grafts lost, 15 were lost within 1 year after transplantation.…

Conclusions: ABO-incompatible living kidney transplantation offers an excellent long-term outcome and is an acceptable treatment for end-stage renal failure.…[Extract.]

Importance

Renal transplantation from a living donor in general offers improved graft survival compared with deceased-donor kidneys and the opportunity for more timely transplantation. The opportunity for direct transplantation between individuals, however, is limited by the prerequisite of compatibility for blood group (ABO) and tissue type (HLA).

Acute intravascular haemagglutination was described in the early 1960s in recipients of non-O donor kidneys in ABO-incompatible (ABOi) transplantation. Thus, the acceptable non-identical blood-group transplant combinations were established (Starzl *et al.*, 1964).

However, in 1981, following the inadvertent transplant of a kidney from a blood-group A donor into a group O recipient, reversal of the acute intravascular thrombosis was achieved by plasma exchange, and normal renal function 20 months later was reported (Slapak *et al.*, 1981). This case offered hope that the limitation of ABOi in live-donor transplantation might potentially be overcome in some instances. Deliberate ABOi transplantation quickly followed, with a variety of immunosuppressive regimens, the majority of which included splenectomy at the time of transplantation. The short-term graft survival rates were acceptable.

This landmark paper was the first to report longer-term outcomes for such transplants with follow-up over an 8-year period of 67 ABOi transplants. There was no detriment to recipient survival, despite the increased immunosuppressive load, and although graft survival was significantly worse up to 4 years after engraftment, it was comparable with ABO compatible grafts thereafter. Thus, ABOi transplantation was established as an important and viable option for patients needing renal transplantation.

Since this time, there has been modification of the protocols for ABOi transplantation with the avoidance of splenectomy in most centres, the use of newer immunosuppressive agents, and a greater understanding of the importance of the blood-group type and antibody titre pre- and post-transplantation on outcomes.

Almost 20 years after the first ABOi transplant, successful HLA-incompatible (HLAi) transplantation was reported (Montgomery *et al.*, 2000). A safer and more cost-effective alternative to live-donor-incompatible transplantation is participation in living-donor exchange programmes. The complexities of such pooled transfers continue to increase, with recently a chain of ten transplants, initiated by a single altruistic donor, over the course of 8 months being completed (Rees *et al.*, 2009).

ABOi transplantation has benefited many hundreds of patients worldwide; together with increasing numbers of successful HLAi procedures, these techniques complement the living-donor exchange programmes in providing renal transplantation for many patients who would otherwise remain on dialysis.

References

Montgomery RA, Zachary AA, Racusen LC, *et al.* (2000). Plasmapheresis and intravenous immune globulin provides effective rescue therapy for refractory humoral rejection and allows kidneys to be successfully transplanted into cross-match-positive recipients. *Transplantation* **70**, 887–895.

Rees MA, Kopke JE, Pelletier RP, *et al.* (2009). A nonsimultaneous, extended, altruistic-donor chain. *New Engl J Med* **360**, 1096–1101.

Slapak M, Naik RB, Lee HA (1981). Renal transplant in a patient with major donor-recipient blood group incompatibility: reversal of acute rejection by the use of modified plasmapheresis. *Transplantation* **31**, 4–7.

Starzl TE, Marchioro TL, Holmes JH, *et al.* (1964). Renal homografts in patients with major donor-recipient blood group incompatibilities. *Surgery* **55**, 195–200.

Chapter 16

Cardiovascular disease

Christopher W. McIntyre

Introduction

The dire cardiovascular consequences of advanced chronic kidney disease (CKD) have been appreciated for nearly 50 years. The first patient treated by chronic dialysis in Seattle was the index case for the seminal NEJM publication by Lindner and colleagues reporting accelerated arterial disease and elevated cardiovascular risk in haemodialysis patients (see paper 19.1). But only in the last 10–15 years has the impact of early CKD on cardiovascular disease been appreciated; and now the multiplicity of pathophysiological processes at work are beginning to be defined. Many risk factors (both disease and treatment specific) are now being implicated in the development of cardiovascular disease in CKD patients, in both the setting of dialysis and with milder degrees of functional impairment.

These new insights have been facilitated by the interrogation of large national registries and health system databases. The appreciation of the importance of bone and mineral abnormalities and the interaction with cardiovascular structure and vascular biology has broadened our view ing of this increased burden of cardiovascular disease previously attributed solely to accelerated atherosclerosis, with higher rates of thrombotic occlusion of unstable plaque. The work of Gerard London and co-workers has defined the role of peripheral arterial compliance and pulse wave propagation (with attendant consequences on central blood pressure) in cardiovascular outcomes. The appreciation that dialysis itself may also contribute to the cardiovascular disease in ESRD patients is even more recent. Such non-traditional risk factors only displace more traditional factors such as blood pressure and lipids by their relative effect. Recent studies of lipid lowering agents have demonstrated some effect on cardiovascular events even at late stages of CKD, although it seems that this effect becomes relatively less important as the contribution of lipids as a risk factor becomes overwhelmed by additional risk factors in dialysis treated patients.

The chosen articles in this chapter are a personal perspective; I have focused on key milestones in expanding our understanding of the individual components of the pathophysiological processes and how they interact. Cardiovascular disease remains the major killer of people with kidney disease, and up to know attempts to ameliorate this (especially in patients receiving dialysis) using therapies developed for treatment in the non uraemic general population have almost universally been ineffective. New targets should result in novel interventions and we are only just entering the era of robust testing of this expanded envelope of therapeutic possibilities.

16.1 Clinical epidemiology of cardiovascular disease in chronic renal disease

Authors

RN Foley, PS Parfrey, MJ Sarnak

Reference

American Journal of Kidney Diseases 1998, **32**, S112–S119.

Summary clinical recommendation

- The risk of cardiovascular disease (CVD) in patients with chronic renal disease (CRD) appears to be far greater than in the general population. For example, among patients treated by hemodialysis (HD) or peritoneal dialysis (PD), the prevalence of coronary artery disease (CAD) is approximately 40% and the prevalence of left ventricular hypertrophy (LVH) is approximately 75%. Among HD and PD patients, total deaths caused by CVD in 1995 were approximately 16,000. CVD mortality in HD and PD patients has been estimated to be approximately 9% per year. Even after stratification by age, gender, race, and presence of diabetes, CVD mortality in HD and PD patients is 10 to 20 times higher than in the general population.

- Patients with CRD should be considered in the highest risk group for subsequent CVD events. Treatment recommendations based on CVD risk stratification should take into account this "highest risk" status of patients with CRD.

- Congestive heart failure (CHF) is more common in CRD than in the general population and is an independent predictor of death in CRD. Among HD and PD patients, the prevalence of CHF is approximately 40%.

- In practice, it is difficult to determine whether CHF reflects left ventricular (LV) dysfunction or extracellular fluid (ECF) volume overload.

- The excess risk of CVD in CRD is caused, in part, by a higher prevalence in these patients of conditions that are recognized as risk factors for CVD in the general population.

- In addition, the excess risk may also be due, in part, to hemodynamic and metabolic factors characteristic of CRD, including proteinuria, increased ECF volume, electrolyte imbalance, anemia, and higher levels of thrombogenic factors and homocysteine than in the general population. Whether other factors unique to CRD also contribute to the excess risk is unknown.

Importance

It is ironic that this pivotal and highly cited article was published within a supplement. Indeed, there is no abstract within the original article, only a list of potential clinical practice recommendations. The key piece of data that has been so heavily cited and generated such impact is actually reproduced from an abstract presented at the American Society of Nephrology annual meeting in 1998 (Sarnak and Levey, 1998).

This article contained several figures derived from US Renal Data System (USRDS) renal-specific data and National Center for Health Statistics (NCHS) general population data. Events were expressed, converted to annual percentage mortality, and shown by sex, ethnicity, and whether or not the patients were on dialysis or not. Very little patient-specific data was obtained, and stratification was based on the International Classification of Diseases (ICD) diagnostic codes.

Cardiovascular mortality was generated from ICD codes specific for arrhythmias, cardiomyopathy, cardiac arrest, myocardial infarction, atherosclerotic heart disease, and pulmonary oedema.

The key figure, which has been widely reproduced subsequently, was plotted across the age range against a non-linear scale for annual mortality. This demonstrated with exquisite clarity the enormous excess of mortality among dialysis patients. This excess (as a proportion) was greater the younger the patients. Those in the 25–35-year age group were experiencing around a 500-fold excess. This increment in mortality risk was maintained all the way up to age >85 years, but the difference between dialysis patients and the general population narrowed incrementally. Although there were some absolute differences in mortality related to sex and black ethnicity, the patterns of mortality were identical.

The article concluded with a series of research recommendations. Many of these were a call for additional natural history studies and improved epidemiological assessment of the entity of cardiovascular disease in the setting of CKD. Rob Foley and his co-workers have gone on to perform many of these studies. Other recommendations such as 'In HD patients, determine the relationships of abnormal cardiac structure and rhythms to underlying CAD, and to the fluid and electrolyte shifts associated with the HD procedure' are yet to receive the kind of rigorous study that they clearly deserve. This article brings into sharp relief the importance of assiduously performed high-quality epidemiological studies (often utilizing registry-based data) to identify correctly areas of importance and frame appropriate research questions *before* novel interventions are developed and tested through the final medium of the prospective randomized controlled trial (RCT).

Reference

Sarnak MJ, Levey AS (1998). *J Am Soc Nephrol* **9**, 160A.

16.2 Outcome and risk factors for left ventricular disorders in chronic uraemia

Authors

PS Parfrey, RN Foley, JD Harnett, GM Kent, DC Murray, PE Barre

Reference

Nephrology Dialysis Transplantation 1996, **11**, 1277–1285.

Abstract

Background: Left ventricular disease occurs frequently in dialysis patients. It may be manifest as concentric LV hypertrophy, LV dilatation with or without LV hypertrophy, or systolic dysfunction. Little is known concerning the clinical outcome and risk factors for these disorders.

Methods: A cohort of 432 end-stage renal disease patients who survived at least 6 months had an echocardiogram on initiation of dialysis therapy. Clinical, laboratory and echocardiographic data was obtained annually during follow-up.

Results: On initiation of ESRD therapy 16% of patients had systolic dysfunction, 41% concentric LV hypertrophy, 28% LV dilatation, and only 16% had normal echocardiograms. Median time to development of heart failure was 19 months in patients with systolic dysfunction, 38 months in concentric LV hypertrophy and 38 months in LV dilatation. The relative risks of heart failure in the three groups were significantly worse than in the normal group, after adjusting for age, diabetes and ischaemic heart disease. Median survival was 38 months in systolic dysfunction, 48 months in concentric hypertrophy, 56 months in LV dilatation, and >66 months in the normal group. Two hundred and seventy-five patients had a follow-up echocardiogram 17 months after starting dialysis therapy together with serial measurement of potential risk factors prior to the echocardiogram. On follow-up echocardiogram the degree of concentric LV hypertrophy was independently related to hypertension while on dialysis, older age, and anaemia while on dialysis; the degree of LV dilatation was related to ischaemic heart disease, anaemia, hypertension and hypoalbuminemia while on dialysis; the degree of systolic dysfunction was associated with ischaemic heart disease and anaemia during follow-up.

Conclusions: Manifestations of left ventricular disease are frequent and persistent in chronic uraemia, and are associated with high risks of heart failure and death. Potentially reversible risk factors include anaemia, hypertension, hypoalbuminaemia and ischaemic heart disease.

Importance

This study is one of a series of important pieces of work coming out of the somewhat remote Canadian Province of Newfoundland. Patrick Parfrey was part of a high- quality team of nephrologists recruited by Henry Gault and has contributed hugely to our understanding of cardiovascular disease. This particular study built on a smaller piece of work published several years earlier looking at the impact of cardiac structure and function on outcomes in patients starting dialysis (Parfrey *et al.*, 1990).

Four hundred and thrity-two patients new to dialysis were studied, largely in Newfoundland, but supplemented with patients from Montreal. Baseline echocardiography was performed within the first year of dialysis, and clinical assessment of the patients, particularly to define their degree of cardiovascular disease, was then performed at yearly intervals.

Only 16% of patients started dialysis with a normal heart. Most of these abnormalities related to left ventricular hypertrophy or dilatation, with only a small proportion having defined systolic dysfunction at baseline. A significant proportion of patients with abnormalities of ventricular morphology went on to develop clinical heart failure. Two hundred and seventy-five patients also underwent follow-up echocardiography. This defined worsening hypertrophy as being driven largely by hypertension, age, and anaemia. Ischaemic heart disease was associated largely with dilatation and the development of systolic contractile dysfunction. Dialysis modality or any details of the dialysis treatment were not reported in this study, and the focus on the factors that might be involved was very firmly on the prevailing belief around that time that aggravated conventional risk factors and therapies were at the centre of these issues. The reliance on conventional echocardiography also limited the assessments that could be made. Both systolic function and left ventricular morphology were measured using methods that required multiple measurement assumptions that are prone to error, particularly in ESRD patients. No detailed consideration of diastolic dysfunction was undertaken. Cardiac magnetic resonance imaging would have addressed many of these issues, but availability was somewhat limited at this time.

This study provided the most comprehensive assessment of the natural history of cardiac abnormalities in late-stage CKD. Despite advances in imaging technology, it is probably still to be bettered. It defined clearly that these abnormalities were common, persistent, and associated with significantly increased risk of death. This study was also important in defining the risks of heart failure development with ventricular hypertrophy being part of a rapidly progressing continuum of cardiac abnormalities.

Reference

Parfrey PS, Griffiths SM, Harnett JD, *et al.* (1990). Outcome of congestive heart failure, dilated cardiomyopathy, hypertrophic hyperkinetic disease, and ischemic heart disease in dialysis patients. *Am J Nephrol* **10**, 213–221.

16.3 Relation between serum phosphate level and cardiovascular event rate in people with coronary disease

Authors

M Tonelli, F Sacks, M Pfeffer, Z Gao, G Curhan, for the Cholesterol And Recurrent Events (CARE) Trial Investigators

Reference

Circulation 2005, **112**, 2627–2633. [Erratum: **116**, e556 (2007).]

Abstract

Background: Higher levels of serum phosphate are associated with adverse cardiovascular outcomes, especially in the setting of overt hyperphosphatemia. Given the biological importance of phosphorus, it is plausible that higher levels of serum phosphate within the normal range.

Methods and results: We performed a post hoc analysis of data from the Cholesterol And Recurrent Events (CARE) study. Baseline serum phosphate levels were measured in 4127 fasting participants who were randomized to receive pravastatin 40 mg daily or placebo and followed up for a median of 59.7 months. We used Cox proportional-hazards models to examine the association between serum phosphate and adverse clinical outcomes after adjustment for potential confounders. During nearly 60 months of follow-up, 375 participants died. A significant association was noted between baseline serum phosphate level and the age-, race-, and sex-adjusted risk of all-cause death (hazard ratio per 1 mg/dL, 1.27; 95% confidence interval, 1.02 to 1.58). After categorization based on baseline phosphate level (<2.5, 2.5 to 3.4, 3.5 to 3.9, and ≥4 mg/dL) and further adjustment, a graded independent relation between phosphate and death was observed (*P* for trend=0.03). For instance, participants with serum phosphate ≥3.5 mg/dL had an adjusted hazard ratio for death of 1.27 (95% confidence interval, 1.02 to 1.59) compared with those with serum phosphate of <3.5 mg/dL. Higher levels of serum phosphate were also associated with increased risk of new heart failure, myocardial infarction, and the composite of coronary death or nonfatal myocardial infarction, but not the risk of stroke.

Conclusions: We found a graded independent relation between higher levels of serum phosphate and the risk of death and cardiovascular events in people with prior myocardial infarction, most of whom had serum phosphate levels within the normal range. Given the ready availability and low cost of serum phosphate assays, this finding may prove clinically useful.

Importance

This article was a crucial milestone in appreciating that metabolic abnormalities associated with CKD could act as cardiovascular risk factors, even while those values remained within the normal range. Serum phosphate had been identified as an independent risk factor in patients receiving dialysis, but this effect had only been demonstrated when patients were clearly hyperphosphataemic (Block *et al.*, 1998). This study tested the hypothesis that, in those individuals with a strong history of adverse cardiovascular events, the actual level of serum phosphate (without levels overtly raised outside the normal range) might still influence outcomes.

Tonelli and co-workers utilized a post-hoc analysis of a previously reported RCT of pravastatin to reduce events in patients who previously had suffered myocardial infarction (many of whom had intercurrent chronic reduction in renal function). The Cholesterol and Recurrent Events

(CARE) study was a RCT of pravastatin versus placebo in 4159 individuals with hyperlipidaemia and a history of myocardial infarction. Serum phosphate and estimated glomerular filtration rate (eGFR) was assessed in all participants, and the effect of serum phosphate was studied against a primary outcome of all-cause mortality, heart failure, and subsequent no fatal cardiac event. Only 5.8% of patients had serum phosphate levels outside the normal range. After full statistical adjustment, patients in the higher parts of the normal range for serum phosphate had an elevated risk of all-cause mortality by about 50% (as compared with the lower part of the normal range). These results were unchanged even if patients with an eGFR of <60 ml/min were included or excluded, or if estimated creatinine clearance (using the Cockcroft–Gault equation) was utilized.

The mean eGFR was around 70 ml/min/1.73 m². Serum phosphate levels were determined partially by renal function, and had a gradated and independent association with all-cause mortality and newly diagnosed congestive heart failure. This study was unable to explore the potential mechanisms behind the association between serum phosphate levels and cardiovascular events.

A similar significant and gradated effect of mild to moderate CKD on subsequent cardiovascular and all-cause mortality was also reported in large population-based studies (Culleton *et al.*, 199; Garg *et al.*, 2002; Go *et al.*, 2004; see also paper 19.10). Combined with other work around this time defining the true prevalence of CKD, these studies helped elevate consideration of renal function to one of the most important potential issues in public health.

References

Block GA, Hulbert-Shearon TE, Levin NW, Port FK (1998). Association of serum phosphorus and calcium × phosphate product with mortality risk in chronic hemodialysis patients: a national study. *Am J Kidney Dis* **31**, 607–617.

Culleton BF, Larson MG, Wilson PW, Evans JC, Parfrey PS, Levy D (1999). Cardiovascular disease and mortality in a community-based cohort with mild renal insufficiency. *Kidney Int* **56**, 2214–2219.

Garg AX, Clark WF, Haynes RB, House AA (2002). Moderate renal insufficiency and the risk of cardiovascular mortality: results from the NHANES I. *Kidney Int* **61**, 1486–1494.

Go AS, Chertow GM, Fan D, McCulloch CE, Hsu CY (2004). Chronic kidney disease and the risks of death, cardiovascular events, and hospitalization. *N Engl J Med* **351**, 1296–1305.

16.4 Coronary-artery calcification in young adults with end-stage renal disease who are undergoing dialysis

Authors

WG Goodman, J Goldin, BD Kuizon, C Yoon, B Gales, D Sider, Y Wang, J Chung, A Emerick, L Greaser, RM Elashoff, IB Salusky

Reference

New England Journal of Medicine 2000, **342**, 1478–1483.

Abstract

Background: Cardiovascular disease is common in older adults with end-stage renal disease who are undergoing regular dialysis, but little is known about the prevalence and extent of cardiovascular disease in children and young adults with end-stage renal disease.

Methods: We used electron-beam computed tomography (CT) to screen for coronary-artery calcification in 39 young patients with end-stage renal disease who were undergoing dialysis (mean [±SD] age, 19±7 years; range, 7 to 30) and 60 normal subjects 20 to 30 years of age. In those with evidence of calcification on CT scanning, we determined its extent. The results were correlated with the patients' clinical characteristics, serum calcium and phosphorus concentrations, and other biochemical variables.

Results: None of the 23 patients who were younger than 20 years of age had evidence of coronary-artery calcification, but it was present in 14 of the 16 patients who were 20 to 30 years old. Among those with calcification, the mean calcification score was 1157±1996, and the median score was 297. By contrast, only 3 of the 60 normal subjects had calcification. As compared with the patients without coronary-artery calcification, those with calcification were older (26±3 vs. 15±5 years, P<0.001) and had been undergoing dialysis for a longer period (14±5 vs. 4±4 years, P<0.001). The mean serum phosphorus concentration, the mean calcium–phosphorus ion product in serum, and the daily intake of calcium were higher among the patients with coronary-artery calcification. Among 10 patients with calcification who underwent follow-up CT scanning, the calcification score nearly doubled (from 125±104 to 249±216, P=0.02) over a mean period of 20±3 months.

Conclusions: Coronary-artery calcification is common and progressive in young adults with end-stage renal disease who are undergoing dialysis.

Importance

This study focused on the increasing importance being given to alternative pathophysiological processes in aggravated cardiovascular risk for patients undergoing dialysis. Coronary artery calcification (CAC) as measured by electron-beam computerized tomography (EBCT) had been utilized to detect atheromatous coronary artery disease (CAD). Although Braun *et al.* (1996) had already reported markedly increased CAC in haemodialysis patients, this was the first study to focus on younger patients and, crucially, the first to track rapid progression in CAC.

This study was undertaken in a small cohort of 39 chronic patients treated with unit-based conventional haemodialysis at the University of California, LA. The study included both young adult (<30 years) and paediatric patients. An even smaller sample of only 22 patients underwent follow-up EBCT assessment 18–24 months later. A comparator patient group (60 patients) with normal renal function were also studied.

Even including the children, 14 versus 25 patients exhibited significant CAC. The CAC scores were extremely high, being several orders of magnitude greater than reported even in the presence of defined CAD in non-CKD patients. CAC scores were related to dialysis vintage and factors related to mineral metabolism (achieved serum phosphate and calcium × phosphate product), as well as daily consumption of calcium in phosphate binders. The ten patients with significant baseline calcification demonstrated a near doubling of CAC at follow-up. The presence of pre-existing vascular calcification has consistently been identified as the strongest risk factor for progressive vascular calcification in all subsequent prospective studies, even if the other factors identified in this initial study have been less consistently confirmed (Sigrist *et al.*, 2007).

This study was unclear how these high CAC scores might relate to underlying angiographically significant disease, but did highlight the early, severe, and rapid burden of cardiovascular disease in haemodialysis patients. Equally important, it helped to focus attention onto calcification, aberrant vascular biology, and potential novel therapeutic targets relating to mineral metabolism. Assessment of vascular calcification became the surrogate of choice for the subsequent study of this interaction, and this study directly informed the design and execution of the pivotal studies of non-calcium-containing phosphate binders. Unfortunately, we are still waiting for conclusive evidence that manipulation of bone and mineral disorder management is capable of reducing cardiovascular events and mortality.

References

Braun J, Oldendorf M, Moshage W, Heidler R, Zeitler E, Luft FC (1996). Electron beam computed tomography in the evaluation of cardiac calcification in chronic dialysis patients. *Am J Kidney Dis* **27**, 394–401.

Sigrist MK, Taal MW, Bungay P, McIntyre CW (2007). Progressive vascular calcification over 2 years is associated with arterial stiffening and increased mortality in patients with stages 4 and 5 chronic kidney disease. *Clin J Am Soc Nephrol* **2**, 1241–1248.

16.5 Arterial calcifications, arterial stiffness, and cardiovascular risk in end-stage renal disease

Authors

J Blacher, AP Guerin, B Pannier, SJ Marchais, GM London

Reference

Hypertension 2001, **38**, 938–942.

Abstract

To test the predictive values of and independent contributions to cardiovascular and all-cause mortality of various arterial parameters exploring characteristics of the arterial wall at different sites, we studied prospectively 110 stable end-stage renal disease patients on hemodialysis. These parameters involved carotid diameter, carotid intima-media thickness, carotid compliance, carotid distensibility, carotid incremental elastic modulus, aortic diameter, aortic pulse wave velocity, and the presence of arterial calcifications measured at the sites of the carotid artery, abdominal aorta, iliofemoral axis, and legs. The presence of calcifications was analyzed semiquantitatively as a score (0 to 4) according to the number of arterial sites with calcifications. During a follow-up of 53±21 months (mean±SD), 25 cardiovascular and 14 noncardiovascular deaths occurred. In univariate analysis, the carotid incremental elastic modulus was the most closely related to prognosis. Risk of death increased with the number of vascular sites involved by calcifications. Moreover, information (in terms of prediction) given by carotid elastic incremental modulus was additive to the presence and extent of vascular calcification-related prediction value. Adjusted hazard ratios of all-cause and cardiovascular mortality for an increase of 1 unit in calcification score were 1.9 (95% confidence interval [CI], 1.4 to 2.6) and 2.6 (95% CI, 1.5 to 4.4), respectively ($P<0.001$ for both). Adjusted hazard ratios of all-cause and cardiovascular mortality for a 1-SD increase in carotid incremental elastic modulus were 1.6 (95% CI, 1.2 to 2.2) and 1.7 (95% CI, 1.2 to 2.4), respectively ($P<0.01$ for both). The results of this study showed that the presence and extent of vascular calcifications were strong predictors of cardiovascular and all-cause mortality. Carotid incremental elastic modulus gave additional predictive value.

Importance

The importance of altered large-vessel structure and function in predicting mortality in patients with ESRD had been identified previously by Gerard London's group. They had performed the first prospective study of arterial stiffness in this patient group (assessed by measuring pulse-wave velocity) and demonstrated that stiffer peripheral conduit arteries were associated with increased mortality (Blacher *et al.*, 1999). Large-vessel vascular calcification, and in particular the medial calcification characteristic of patients with CKD, had been identified for some time. This study was the first to effectively highlight that an increasing burden of vascular calcification was associated with incremental increases in mortality, and that this added an additional degree of prediction beyond just the effect of arterio- and atherosclerotic arterial disease on arterial stiffness.

A hundred and ten haemodialysis patients were subjected to a detailed study of their arterial tree and followed up for almost 5 years. This included direct measurement of pulse-wave velocity (utilizing a Doppler ultrasound-based system to study the carotid artery including carotid intimal medial thickness). The presence of calcifications was assessed semi-quantitatively from plain radiology at multiple sites. A score was then provided based on the number of sites affected. No quantification of the severity at any particular site was possible with this technique.

The key findings were that each increment in the number of arterial sites exhibiting calcification was associated with an incremental reduction in survival. The most heavily calcified patients had only around 10% survival at the end of the observation period. This information was additive to carotid elastic incremental modulus (measuring arterial compliance) in predicting the risk of death. The increased mortality risk was directed at both cardiovascular and all-cause mortality. This stressed the important point that cardiovascular pathophysiology is still able to impact on the risk of death from non-directly cardiovascular causes, presumably from the consequences of impaired cardiovascular resilience and reserve.

This group of studies was used extensively in transferring focus onto the prevention of worsening vascular calcification as a principal therapeutic aim in the management of patients receiving dialysis. These observations allowed vascular calcification progression to be justified as a reasonable surrogate end point in the study of therapeutic agents directed at bone and mineral metabolism. This study stressed that vascular calcification resulted in arterial stiffness, but was not the sole determinant, with non-calcific reduction in compliance also being characteristic of CKD patients.

Reference

Blacher J, Guerin AP, Pannier B, Marchais SJ, Safar ME, London GM (1999). Impact of aortic stiffness on survival in end-stage renal disease. *Circulation* **99**, 2434–2439.

16.6 Chronically decreased aortic distensibility causes deterioration of coronary perfusion during increased left ventricular contraction

Authors

S Ohtsuka, M Kakihana, H Watanabe, Y Sugishita

Reference

Journal of the American College of Cardiology 1994, **24**, 1406–1414.

Abstract

Objectives: This study investigated the long-term effects of decreased aortic distensibility on the heart in relation to coronary perfusion.

Background: Aortic distensibility is decreased in patients with atherosclerosis and hypertension and in the elderly. However, the effect of a long-term decrease in aortic distensibility on coronary perfusion has not been fully investigated.

Methods: Twelve anesthetized dogs underwent thoracotomy and were allocated to two groups: Group I included six control dogs with a normal aorta; Group II included six dogs with decreased aortic distensibility produced by banding the descending aorta. After 4 to 6 weeks, the dogs had a second operation to measure coronary artery flow and transmural flow distribution. Measurements were performed at baseline and during isoproterenol infusion.

Results: At baseline, arterial compliance was reduced by 35% in Group II. Hemodynamic variables, regional wall motion and coronary flow were also similar in both groups. However, during isoproterenol infusion, coronary flow increased more in Group II than in Group I ($p < 0.01$), and the coronary flow reserve ratio decreased more in Group II than in Group I (mean [$\pm$ SD] 1.9 ± 0.4 vs. 2.4 ± 0.3, $p < 0.05$). During isoproterenol infusion the endocardial flow increased less in Group II than in Group I ($p < 0.05$), and the endocardial/epicardial flow ratio was significantly decreased in Group II compared with Group I (mean [$\pm$ SD] 0.70 ± 0.18 vs. 0.99 ± 0.22, $p < 0.05$). The subendocardial electrocardiogram showed ST segment elevation during isoproterenol infusion in Group II ($p < 0.05$) but not in Group I.

Conclusions: These results demonstrate that during increased ventricular contraction, chronically decreased aortic distensibility contributes to a further decrease in the coronary flow reserve ratio, impairs endocardial blood flow and may induce subendocardial ischemia even in the absence of coronary artery stenosis.

Importance

This set of experiments in dogs was the second of two studies relating to the impact of peripheral atrial compliance on myocardial perfusion performed by the same Japanese research group. They had already demonstrated that, in animals with restricted large-vessel coronary flow, the addition of reducing aortic arterial compliance resulted in both a reduction in fractional flow reserve and clear evidence of subsequent demand myocardial ischaemia (Watanabe *et al.*, 1992). This particular study went further to investigate whether increasing conduit arterial stiffness alone was sufficient to generate cardiac ischaemia in the absence of coronary large-vessel lesions.

Dogs underwent thoracotomy under anaesthesia and had their aortas effectively stiffened by the application of non-compliant external bandaging. After a 4–6-week recovery period, dogs with both normal aortas (but mock operated on) and those with surgically reduced aortic distensibility were assessed for coronary-artery blood flow and transmural flow distribution. This was performed both at rest and during inotropic stimulation (using isoproterenol infusion).

The coronary flow reserve was reduced in the treatment animals, with myocardial blood flow normal at rest. However, after ventricular stimulation, the animals with reduced arterial compliance demonstrated significant reductions in the ratio of endocardial/epicardial blood flow, and endocardial intracardiac ECG demonstrated convincing evidence of myocardial ischaemia in that territory.

This study provided direct experimental evidence that altering peripheral arterial physical characteristics was able to generate potential myocardial ischaemia, even without the need for additional large-vessel coronary disease. This presumably was a result of the increased pulse-wave velocity altering central arterial pulse waveform. The rapidly returning peripheral reflectance wave reinforces the systolic peak (increasing cardiac work) but fails to reinforce the diastolic portion (relatively reduced coronary perfusion pressure in diastole). This provided a coherent pathophysiological paradigm to assist our emerging understanding of the importance of increased arterial stiffness (and vascular calcification) in CKD. Such elegant experimental data provided the initial biological plausibility to start to appreciate the lower relative importance of a conventional coronary-artery disease/large-vessel atheroma model in understanding the hugely elevated rates of cardiovascular attrition in CKD patients.

Reference

Watanabe H, Ohtsuka S, Kakihana M, Sugishita Y (1992). Decreased aortic compliance aggravates subendocardial ischaemia in dogs with stenosed coronary artery. *Cardiovasc Res* **26**, 1212–1218.

16.7 Increased infarct size in uremic rats: reduced ischemia tolerance?

Authors

R Dikow, LP Kihm, M Zeier, J Kapitza, J Törnig, K Amann, C Tiefenbacher, E Ritz

Reference

Journal of the American Society of Nephrology 2004, **15**, 1530–1536.

Abstract

In patients with renal failure, myocardial infarction (MI) is more frequent and the rate of death from acute MI is very high. It has been argued that ischemia tolerance of the heart is reduced in uremia, but direct evidence for this hypothesis has not been provided. It was the purpose of this study (*1*) to ligate the left coronary artery and to measure the nonperfused area (risk area: total infarction plus penumbra) as well as the area of total infarction in subtotally nephrectomized (SNX) rats compared with sham-operated pair-fed control rats and (*2*) to examine the effects of potential confounders such as BP, sympathetic overactivity, and salt retention. The left coronary artery was ligated for 60 min, followed by reperfusion for 90 min. For visualizing perfused myocardium, lissamine green ink was injected. The nonperfused area (lissamine exclusion) and the area of total infarction (triphenyltetrazolium chloride stain) were assessed in sections of the left ventricle using image analysis. Groups of SNX rats also received: antihypertensive treatment (nadolol plus hydralazine); moxonidine; high salt diet or low salt diet (1.58% *versus* 0.015%). In surviving animals, the nonperfused area at risk (as the proportion of total left ventricular area), presumably determined by the geometry of vascular supply, was similar in sham-operated and SNX animals (0.38 ± 0.13 versus 0.45 ± 0.09; NS). In contrast, the infarcted area, given as a proportion of the nonperfused risk area, was significantly ($P < 0.003$) higher in SNX (0.68 ± 0.09) compared with sham-operated (0.51 ± 0.11) rats and was not altered by any of the above interventions. The finding that a greater proportion of nonperfused myocardium undergoes total necrosis is consistent with the hypothesis of reduced ischemia tolerance of the heart in renal failure. The findings could explain the high rate of death from MI in patients with impaired renal function.

Importance

The increased risk of cardiovascular mortality associated with advanced CKD was relatively well appreciated by the time of this publication. CKD patients were at increased risk of myocardial infarction, compared with non-uraemic subjects, and there was also an increase in the associated mortality (Shlipak *et al.*, 2002). The group in Heidelberg had already reported a number of studies relating to abnormal cardiac structure and capillary density reduction in uraemic animal models (Amann *et al.*, 1992, 2003). This study reported the results of an important set of rodent-based experiments relating directly to the possibility that uraemia resulted directly in reduced ischaemic tolerance.

Rats were rendered moderately uraemic after two-step subtotal nephrectomy. The uraemic interval was also quite short, with the final stage of the experiments being performed 3 weeks later. Experiments were controlled using mock-operated animals. Myocardial infarction was induced by coronary artery ligation. The animals were subsequently sacrificed and the total underperfused area (lissamine ink exclusion) and the myocardial area (triphenyltetrazolium chloride staining) were assessed. Both areas were quantified from direct examination of the hearts after full sectioning, which also allowed accurate measurement of ventricular mass. Additional animals were also exposed to a series of interventions designed to compensate for hypertension, salt retention, and sympathetic overactivity resulting from the reduction in renal mass.

A standardized territory of the left ventricle sustained infarction. The area that was at risk with underperfusion was similar between nephrectomized and mock-operated animals (corrected for left ventricular mass changes). However, the infarct size as a proportion of the underperfused area was significantly greater in the uraemic animals compared with the controls with normal renal function. None of the interventions tested (salt restriction, β-blockade, hydralazine, or moxonidine) altered this finding. There was an appreciable rate of death from ventricular fibrillation after coronary ligation in the nephrectomized animals and this was reduced by β-blockade.

Although extrapolation from such animal studies into human disease is often problematical, this well-conceived and expertly performed series of experiments provided crucial direct evidence that uraemia itself was capable of priming the heart to be particularly sensitive to demand ischaemia. This effect did not appear to be amenable to any of the tested interventions, and this study was unable to perform any further investigation of the pathophysiological mechanisms.

References

Amann K, Wiest G, Zimmer G, Gretz N, Ritz E, Mall G (1992). Reduced capillary density in the myocardium of uremic rats—a stereological study. *Kidney Int* **42**, 1079–1085.

Amann K, Tyralla K, Gross ML, *et al.* (2003). Cardiomyocyte loss in experimental renal failure: prevention by ramipril. *Kidney Int* **63**, 1708–1713.

Shlipak MG, Heidenreich PA, Noguchi H, Chertow GM, Browner WS, McClellan MB (2002). Association of renal insufficiency with treatment and outcomes after myocardial infarction in elderly patients. *Ann Intern Med* **137**, 555–562.

16.8 Atorvastatin in patients with type 2 diabetes mellitus undergoing hemodialysis

Authors

C Wanner, V Krane, W März, M Olschewski, JF Mann, G Ruf, E Ritz, for the German Diabetes and Dialysis Study Investigators

Reference

New England Journal of Medicine 2005, **353**, 238–248.

Abstract

Background: Statins reduce the incidence of cardiovascular events in persons with type 2 diabetes mellitus. However, the benefit of statins in such patients receiving hemodialysis, who are at high risk for cardiovascular disease and death, has not been examined.

Methods: We conducted a multicenter, randomized, double-blind, prospective study of 1255 subjects with type 2 diabetes mellitus receiving maintenance hemodialysis who were randomly assigned to receive 20 mg of atorvastatin per day or matching placebo. The primary end point was a composite of death from cardiac causes, nonfatal myocardial infarction, and stroke. Secondary end points included death from all causes and all cardiac and cerebrovascular events combined.

Results: After four weeks of treatment, the median level of low-density lipoprotein cholesterol was reduced by 42 percent among patients receiving atorvastatin, and among those receiving placebo it was reduced by 1.3 percent. During a median follow-up period of four years, 469 patients (37 percent) reached the primary end point, of whom 226 were assigned to atorvastatin and 243 to placebo (relative risk, 0.92; 95 percent confidence interval, 0.77 to 1.10; $P = 0.37$). Atorvastatin had no significant effect on the individual components of the primary end point, except that the relative risk of fatal stroke among those receiving the drug was 2.03 (95 percent confidence interval, 1.05 to 3.93; $P = 0.04$). Atorvastatin reduced the rate of all cardiac events combined (relative risk, 0.82; 95 percent confidence interval, 0.68 to 0.99; $P = 0.03$, nominally significant) but not all cerebrovascular events combined (relative risk, 1.12; 95 percent confidence interval, 0.81 to 1.55; $P = 0.49$) or total mortality (relative risk, 0.93; 95 percent confidence interval, 0.79 to 1.08; $P = 0.33$).

Conclusions: Atorvastatin had no statistically significant effect on the composite primary end point of cardiovascular death, nonfatal myocardial infarction, and stroke in patients with diabetes receiving hemodialysis.

Importance

The German Diabetes Dialysis Study (4D) study was undertaken to examine the possibility that it was reasonable to extend cardiovascular protective interventions, largely developed in the general population, and expect to receive similar or even greater benefit in the high-event-rate haemodialysis population. Dialysis patients were well known to have a characteristic pattern of dyslipidaemia, with lower levels of low-density lipoprotein (LDL) cholesterol and a relative preponderance of very-low-density particles. The high event rate was well established, and much of this increased risk was attributed largely to an acceleration and aggravation of conventional large-vessel atheromatous disease with thrombotic occlusion at the final event, complicating plaque rupture.

In total, 1255 patients with established type 2 diabetes mellitus and receiving haemodialysis were recruited and randomized on a 1:1 basis to either atorvastatin or placebo, in a prospective double-blind RCT. The primary end point was a composite of terminal stroke, myocardial infarction or non-fatal event. Only one event was allowed per patient. The two groups were well balanced, and intervention with atorvastatin resulted in good and sustained separation in achieved LDL cholesterol levels. The key finding, however, was no effect on the primary end point. This relative lack of effect had also been reported in the AURORA study of rosuvastatin in 2776 subjects on haemodialysis between the ages of 50 and 80 years (Fellstrom *et al.*, 2009). This study also demonstrated consistent reduction in LDL cholesterol but no effect on either the composite end point or any of the individual components. The subsequent SHARP study did report a reduction in a primary end point largely made up of revascularization events, but this did not impact on coronary events and both pre-dialysis and haemodialysis patients were studied (Baigent *et al.*, 2011). Although the analysis is difficult to dissect from the published final study, it would appear that the majority of this effect was in these pre-dialysis patients.

These studies were crucial components in the important paradigm shift of thinking about elevated cardiovascular mortality not necessarily being an amplification of general risk factors and their clinical consequences but as a result of a wide variety of 'non-classical' factors, working through previously underappreciated pathomechanisms and requiring unconventional therapeutic strategies.

References

Baigent C, Landray MJ, Reith C, *et al.* (2011). The effects of lowering LDL cholesterol with simvastatin plus ezetimibe in patients with chronic kidney disease (Study of Heart and Renal Protection): a randomised placebo-controlled trial. *Lancet* **377**, 2181–2192.

Fellstrom BC, Jardine AG, Schmieder RE, *et al.* (2009). Rosuvastatin and cardiovascular events in patients undergoing hemodialysis. *N Engl J Med* **360**, 1395–1407.

16.9 Haemodialysis induced cardiac dysfunction is associated with an acute reduction in global and segmental myocardial blood flow

Authors

CW McIntyre, JO Burton, NM Selby, L Lecciscotti, S Korsheed, CS Baker, PG Camici

Reference

Clinical Journal of the American Society of Nephrology 2008, **3**, 19–26.

Abstract

Background and objectives: Hemodialysis is associated with hemodynamic instability, acute cardiac ischemia and the development of regional wall motion abnormalities (RWMAs). This study used serial intradialytic $H_2^{15}O$ positron emission tomography scanning to confirm that the development of dialysis-induced RWMAs was associated with reduction in myocardial blood flow (MBF).

Design, setting, participants and measurements: Four prevalent hemodialysis patients without angiographically significant coronary artery disease had measurements of MBF during standard hemodialysis and biofeedback dialysis. All patients underwent serial measurements of MBF using positron emission tomography. Concurrent echocardiography was used to assess left ventricular function and the development of RWMAs. Hamodynamic variables were measured using continuous pulse wave analysis.

Results: Mean prehemodialysis MBF was within the normal range. Global MBF was acutely reduced during hemodialysis. Segmental MBF was reduced to a significantly greater extent in areas that developed RWMAs compared with those that did not. Not all regions with reduced MBF were functionally affected, but a reduction in myocardial blood flow of > 30% from baseline was significantly associated with the development of RWMAs. No significant differences in hemodynamic tolerability, RWMA development or MBF between dialysis modalities were observed.

Conclusions: Hemodialysis is associated with repetitive myocardial ischaemia, which, in the absence of coronary artery disease, may be due to coronary microvascular dysfunction. Stress-induced segmental left ventricular dysfunction correlates with matched reduction in MBF. Functional poststress recovery is consistent with myocardial stunning induced by hemodialysis. This process may be important in the development of heart failure in long-term hemodialysis patients.

Importance

The selection of this particular study is obviously a very personal choice. Although personally a little uncomfortable with its inclusion, it represents the initial experimental evidence that, in humans, conventional haemodialysis with ultrafiltration is able to produce a significant segmental reduction in myocardial perfusion. This study and interrelated series of studies (summarized by McIntyre, 2010) have identified that systemic circulatory stress is a common consequence of conventional haemodialysis, and that it is capable of producing recurrent ischaemia in a variety of vulnerable vascular beds, driving end-organ injury and mortality risk.

This particular study utilized cardiac positron emission tomography (PET) scanning combined with radioactive water as the imaging isotope. The study presented a number of significant technical challenges to allow the assessment of segmental myocardial blood flow (MBF) in real time under the stress of haemodialysis. The patients were recruited from our home unit but were studied 120 miles away. The radioactive water (necessary to have a rapid equilibration of imaging isotope into myocardial tissue) needed an adjacent cyclotron to produce a sterile isotope for immediate administration. This was added to the complexity needed to build a haemodialysis set-up in the PET scanner. The patients were then subjected to repeat assessment utilizing biofeedback-controlled dialysis to examine the possibility that improving haemodynamic stress during treatment might eliminate the cardiac injury. All patients had undergone coronary angiography and none had significant large-vessel coronary disease.

We were able to demonstrate that dialysis was capable of inducing a reduction in MBF of a similar magnitude to that associated with acute coronary syndromes. This recovered after dialysis was discontinued. The areas of the ventricle that suffered reductions in contractile function (myocardial stunning) co-localized to the areas of maximum reduction in MBF. Where intradialytic blood pressure was maintained best by biofeedback dialysis, there was a significant increase in the minimum MBF seen. These results were largely reproduced in a subsequent dialysis PET study performed in Groenigen in the Netherlands by Casper Franssen and co-workers (Dasselaar *et al.*, 2009). This utilized a different isotope and identified reduction in MBF at an early stage of the haemodialysis procedure.

The appreciation of the ischaemia-inducing potential of dialysis has now led to extension of this concept into recurrent gut ischaemia (driving translocation of endotoxin and systemic inflammation), renal injury (damaging residual renal function), and recurrent brain injury (potentially providing a biological basis for cognitive decline and increasing levels of depression).

References

Dasselaar JJ, Slart RH, Knip M, *et al.* (2009). Haemodialysis is associated with a pronounced fall in myocardial perfusion. *Nephrol Dial Transplant* **24**, 604–610.

McIntyre CW (2010). Recurrent circulatory stress: the dark side of dialysis. *Semin Dial* **23**, 449–451.

16.10 Effect of frequent nocturnal hemodialysis versus conventional hemodialysis on left ventricular mass and quality of life: a randomized controlled trial

Authors

BF Culleton, M Walsh, SW Klarenbach, G Mortis, N Scott-Douglas, RR Quinn, M Tonelli, S Donnelly, MG Friedrich, A Kumar, H Mahallati, BR Hemmelgarn, BJ Manns

Reference

Journal of the American Medical Association 2007, **19**, 1291–1299.

Abstract

Context: Morbidity and mortality rates in hemodialysis patients remain excessive. Alterations in the delivery of dialysis may lead to improved patient outcomes.

Objective: To compare the effects of frequent nocturnal hemodialysis vs conventional hemodialysis on change in left ventricular mass and health-related quality of life over 6 months.

Setting, design, and participants: A 2-group, parallel, randomized controlled trial conducted at 2 Canadian university centers between August 2004 and December 2006. A total of 52 patients undergoing hemodialysis were recruited.

Intervention: Participants were randomly assigned in a 1:1 ratio to receive nocturnal hemodialysis 6 times weekly or conventional hemodialysis 3 times weekly.

Main outcome measures: The primary outcome was change in left ventricular mass, as measured by cardiovascular magnetic resonance imaging. The secondary outcomes were patient-reported quality of life, blood pressure, mineral metabolism, and use of medications.

Results: Frequent nocturnal hemodialysis significantly improved the primary outcome (mean left ventricular mass difference between groups, 15.3 g, 95% confidence interval [CI], 1.0 to 29.6 g; $P = .04$). Frequent nocturnal hemodialysis did not significantly improve quality of life (difference of change in EuroQol 5-D index from baseline, 0.05; 95% CI, −0.07 to 0.17; $P = .43$). However, frequent nocturnal hemodialysis was associated with clinically and statistically significant improvements in selected kidney-specific domains of quality of life ($P = .01$ for effects of kidney disease and $P = .02$ for burden of kidney disease). Frequent nocturnal hemodialysis was also associated with improvements in systolic blood pressure ($P = .01$ after adjustment) and mineral metabolism, including a reduction in or discontinuation of antihypertensive medications (16/26 patients in the nocturnal hemodialysis group vs 3/25 patients in the conventional hemodialysis group; $P < .001$) and oral phosphate binders (19/26 patients in the nocturnal hemodialysis group vs 3/25 patients in the conventional dialysis group; $P < .001$). No benefit in anemia management was seen with nocturnal hemodialysis.

Conclusion: This preliminary study revealed that, compared with conventional hemodialysis (3 times weekly), frequent nocturnal hemodialysis improved left ventricular mass, reduced the need for blood pressure medications, improved some measures of mineral metabolism, and improved selected measures of quality of life.

Importance

This study was the first prospective RCT of extended dialysis schedules. Up to this point, experience relating to the potential beneficial effects of extended dialysis schedules had been gleaned from extended case series alone. However, this study represented a coming of age in dialysis-based cardiovascular research. It tested the hypothesis that increasing dialysis frequency, in the setting of in-centre nocturnal dialysis therapy, is capable of altering left ventricular structure (assessed by cardiac magnetic resonance imaging, the 'gold standard') as a well-accepted surrogate of cardiovascular risk.

This study was performed in ten dialysis units based around two Canadian academic institutions. Fifty-two patients were recruited from the existing unit and home-based dialysis patient pool and randomized on a 1:1 basis to either three time per week conventional treatment (10–13.5 h of dialysis per week) or nocturnal therapy (30–48 h performed over five to six sessions per week). The primary end point of this study was the detection of a reduction of left ventricular mass (LVM) using cardiac magnetic resonance imaging, over a 6-month period. A careful suite of health-related quality-of-life (HRQOL) measures were also undertaken, as well as monitoring of blood pressure, anaemia, mineral status, and hospitalization/vascular access complications.

The headline result was a reduction in LVM of nearly 16 g, even in those patients who were already well established on haemodialysis. It is biologically plausible that this magnitude of change will be associated with a significant decrease in cardiovascular risk. Blood pressure and mineral control both improved, allowing a significant reduction in pill burden directed at both of those issues. Anaemia, hospitalization, and vascular access complications were no different between the two groups. There was a significant improvement in two out of four kidney disease-specific domains of HRQOL measures. The lack of significant effect in other domains was probably influenced by low patient numbers and the poor sensitivity of these quality-of-life evaluation instruments within the dialysis population.

More frequent dialysis appears to possess the potential to address many of the problems that are attributed to conventional haemodialysis therapy. The expanded envelope of cost and patient acceptability are clearly challenges, and this study provided the justification and much of the framework for the subsequent frequent nocturnal haemodialysis studies (Rocco *et al.*, 2011; see also paper 12.10) to provide data of sufficient quality to inform meaningfully the debate relating to expenditure to support ESRD programmes. Although important and largely successful, unfortunately these studies remain an incremental step on that journey.

Reference

Rocco MV, Lockridge RS Jr, Beck GJ *et al.* (2011). The effects of frequent nocturnal home hemodialysis: the Frequent Hemodialysis Network Nocturnal Trial. *Kidney Int* **80**, 1080–1091.

Chapter 17

Bone and mineral metabolism in chronic kidney disease

John Cunningham

Introduction

The papers chosen for this chapter bring us from the era when it was not understood why parathyroidectomized animals died of tetany, or how exposure to sunlight was capable of healing rickets, to more recent landmark events such as the identification of the calcium-sensing receptor and the demonstration that disorders of fibroblast growth factor 23 (FGF23) regulation and action are central to the pathogenesis of tumour-induced osteomalacia and other phosphate wasting syndromes. Along the way, we see outstanding, prescient accounts of the role of phosphate in the genesis of the mineral disturbances that accompany chronic kidney disease (CKD) and the consequences of a progressive reduction of nephron number leading to the 'intact nephron hypothesis', as espoused by Bricker and colleagues in 1960. The review by Stanbury from 1968 lamented the lack of focus on the skeleton up to that time and predicted a continuing lack of focus in the future—a fair point, in that over the past two or three decades the enormous research effort that has been drawn towards the parathyroids and the vitamin D system has probably been at the expense of the bone itself. In the early 1970s, two groups, led by Fraser and Kodicek and by DeLuca, demonstrated the structure of 1,25-dihydroxyvitamin D and the importance of the kidney as the principal site of its production. It was not long before Bricker, Coburn, and Norman reported the first studies of 1,25-dihydroxyvitamin D (calcitriol) used as a treatment in uraemic subjects, a paper demonstrating spectacular effects on hyperparathyroidism, as well as giving early warning of some of the less desirable tendency of vitamin D compounds to cause hypercalcaemia and hyperphosphataemia. Later, the group of Thadhani working at Harvard published the first of a series of papers looking at the effects of treatment with active vitamin D receptor ligands on the survival of patients with CKD, showing apparent benefit attributable to vitamin D compounds. The identification and cloning of the extracellular calcium-sensing receptor in bovine parathyroid tissue by Brown and colleagues in the early 1990s constituted another dramatic step forward and quickly led to the development of compounds capable of modifying the action of this receptor, one of which, cinacalcet, has already seen the light of day as a pharmaceutical agent used to treat hyperparathyroidism. The elapsed time between the cloning of the receptor and the first papers describing the action of calcimimetics was remarkably short. Finally, FGF23, something of a 'new kid on the block', was identified as the central cause of a variety of phosphate wasting syndromes. As an important phosphate-regulating hormone in both physiological and pathophysiological scenarios, extreme elevation of FGF23 as seen in CKD may prove to be a sensitive and potent marker for adverse cardiovascular outcomes in these patients.

One can only presume that this blistering pace of development will continue in the future, although, as in the past, it is difficult to predict from where the truly radical developments will emerge.

17.1 The extraction of a parathyroid hormone which will prevent or control parathyroid tetany and which regulates the level of blood calcium

Author

JB Collip

Reference

Journal of Biological Chemistry 1925, **63**, 395–438.

Abstract

1. An extract has been made from the parathyroid glands of oxen by the use of which parathyroid tetany in dogs can be prevented or controlled.

2. The active principle in this extract produces its effect by causing the calcium content of the blood serum to be restored within normal limits.

3. A very close parallelism has been observed between the clinical condition of experimental animals and the calcium content of the blood serum. Coincident with the marked improvement observed following the use of the active extract a rise in blood calcium has been noted.

4. Overdosage effects have been observed and the blood findings in this condition invariably show a condition of hypercalcemia.

5. The symptoms of hypercalcemia are anorexia, vomiting, apathy, drowsiness verging into coma, and a failing circulation.

6. Hypercalcemia in parathyroidectomized dogs is a fatal condition if allowed to persist.

7. Sodium bicarbonate has been observed to reduce the calcium content of the blood serum in hypercalcemia.

8. Tetania parathyreopriva has been prevented or controlled in dogs receiving no preoperative preparation and which have been placed on a heavy meat diet immediately following recovery from the operative procedure. Animals in which tetany has been prevented from occurring by prophylactic treatment have been thrown into tetany by temporary withdrawal of the treatment.

9. One to two treatments per day are sufficient to prevent tetany in parathyroidectomized dogs.

10. The extract containing the active principle has been found to be effective by each of three modes of administration; namely, by the oral route, by intravenous injection, and by subcutaneous injection.

11. A rise in the level of blood calcium in the normal dog has been observed following the injection of parathyroid extract.

Importance

Collip's paper is remarkable in several respects. The studies described collectively represented an enormous step forward in the understanding of the regulation of extracellular fluid calcium concentration and the critical role of the parathyroids in this regulation. Total parathyroidectomy had long been known to lead to fatal tetany. Cross-circulation experiments had shown that blood from an animal in tetany increased the neural excitability in a normal limb. In 1907, a palliative effect of calcium on tetany was identified, and in 1913 low blood calcium in tetanic animals was documented, followed in 1918 by the establishment of a normal range of serum calcium (9.2–11.3 mg/dl, 2.3–2.8 mmol/l) to be compared with serum calcium in tetanic patients, which was typically about 4–6 mg/dl (1–1.5 mmol/l). Finally, it was found that parathyroidectomized animals could be kept alive for long periods when fed on calcium-enriched diets containing lactose—a combination now known to facilitate intestinal calcium absorption—with other studies at about the same time showing similar amelioration of tetany by intravenous administration of calcium. With considerable difficulty, Collip developed a bovine parathyroid extract capable of preventing tetany in totally parathyroidectomized animals (dogs) with a close parallelism between their clinical state and serum calcium concentration. It was further noted that excessive doses of the parathyroid extract led to hypercalcaemia.

This paper is also notable for the extraordinary amount of experimental detail in what, by modern standards at least, was an exceptionally long paper providing an important bedrock upon which the future understanding of parathyroid disorders was built. It was also in 1925 that the phosphaturic action of parathyroid hormone (PTH) extract on the kidney was identified. Among the most important later developments were the discovery by Chase and Auerbach (1967) of the role of adenylate cyclase and cyclic AMP as an intracellular second messenger in the mediation of PTH effects on its target organs, the structural analysis of PTH (Brewer and Ronan, 1970), and the demonstration that the biological activity resided at the amino terminal end (Potts *et al.*, 1971), and with that the development of radioimmune assays sensitive enough to assay the hormone in clinical practice (Berson and Yalow, 1968). Without this earlier work, none of our understanding of the critical role of PTH in the maintenance of normal serum calcium in the face of developing CKD, and also the development of secondary hyperparathyroidism and its consequences in that clinical scenario, could have been realized.

References

Berson SA, Yalow RS (1968). Immunochemical heterogeneity of parathyroid hormone in plasma. *J Clin Endocrinol Metab* **28**, 1037–1047.

Brewer HB, Ronan R (1970). Bovine parathyroid hormone: amino acid sequence. *Proc Nat Acad Sci USA* **67**, 1862–1869.

Chase LR, Auerbach CD (1967). Parathyroid function and the renal excretion of 3′,5′-adenylic acid. *Proc Nat Acad Sci USA* **58**, 518–525.

Potts JT, Tregear GW, Keutmann H, *et al.* (1971). Synthesis of a biologically active N-terminal tetratriacontapeptide of parathyroid hormone. *Proc Nat Acad Sci* **68**, 63–67.

17.2 The pathologic physiology of chronic Bright's disease. An exposition of the 'intact nephron hypothesis'

Authors

NS Bricker, PA Morrin, SW Kime Jr

Reference

American Journal of Medicine 1960, **28**, 77–98.

Abstract

The course of advancing chronic renal disease is characterized by the development of a constellation of clinical, biochemical and physiologic derangements. These derangements may ultimately involve many organs and organ systems; however, the fundamental event underlying their development is the progressive destruction of nephrons. Although the causal relationship between intrinsic renal disease and the complex abnormalities of the uremic state was recognized by Bright more than twelve decades ago, the precise nature of the events leading from the initial destruction of nephrons to the picture of terminal uremia is yet to be fully understood. Until it becomes possible to prevent the various forms of chronic renal disease or to interrupt their inexorable progression, a major requisite to effective concepts of therapy is the clarification of the sequential events in pathologic physiology. In this regard it is essential to define clearly the functional capacity, range of operation and limitations of the diseased kidney. The present discussion consists of a review of recent experimental observations relating to these considerations.

Importance

A notable feature of this article is the extent to which, despite being published in a journal devoted principally to clinical internal medicine and its subspecialties, it delves deeply into renal physiology, and references most of the figures who contributed to the 'state of the art' of renal pathophysiology during the 15 years following World War II. Early in the paper, Bricker, who was a renal physiologist, stated that '…until it becomes possible to prevent the various forms of chronic renal disease or to interrupt their inexorable progression, a major requisite to effective concepts of therapy is the clarification of the sequential events in pathologic physiology. In this regard it is essential to define clearly the functional capacity, range of operation and limitations of the diseased kidney…' This powerfully makes a general point that clinical medicine will rarely advance except when underpinned by an understanding of the relevant pathophysiology. The article reviewed, with great lucidity, the literature covering the renal handling of water, sodium, potassium, and phosphate. Central to the discussion was the notion that, in most pathologies associated with chronic renal insufficiency, there is a tendency for nephrons to 'drop out' in an 'all-or-nothing' fashion. Although direct measurement of single-nephron glomerular filtration rate (GFR) was still some way off, the necessity for residual nephrons to 'up their game' by increasing their GFR, and also adapting their handling of water and solute, was a central plank of Bricker's thinking at this time. For example, a nephron that is already in a highly phosphaturic state under the influence (as we know now) of PTH and FGF23 has little capacity to reduce further the tubular reabsorption of phosphate, a concept that would have been readily appreciated in the early 1950s

(Goldman and Bassett, 1954). Thus, the clinical sequelae of CKD are inevitably associated with a striking reduction in the adaptive capacity of the kidney on many fronts. The application of these principles to the management of moderate and severe renal failure in the pre-dialysis era focused initially on water, sodium, potassium, and later phosphate (Platt, 1952; Goldman and Bassett, 1954; Schwartz, 1955).

Bricker acknowledged that the observations of Bright (see papers 3.1 and 5.3), establishing the relationship between chronic renal disease and the uraemic state, set the stage for much of his work and this is reflected in his use of the term 'chronic Bright's disease' in this article.

References

Goldman R, Bassett SH (1954). Phosphorus excretion in renal failure. *J Clin Invest* **33**, 1623–1625.

Platt R (1952). Structural and functional adaptation in renal failure. *Brit Med J* **1**, 1313–1317.

Schwartz B (1955). Potassium and the kidney. *New Engl J Med* **253**, 601–608.

17.3 Bone disease in uremia

Authors

SW Stanbury

Reference

American Journal of Medicine 1968, **44**, 714–724.

Summary & Importance

While the focus of *Landmarks in Nephrology* is on original articles, here a review paper has been selected because it is far reaching and prescient. Stanbury opens with a key summary statement. '...it is necessary to emphasise that one cannot understand bone disease without studying the involved bone itself and that much of the confusion that enveloped azotemic osteodystrophy in the past stemmed from neglect of this...' Furthermore '...that history may repeat itself in the osteodystrophy complicating chronic hemodialytic therapy unless systemic studies are made of biopsy specimens of bone using the many techniques that are now available...' These predictions were right—the number of bone biopsies performed for diagnostic or research purposes in uraemic patients has always lagged behind that required to define the underlying pathology properly, and current clinical guidelines continue to lament the impoverished state of our knowledge of what is really going on in the bones of dialysis patients.

Stanbury's influence in the field peaked around the inception of maintenance haemodialysis, a time at which the type of renal osteodystrophy seen moved from that associated with progressive CKD to that associated with long-term haemodialysis. Stanbury was a strong believer in the central importance of defective mineralization in the genesis of renal osteodystrophy (Stanbury and Lumb, 1962), in this respect finding himself, not for the only time, somewhat at odds with at least one of the other major opinion leaders of his time, Fuller Albright (Albright *et al.*, 1937), who emphasized hyperparathyroid bone disease ('azotemic hyperparathyroidism'). The studies of uraemic bone at the time preceded the full characterization of the vitamin D endocrine system, and vitamin D therapies were largely confined to extraordinarily high doses of native vitamin D_2 (ergocalciferol).

The article also touched on another burning argument of the day—the potential role of metabolic acidosis in azotemic osteodystrophy and hence also that of correction of acidosis. The paper ranges over the important issues of vitamin D resistance, calcium balance, and also hyperparathyroidism. Stanbury also described what was almost certainly nodular hyperplasia of the parathyroid glands with 'apparently adenomatous transformation in the glands'. He even referred to autonomous hyperparathyroidism (effectively the phenotype of primary hyperparathyroidism) following renal transplantation (Stanbury *et al.*, 1960).

Throughout, Stanbury's opinions are expressed strongly, suggesting that behind the scenes he was fighting significant academic battles. The paper is, however, a masterly and far-reaching discussion of the state of play that existed at that time.

References

Albright F, Drake TG, Sulkowitch HW (1937). Renal osteitis fibrosa cystica; report of a case with discussion of metabolic aspects. *Bull Johns Hopkins Hosp* **60**, 377–399.

Stanbury SW, Lumb GA (1962). Metabolic studies of renal osteodystrophy. I. Calcium, phosphorus and nitrogen metabolism in rickets, osteomalacia and hyperparathyroidism complicating chronic uraemia and in the osteomalacia of the adult Fanconi syndrome. *Medicine* **41**, 1–34.

Stanbury SW, Lumb GA, Nicholson WF (1960). Elective sub-total parathyroidectomy for renal hyperparathyroidism. *Lancet* **1**, 793–799.

17.4 Calcium, phosphorus and bone in renal disease and transplantation

Authors

NS Bricker, E Slatopolsky, E Reiss, LV Avioli

Reference

Archives of Internal Medicine 1969, **123**, 543–553.

Abstract

Calcium-phosphate-bone interrelationships become disrupted progressively in advancing renal disease. Parathyroid hormone (PTH) release, normally attuned to calcium homeostasis requirements, becomes dominated by alterations in phosphate balance. With each wave of nephron destruction, there is believed to occur transient hyperphosphatemia, transient hypocalcemia, and a step-wise rise in PTH levels. When the glomerular filtration rate falls below 25 to 30 ml per minute, hyperphosphatemia persists, hypocalcemia tends to persist, and the stimulus to PTH release is exaggerated. Vitamin D resistance contributes both to hypocalcemia (thus to accelerated PTH secretion) and to osteomalacia. In patients receiving long-term hemodialysis, if hyperphosphatemia and hypocalcemia persist, PTH levels may remain high and osteitis fibrosa may progress. Successful renal transplantation typically leads to regression of hyperparathyroidism and restoration of vitamin D sensitivity; however, hyperparathyroidism may regress slowly, and severe hypercalcemia must be guarded against. True autonomy of PTH release apparently occurs rarely in chronic renal disease.

Importance

The studies described in this paper gave rise to the concept that became known as the 'trade-off hypothesis'. Building on their earlier work (Slatopolsky *et al.*, 1968), the trade-off hypothesis focused specifically on the necessity for the kidney to adapt its handling of phosphate in the face of falling GFR and the mechanisms necessary for the kidney to achieve this. A powerful role for PTH was identified, with progressive elevation of PTH seen over time in dogs subjected to subtotal nephrectomy. This paper further demonstrated that the progressive reduction of the tubular reabsorption of phosphate, apparently driven by PTH, was greatly attenuated if the animals were subjected to a proportional reduction of dietary phosphate. The really significant outcome was the attenuation of secondary hyperparathyroidism and with that the attenuation of an important consequence of hyperparathyroidism, increased osteoclastic bone resorption. The other side of the coin was nicely demonstrated by Lemann's group, who showed that profound renal phosphate retention was generated by healthy volunteers on low-phosphate diets (Dominguez *et al.*, 1976).

We must remember that these studies were undertaken in the 1960s, and a role for vitamin D was probably not considered seriously at the time. Looking back, we can now see that FGF23 was almost certainly a significant component of these adaptive responses and that the modification to the tubular reabsorption of phosphate was probably driven by both PTH and FGF23 acting in concert (Gutierrez *et al.*, 2005). An important clinical spin off from this work was heightened awareness of the importance of controlling hyperphosphataemia in patients with advanced CKD.

Subsequent studies in man, using similar experimental protocols, yielded consistent, although not always identical, findings to those from the original animal work.

An additional piece of the jigsaw, again not appreciated at the time, was the impact of hyperphosphataemia on vitamin D metabolism and specifically the production of 1,25-dihydroxyvitamin D. In the 1970s, it was shown convincingly that phosphate was an important regulator of the 1-α hydroxylase enzyme, and more recently a role for FGF23 in that regulation has been established, as FGF23, elevated in response to hyperphosphataemia, powerfully down regulates 1-α hydroxylase, an action that is counter-regulatory to that of PTH (Gutierrez *et al.*, 2005). The early implications of this work were discussed in detail in an excellent review in the *New England Journal of Medicine* by Bricker (1972), and a contemporary view is offered by Slatopolsky in *Kidney International* (2011).

References

Bricker NS (1972). On the pathogenesis of the uremic state. An exposition of the 'trade-off hypothesis'. *N Engl J Med* **286**, 1093–1099.

Dominguez JH, Gray RW, Lemann J Jr (1976). Dietary phosphate deprivation in women and men: effects on mineral and acid balances, parathyroid hormone and the metabolism of 25-OH-vitamin D. *J Clin Endocrinol Metab* **43**, 1056–1068.

Gutierrez O, Isakova T, Rhee E *et al.* (2005). Fibroblast growth factor-23 mitigates hyperphosphatemia but accentuates calcitriol deficiency in chronic kidney disease. *J Am Soc Nephrol* **16**, 2205–2215.

Slatopolsky E (2011). The intact nephron hypothesis: the concept and its implications for phosphate management in CKD-related mineral and bone disorder. *Kidney Int* (Suppl.) **79**, S3–S8.

Slatopolsky E, Robson AM, Elkan I, Bricker NS (1968). Control of phosphate excretion in uremic man. *J Clin Invest* **47**, 1865–1874.

17.5 Isolation and identification of 1,25-dihydroxycholecalciferol. A metabolite of vitamin D active in intestine

Authors

MF Holick, HK Schnoes, HF DeLuca, T Suda, RJ Cousins

Reference

Biochemistry 1971, **10**, 2799–2804.

Abstract

A metabolite of vitamin D_3, thought to be the "tissue-active" form of the vitamin in the intestine, has been isolated from chicken intestines in pure form as the monotriethylsilyl ether derivative. The structure of this metabolite has been identified as 1,25 dihydroxycholecalciferol by means of mass spectrometry, ultraviolet absorption spectophotometry, and specific chemical reactions.

Importance

It is difficult to overestimate the significance of the discovery and characterization of 1,25-dihydroxyvitamin D, the physiological hormonal form of vitamin D. This work was done by the group headed by Hector DeLuca at the University of Wisconsin and was enabled by crucial technical developments in 1966. High-specific-activity vitamin D compounds became available for the first time, allowing tracking of the pathways of vitamin D metabolism (Neville and DeLuca, 1966). This group subsequently spawned a large number of individuals who were to become prominent in the vitamin D field. Several of these are authors on the *Biochemistry* paper discussed here. This was the first detailed description of the chemical structure of the active form of vitamin D determined by mass spectrometry, along with evidence of its particular tissue effects. The hormone was extracted from the intestines of chicks labelled with tritiated vitamin D_3. This paper is nicely complemented by that of Fraser and Kodicek (1970) working in Cambridge, UK, who demonstrated the synthesis of a metabolite (subsequently shown to be 1,25-dihydroxyvitamin D) by kidney homogenates. In the studies by Fraser and Kodicek, a number of organs were investigated empirically and only in the kidney was substantial production of the more polar 1,25-dihydroxyvitamin D compound seen. These authors also speculated that the failure of renal biosynthesis of 1,25-dihydroxyvitamin D was the immediate cause of vitamin D resistance seen in chronic renal failure. Writing later, Fraser modestly stated that '…despite its popularity, this *Nature* paper is not of special importance…', an assertion with which many would disagree.

Nevertheless, these two papers are perfectly complementary and together constituted an enormous step forward in our understanding of the actions of vitamin D, and how these actions are modified in chronic renal disease. It is notable that these studies took place almost exactly half a century after the seminal observations of Mellenby (1919), who discovered that cod liver oil could cure rickets, and Huldschinsky (1919), who showed that ultraviolet irradiation of a single limb would cure rickets in all limbs, thereby satisfying the criteria for a hormone: synthesized at one site and active at a remote site.

Collectively, this work provided the basis for an emerging understanding of the regulation of vitamin D metabolism, its role in controlling skeletal and mineral homeostasis, and as a treatment for vitamin D-deficient states, particularly those associated with vitamin D resistance.

References

Fraser D R, Kodicek E (1970). Unique biosynthesis by kidney of a biologically active vitamin D metabolite. *Nature* **228**, 764–766.

Huldschinsky K (1919). Heilung von Rachitis durch kunstliche Hobensonne. *Deutsch Med Wochenschr* **41**, 712–713.

Mellanby E (1919). An experimental investigation on rickets. *Lancet* **1**, 407–412.

Neville PF, DeLuca HF (1966). The synthesis of [1,2–3H] vitamin D3 and the tissue localization of a 0.25-μg (10 IU) dose per rat. *Biochemistry* **5**, 2201–2207.

17.6 Action of 1,25-dihydroxycholecalciferol, a potent kidney produced metabolite of vitamin D$_3$, in uremic man

Authors

Brickman, AS, JW Coburn AW Norman

Reference

New England Journal of Medicine 1972, **287**, 891–895.

Abstract

Only the kidney is capable of producing 1,25-dihydroxycholecalciferol (1,25diOHC), the probable active form of vitamin D. The possibility that parenchymal damage in chronic renal disease impairs production of 1,25diOHC and accounts for 'vitamin-D resistant' uremia prompted our evaluation of its effects in uremic man. Three patients with advanced renal failure showed significant responses to daily treatment with only 100 U (2.7 μg) of 1,25diOHC for six to 10 days: serum calcium and phosphorus rose; intestinal radioactive calcium (^{47}Ca) absorption increased by 30 to 220 per cent; and fecal calcium decreased by 25 to 71 per cent in those undergoing balance studies. In contrast, 40,000 U (1 mg) of vitamin D caused no change in serum calcium and phosphorus and had negligible effects on ^{47}Ca absorption. Thus, 1,25diOHC is highly active in uremic man, and its impaired production may account for certain abnormalities of calcium homeostasis in uremia. The agent may hold future promise in management of disordered calcium metabolism in uremia.

Importance

This publication, a landmark in that it was the first description of the use of 1,25-dihydroxyvitamin D as treatment for the vitamin D resistance of uraemia, built on the early understanding that calcitriol was the probable hormonal form of vitamin D, and that failure of its synthesis underpinned the vitamin D resistance seen in uraemia. It also reflected the early demonstration that this hormone localized to certain classical target tissues of vitamin D (Norman *et al.*, 1971) and that the kidney was the organ responsible for synthesizing almost all of the circulating 1,25-dihydroxyvitamin D (Fraser and Kodicek; 1970). Only three patients with advanced renal failure were studied, in whom large doses (1 mg) of native vitamin D had already been shown to have negligible effects on calcium absorption or serum calcium and phosphorus. In contrast, the 1,25-dihydroxyvitamin D, when given at doses of only 2.7 μg daily for 6–10 days, elevated serum calcium and phosphorus and decreased faecal calcium. Confirmatory studies followed in short order, one of these utilizing the pro-drug alfacalcidol, which generated similar biological responses in uraemic patients (Davie *et al.*, 1976). The arrival of increasingly reliable assays for PTH was soon applied to studies of this type, and showed a striking reduction of PTH in patients treated with 1,25-dihydroxyvitamin D or alfacalcidol (Brownjohn *et al.*, 1977). These medications proved highly effective in the treatment of hyperparathyroidism, by far the commonest and most damaging form of metabolic bone disease in uraemia at that time. Substantial skeletal healing was documented, manifest by radiological improvement and reduction of elevated alkaline phosphatase. On the down side, the narrow therapeutic window of active vitamin D compounds quickly became apparent with hypercalcaemia and hyperphosphataemia recognized as important adverse events. At that time, there was no perception that PTH could be oversuppressed, and the general mantra was 'low is good and lower is better'. So spectacular were the early responses to the new active vitamin D compounds that the secondary problem of augmenting intestinal phosphate absorption was not fully appreciated, not least because most of the early studies were of short duration. Even now, some 40 years later, there remains a surprising amount of uncertainty as to how best to deploy these compounds (Wetmore and Quarles, 2008).

References

Brownjohn AM, Goodwin FJ, Hately W, Marsh FP, O'Riordan JL, Papapoulos SE (1977). 1-alpha-hydroxycholecalciferol for renal osteodystrophy. *Brit Med J* **2**, 721–723.

Davie MWJ, Chalmers TM, Hunter UO, Pelc B, Kodicek E (1976). 1-Alphahydroxycholecalciferol in chronic renal failure. Studies of the effect of oral doses. *Ann Intern Med* **84**, 281–285.

Fraser DR, Kodicek E (1970). Unique biosynthesis by kidney of a biologically active vitamin D metabolite. *Nature* **228**, 764–766.

Norman AW, Myrtle JF, Midgett RJ, Nowicki HG, Williams V, Popjak G (1971). 1,25-dihydroxy cholecalciferol: identification of the proposed active form of vitamin D3 in the intestine. *Science* **173**, 51–54.

Wetmore JB, Quarles LD (2008). Calcimimetics or vitamin D analogs for suppressing parathyroid hormone in end-stage renal disease: time for a paradigm shift? *Nat Clin Pract Nephrol* **5**, 24–33.

17.7 The dialysis encephalopathy syndrome. Possible aluminum intoxication

Authors

AC Alfrey, GR LeGendre, WD Kaehny

Reference

New England Journal of Medicine 1976, **294**, 184–188.

Abstract

The aluminum content of muscle, bone and brain was measured in control subjects and in uremic patients on dialysis who had been maintained on phosphate-binding aluminum gels. The mean muscle aluminum was 14.8 ppm, and the trabecular-bone aluminum 98.5 ppm in the patients on dialysis, as compared with 1.2 and 2.4 in control subjects (P < 0.05). Brain gray-matter aluminum values in a group of uremic patients on dialysis who died of a neurologic syndrome of unknown cause were 25 ppm as compared with 6.5 ppm in a group of uremic patients on dialysis who died of other causes and 2.2 ppm in control subjects. The fact that brain gray-matter aluminum was higher in all patients with the dialysis-associated encephalopathy syndrome than any of the control subjects or other uremic patients on dialysis suggests that this syndrome may be due to aluminum in intoxication.

Importance

During the early 1970s, an hitherto unrecognized syndrome of rapidly progressive encephalopathy emerged in patients with renal failure. The paper by Alfrey and colleagues provided convincing, if not conclusive, evidence that aluminium was the principle aetiological factor. Brain aluminium content was increased substantially in affected patients and was much higher than those in 'control' uraemic subjects without encephalopathy. These, in turn, were much higher than the brain aluminium content in non-uraemic individuals.

Others, principally groups in Sheffield (see paper 12.6) and Newcastle (Ward *et al.*, 1978) also described this syndrome and reported that patchy distribution of cases was associated with variations in water borne aluminium. The Newcastle and Sheffield groups further identified aluminium as the principle aetiological factor in an unusually symptomatic form of osteomalacia found in dialysis patients. Although aluminium was present in serum at extremely low concentration, it was selectively taken up at the mineralization front in bone; studies by Faugere and Malluche (1986) elegantly showed that the patchy linear deposition of aluminium coincided precisely with areas of mineralization failure. These findings were of enormous importance to dialysis patients who had been facing a frightening epidemic of uncertain aetiology without a coherent preventative strategy. The effects on clinical practice were dramatic, and centred initially around the routine use of deionized water for dialysis and subsequently the progressive withdrawal of aluminium-based phosphate binders in the face of clear evidence that oral aluminium could be a significant and sometimes dominant contributor to overall aluminium burden (Felsenfeld *et al.*, 1982). The initial move to calcium-based phosphate binders itself brought difficulties with recurrent hypercalcaemia seen quite commonly and a later appreciation that high oral calcium intake probably contributed to accelerated vascular calcification and possibly to increased morbidity and mortality

(Braun *et al.*, 1996). Thus, the withdrawal of a toxic phosphate binder was immediately followed by the introduction of another suboptimal agent, albeit a less toxic one.

References

Braun J, Oldendorf M, Moshage W, Heidler R, Zeitler E, Luft FC (1996). Electron beam computed tomography in the evaluation of cardiac calcification in chronic dialysis patients. *Am J Kidney Dis* **27**, 394–401.

Faugere MC, Malluche HH (1986). Stainable aluminum and not aluminum content reflects bone histology in dialyzed patients. *Kidney Int* **30**, 717–722.

Felsenfeld AJ, Gutman RA, Llach F, Harrelson JM (1982). Osteomalacia in chronic renal failure: a syndrome previously reported only with maintenance dialysis. *Am J Nephrol* **2**, 147–154.

Ward MK, Feest TG, Ellis HA, Parkinson IS, Kerr DNS (1978). Osteomalacic dialysis osteodystrophy: evidence for a water-borne aetiological agent, probably aluminium. *Lancet* **1**, 841–845.

17.8 Cloning and characterization of an extracellular Ca²⁺-sensing receptor from bovine parathyroid

Authors

EM Brown, G Gamba, D Riccardi, M Lombardi, R Butters, O Kifor, A Sun, MA Hediger, J Lytton, SC Hebert

Reference

Nature 1993, **366**, 575–580.

Abstract

Maintenance of a stable internal environment within complex organisms requires specialized cells that sense changes in the extracellular concentration of specific ions (such as Ca^{2+}). Although the molecular nature of such ion sensors is unknown, parathyroid cells possess a cell surface Ca^{2+}-sensing mechanism that also recognizes trivalent and polyvalent cations (such as neomycin) and couples by changes in phosphoinositide turnover and cytosolic Ca^{2+} to regulation of parathyroid hormone secretion. The latter restores normocalcaemia by acting on kidney and bone. We now report the cloning of complementary DNA encoding an extracellular Ca^{2+}-sensing receptor from bovine parathyroid with pharmacological and functional properties nearly identical to those of the native receptor. The novel approximately 120K receptor shares limited similarity with the metabotropic glutamate receptors and features a large extracellular domain, containing clusters of acidic amino-acid residues possibly involved in calcium binding, coupled to a seven-membrane-spanning domain like those in the G-protein-coupled receptor superfamily.

Importance

When looking at the development of our understanding of parathyroid physiology and pathophysiology, there are three defining issues that have set the framework for this field. The first was the appreciation that the parathyroid glands dominated the control of extracellular fluid calcium concentration, and that without them lethal tetany supervened. Secondly, the identification of PTH as the functionally critical output from the parathyroid glands, coupled with the ability to measure it reliably and to understand the function of its receptor in target tissue, generated an enormous acceleration in our understanding of the role of this gland and its hormone. Finally, the work described in this *Nature* paper by Brown and colleagues defined the structure of the calcium-sensing receptor (CaSR) on parathyroid and other cells and simultaneously advanced our understanding of the functionality of this receptor. This paper effectively fired the starting gun for an extraordinarily rapid development of understanding of the physiology and pathophysiology of the parathyroid glands and the development of therapeutic tools based on their ability to manipulate the behaviour of the CaSR. These developments have moved apace, with the rapid identification of activating and inactivating mutations of the CaSR underlying, respectively, the clinical syndromes of autosomal dominant hypocalcaemia and familial hypocalciuric hypercalcaemia (Pollak *et al.*, 1993). Immune-mediated diseases may also operate via the CaSR, which may be a target of cell- and antibody-mediated attack in idiopathic autoimmune hypoparathyroidism (Kifor *et al.*, 2004). This paper described the cloning and characterization of the

CaSR from bovine parathyroid tissue. Related studies showed that extracellular divalent and tri-valent cations operated through a cell-surface-sensing mechanism that demonstrably coupled to changes in cytosolic calcium and phosphoinositide turnover, which regulated PTH secretion in a manner that, in the case of low extracellular calcium concentration, restored normocalcaemia by actions on bone and kidney (Brown and MacLeod, 2001).

Another crucial and remarkably rapid development of the work described in this paper has been the development of small molecules targeting the CaSR. Prominent among these have been the phenylalkylamine derivatives with calcimimetic activity, which act as positive allosteric modifiers of the CaSR and increase its sensitivity to its ligands. Calcimimetics have now found an important role in the treatment of hyperparathyroid disorders (Steddon and Cunningham, 2005).

References

Brown EM, MacLeod RJ (2001). Extracellular calcium sensing and extracellular calcium signaling. *Physiol Rev* **81**, 239–297.

Kifor O, McElduff A, LeBoff MS, *et al.* (2004). Activating antibodies to the calcium-sensing receptor in two patients with autoimmune hypoparathyroidism. *J Clin Endocrinol Metab* **89**, 548–556.

Pollak MR, Brown EM, Chou YH, *et al.* (1993). Mutations in the human Ca2+-sensing receptor gene cause familial hypocalciuric hypercalcemia and neonatal severe hyperparathyroidism. *Cell* **75**, 1297–1303.

Steddon S, Cunningham J (2005). Calcimimetics and calcilytics—fooling the calcium receptor. *Lancet* **365**, 2237–2239.

17.9 Survival of patients undergoing hemodialysis with paricalcitol or calcitriol therapy

Authors

M Teng, M Wolf, E Lowrie, N Ofsthun, JM Lazarus, R Thadhani

Reference

New England Journal of Medicine 2003, **349**, 446–456.

Abstract

Background: Elevated calcium and phosphorus levels after therapy with injectable vitamin D for second-ary hyperparathyroidism may accelerate vascular disease and hasten death in patients undergoing long-term hemodialysis. Paricalcitol, a new vitamin D analogue, appears to lessen the elevations in serum calcium and phosphorus levels, as compared with calcitriol, the standard form of injectable vitamin D.

Methods: We conducted a historical cohort study to compare the 36-month survival rate among patients undergoing long-term hemodialysis who started to receive treatment with paricalcitol (29,021 patients) or calcitriol (38,378 patients) between 1999 and 2001. Crude and adjusted survival rates were calculated and stratified analyses were performed. A subgroup of 16,483 patients who switched regimens was also evaluated.

Results: The mortality rate among patients receiving paricalcitol was 3417 per 19,031 person-years (0.180 per person-year), as compared with 6805 per 30,471 person-years (0.223 per person-year) among those receiving calcitriol (P<0.001). The difference in survival was significant at 12 months and increased with time (P<0.001). In the adjusted analysis, the mortality rate was 16 percent lower (95 percent confidence interval, 10 to 21 percent) among paricalcitol-treated patients than among calcitriol-treated patients. A significant survival benefit was evident in 28 of 42 strata examined, and in no stratum was calcitriol favored. At 12 months, calcium and phosphorus levels had increased by 6.7 and 11.9 percent, respectively, in the paricalcitol group, as compared with 8.2 and 13.9 percent, respectively, in the calcitriol group (P<0.001). The two-year survival rate among patients who switched from calcitriol to paricalcitol was 73 percent, as compared with 64 percent among those who switched from paricalcitol to calcitriol (P=0.04).

Conclusions: Patients who receive paricalcitol while undergoing long-term hemodialysis appear to have a significant survival advantage over those who receive calcitriol. A prospective, randomized study is criti-cal to confirm these findings.

Importance

This paper proved to be the first of an exciting cascade of studies that appeared to show a survival advantage for maintenance haemodialysis patients according to the type of vitamin D treatment used, and subsequently whether any vitamin D at all had been given. A historical cohort design was used to demonstrate that, in patients who had received paricalcitol, the adjusted mortal-ity rate was 15% lower than that in calcitriol-treated patients. Subsequent studies by the same Harvard-based group used a similar design to compare survival in patients who had, and had not, at any time received injectable active vitamin D treatment with calcitriol or paricalcitol (Teng *et al.*, 2005). Here, substantially lower mortality was seen in patients who had received active vitamin D treatment, with the somewhat counterintuitive observation that this benefit appeared to be maintained even in those with low PTH, high calcium, and high phosphate, in whom active vitamin D treatment would normally be relatively contraindicated.

These studies sparked an enormous interest in the role of vitamin D beyond its classical actions related to bone and mineral metabolism, and in particular focused on vitamin D action on the heart and vasculature. Studies of a similar design in South American cohorts showed broadly similar results in patients treated with oral active vitamin D compounds, demonstrating that the effect was not confined to those who were treated parenterally. These latter studies also showed an inverse dose response relationship, whereby the highest mortality was seen in patients who had received no vitamin D and the lowest mortality seen in those who had received the smallest doses of vitamin D, with higher dose vitamin D-treated patients occupying an intermediate position (Naves-Diaz *et al.*, 2008).

Much work has flowed directly and indirectly from these observations. Experimental studies using vitamin D receptor and 1α-hydroxylase knockout mice (Zhou *et al.*, 2008) and clinical studies in patients with CKD (London *et al.*, 2007) suggested that activation of the vitamin D receptor is associated with higher levels of vascular health. Compelling work in a human *ex vivo* model have suggested a U-shaped relationship between vitamin D exposure and vascular calcification, whereby no exposure, and high exposure, to active vitamin D are both more likely to be associated with vascular calcification than intermediate-level exposure (Schroff *et al.*, 2010). Interesting though these observations are, there remains a distinct paucity of high-quality clinical trial data to support them, and current management recommendations are still underpinned by a mixture of belief and fact.

References

London GM, Guérin AP, Verbeke FH, *et al.* (2007). Mineral metabolism and arterial functions in end-stage renal disease: potential role of 25-hydroxyvitamin D deficiency. *J Am Soc Nephrol* **18**, 613–620.

Naves-Diaz M, Alvarez-Hernandez D, Passlick-Deetjen J, *et al.* (2008). Oral active vitamin D is associated with improved survival in hemodialysis patients. *Kidney Int* **74**, 1070–1078.

Schroff R, Knott C, Rees L (2010). The virtues of vitamin D—but how much is too much? *Ped Nephrol* **25**, 1607–1620.

Teng M, Wolf M, Ofsthun MN, *et al.* (2005). Activated injectable vitamin D and hemodialysis survival: a historical cohort study. *J Am Soc Nephrol* **16**, 1115–1125.

Zhou C, Lu F, Cao K, Xu D, Goltzman D Miao D (2008). Calcium-independent and 1,25(OH)2D3-dependent regulation of the renin–angiotensin system in 1α-hydroxylase knockout mice. *Kidney Int* **74**, 170–179.

17.10 Cloning and characterization of FGF23 as a causative factor of tumor-induced osteomalacia.

Authors

T Shimada, S Mizutani, T Muto, T Yoneya, R Hino, S Takeda, Y Takeuchi, T Fujita, S Fukumoto, T Yamashita

Reference

Proceedings of the National Academy of Sciences USA 2001, **98**, 6500–6505.

Abstract

Tumor-induced osteomalacia (TIO) is one of the paraneoplastic diseases characterized by hypophosphatemia caused by renal phosphate wasting. Because removal of responsible tumors normalizes phosphate metabolism, an unidentified humoral phosphaturic factor is believed to be responsible for this syndrome. To identify the causative factor of TIO, we obtained cDNA clones that were abundantly expressed only in a tumor causing TIO and constructed tumor-specific cDNA contigs. Based on the sequence of one major contig, we cloned 2,270-bp cDNA, which turned out to encode fibroblast growth factor 23 (FGF23). Administration of recombinant FGF23 decreased serum phosphate in mice within 12 h. When Chinese hamster ovary cells stably expressing FGF23 were s.c. implanted into nude mice, hypophosphatemia with increased renal phosphate clearance was observed. In addition, a high level of serum alkaline phosphatase, low 1,25-dihydroxyvitamin D, deformity of bone, and impairment of body weight gain became evident. Histological examination showed marked increase of osteoid and widening of growth plate. Thus, continuous production of FGF23 reproduced clinical, biochemical, and histological features of TIO *in vivo*. Analyses for recombinant FGF23 products produced by Chinese hamster ovary cells indicated proteolytic cleavage of FGF23 at the RXXR motif. Recent genetic study indicates that missense mutations in this RXXR motif of FGF23 are responsible for autosomal dominant hypophosphatemic rickets, another hypophosphatemic disease with similar features to TIO. We conclude that overproduction of FGF23 causes TIO, whereas mutations in the FGF23 gene result in autosomal dominant hypophosphatemic rickets possibly by preventing proteolytic cleavage and enhancing biological activity of FGF23.

Importance

This study established disturbed phosphate regulation by FGF23 as the underlying cause of tumour-induced osteomalacia. This condition, in which a tumour (usually of mesenchymal origin) is associated with a renal phosphate wasting syndrome that is cured by complete resection of the tumour, had for some time been thought to be the result of a circulating phosphaturic factor. A similar scenario was thought to exist in some other phosphate wasting conditions, notably X-linked hypophosphataemia (Bowe *et al.*, 2001). Much experimental work had been conducted in the latter, facilitated by the existence of a murine homologue (the Hyp mouse). Cross-circulation and transplantation studies using Hyp mice eventually established the role of a humoral factor—from the transplantation studies, it was apparent that the abnormality resided in the animal and not in the transplanted kidney (Nesbitt *et al.*, 1992). In this paper, cDNA clones extracted from a tumour apparently causing phosphate wasting osteomalacia were found to encode FGF23. Further support for the role of FGF23 was obtained from implantation of Chinese hamster ovary cells expressing FGF23 into nude mice, who developed hypophosphataemia within hours. The mouse phenotype also included low plasma calcitriol concentrations, especially when taken in the context of the prevailing hypophosphataemia, which, in other circumstances, would be expected to upregulate calcitriol production. This phenotype is remarkably similar to that of human X-linked hypophosphataemia, as well as that seen in the Hyp mouse.

This study provided an excellent example of the careful study of a single patient with a precisely defined phenotype, generating a large leap forward in our understanding of a clinical condition. Later, the same group established the critical role of Klotho in reconstituting the FGF receptor 1, enabling activity of FGF23 on selected cell types by this method (Urakawa *et al.*, 2006). FGF23 knockout mice and patients with hyperphosphataemic tumoural calcinosis are hyperphosphataemic and have high renal tubular phosphate reabsorption and high serum calcitriol levels (Lyles *et al.*, 1988). The later identification of an association between FGF23 and cardiovascular morbidity and mortality in the CKD population (Faul *et al.*, 2011) further drew together the linked roles of phosphate, vitamin D metabolism, and FGF23 in the maintenance or otherwise of vascular health.

References

Bowe AE, Finnegan R, Jan de Beur SM, *et al.* (2001). FGF-23 inhibits renal tubular phosphate transport and is a PHEX substrate. *Biochem Biophys Res Commun* **284**, 977–981.

Lyles KW, Halsey DL, Friedman NE, Lobaugh B (1988). Correlations of serum concentrations of 1,25-dihydroxyvitamin D, phosphorus, and parathyroid hormone in tumoral calcinosis. *J Clin Endocrinol* **67**, 88–92.

Nesbitt T, Coffman TM, Griffiths R, Drezner MK (1992). Crosstransplantation of kidneys in normal and Hyp mice. Evidence that the Hyp mouse phenotype is unrelated to an intrinsic renal defect. *J Clin Invest* **89**, 1453–1459.

Faul C, Amaral AP, Oskoeui B, *et al.* (2011). FGF23 induces left ventricular hypertrophy. *J Clin Invest* **121**, 4393–4408.

Urakawa I, Yamazaki Y, Shimada T, *et al.* (2006). Klotho converts canonical FGF receptor into a specific receptor for FGF23. *Nature* **444**, 770–774.

Chapter 18

Renal anaemia

Christopher G. Winearls

Introduction

It was Robert Christison who first observed the association of anaemia and renal disease, writing, 'I am acquainted with no natural disease at least of a chronic nature, which so closely approaches haemorrhage in its power of impoverishing the red particles of the blood.' He observed too the 'leukophlegmatic waxiness of the complexion' and the 'brown tinge' so familiar to nephrologists (see paper 5.5). The endocrine functions of the kidney dawned on physiologists rather late. What might have been a curiosity became a clinical challenge when the first patients with irreversible kidney failure were prevented from dying of electrolyte derangement by dialysis but gradually manifested the consequences of endocrine deficiency, most particularly anaemia and 'renal rickets'. Indeed, Homer Smith's classic book on the kidney makes no mention of the relationship of erythropoiesis and the kidney (Smith, 1951). The story of renal anaemia starts with the final proof of the existence of an erythropoieitic substance by Erslev (1953) then discovering that the kidney was the major organ of origin, purifying it, measuring it, cloning its gene, producing it by recombinant DNA technology, and then showing that it reversed the anaemia of uraemic subjects. This was thought to be the end of the matter, but it was not. The anaemia was found to be more than an endocrine deficiency state and its effects, and those of its reversal, proved rather complex.

References

Erslev A (1953). Humoral regulation of red cell production. *Blood* **8**, 349–357.

Smith HW (1951). *The Kidney Structure and Function in Health and Disease*. Oxford University Press, New York.

18.1 Role of the kidney in erythropoiesis

Authors

LO Jacobson, E Goldwasser, W Fried, L Pizak

Reference

Nature 1957, **179**, 633–634.

Summary

This letter reports that plasma derived from nephrectomized rats treated with cobalt or phlebotomy had no increase in erythropoietic activity, which was assayed by injecting their plasma into starved rats and measuring the uptake of iron-59 into the recipient rats' erythrocytes. Uptake was similar to that found in unstimulated controls with intact kidneys. In contrast, rats not subjected to nephrectomies, adrenalectomized rats (with surgical stress and post-operative haemoglobin levels comparable to the nephrectomized rats), and rats with ligated ureters (resulting in uraemia comparable to those subjected to nephrectomy) retained the ability to drive erythropoiesis.

Importance

This much cited paper implicated the kidneys in erythropoietin production and provided an explanation to nephrologists as to why their patients were anaemic. The authors considered the possibility that the kidney might activate erythropoietin produced elsewhere but argued that this was unlikely as the assay was performed in animals with intact kidneys. They also acknowledged the possibility that the kidneys produced an inactive precursor of erythropoietin that was subsequently activated by a different organ but felt that if this was the case the kidney still had a central role in erythropoiesis.

What is not clear is why the authors investigated the kidneys so late in their search for the site of erythropoietin production; they had already tested the effects of hypophysectomy, thyroidectomy, gonadectomy, splenectomy, gastrectomy, seven-eighths hepatectomy, gastrectomy, adrenalectomy, and removal of the intestine. Prior to this publication, the authors had already established that the balance of the erythron depended on the relationship of oxygen supply to the demand for its use, but the authors did not speculate on why the kidney should be the organ that sensed this oxygen supply/demand relationship (Kurtz and Eckardt, 1991). They observed that ureteric ligation, which they correctly noted acutely abolished excretory function but not endocrine function, reduced the response to cobalt but not as much as nephrectomy. However, they did not draw the inference that the reduction in oxygen demand, due to the absence of a need to reabsorb the filtered load, might contribute to this intermediate result.

Subsequent work has shown that erythropoietin is produced, albeit in small quantities, in many other organs (Maxwell *et al.*, 1997), and in the fetus, it is the liver that makes the major contribution. The work of many groups has identified the oxygen-sensing system, the identification of interstitial fibroblasts as the erythropoietin-producing cells, and the effects of kidney injury on their phenotype consistent with these original experiments (Koury *et al.*, 1988; Ratcliffe *et al.*, 1997; Maxwell *et al.*, 1997).

References

Koury ST, Bondurant MC, Koury MJ (1988). Localization of erythropoietin synthesizing cells in murine kidneys by *in situ* hybridisation. *Blood* **71**, 524–527.

Kurtz A, Eckardt KU (1991). Renal function and oxygen sensing. In: *Erythropoietin Molecular, Cellular and Clinical Biology*, pp. 79–98. Edited by AJ Erslev, JW Adamson, JW Eschbach, CG Winearls. The John Hopkins University Press, Baltimore/London.

Maxwell PH, Ferguson DJ, Nicholls LG, *et al.* (1997). Sites of erythropoietin production. *Kidney Int* **51**, 393–401.

Maxwell PH, Ferguson DJ, Nicholls LG, Johnson MH, Ratcliffe PJ (1997). The interstitial response to renal injury: fibroblast-like cells show phenotypic changes and have reduced potential for erythropoietin gene expression. *Kidney Int* **52**, 715–724.

Ratcliffe PJ, Ebert BL, Firth JD, *et al.* (1997). Oxygen regulated gene expression: erythropoietin as a model system. *Kidney Int* **51**, 514–526.

18.2 Bioassay of erythropoietin in mice made polycythaemic by exposure to air at a reduced pressure. A bioassay for erythropoietin

Authors

PM Cotes, DR Bangham

Reference

Nature 1961, **191**, 1065–1067.

Summary

The test animals were female mice that had been maintained in a tank for 14 days with air at a pressure of half an atmosphere and a CO_2 concentration of <1%. Iron incorporation was measured 20 h after the intravenous injection of 0.1 μCi iron-59 citrate. Animals returned to normal pressure showed suppression of iron incorporation to <10% of normal mice. For the measurement of the erythropoietic activity of test material, it was injected on days 1 and 2 or 3 and 4, after the mice returned to normoxia. The iron-59 was injected on day 3 or 5, and the mice were sacrificed on day 4 or 6. The response was taken as the percentage of the administered iron-59 present in the blood 20 h after the injection. There was a log linear relationship between the dose of the test substance and iron incorporation. The assay performed better when the animals were given the extra 2 days at normoxia before the assay was started. The assay detected rabbit, sheep, monkey, and human eythropoietic activity, and the slopes of the regression curves did not differ significantly.

Importance

'If you can not measure it, you can not improve it.'
Lord Kelvin

This paper described meticulous experiments to measure the intangible substance erythropoietin in the era before radio-immunoassays, HPLC, and RNase protection assays. There was no clean material that could be measured in molar terms. For such a numerical measurement to have any meaning, it would have to be related to the activity of the hormone. This bioassay, which was an improvement on predecessors, provided the platform for defining reference material described later (Cotes and Bangham, 1966) and the development of a radioimmunoassay (Cotes, 1982). Even today, measurements of serum erythropoietin are expressed as units/ml based on this biological activity. Erythropoietin is characterized by its ability to induce an increase in red-cell mass. It would have been too cumbersome and would have required repeated injections and a long time to see the effect on red-cell mass itself. Instead, the first step was to choose a surrogate measure of increased red-cell production, and incorporation of iron-59 into red cells was likely to be the most reproducible. To produce a low background required suppression of endogenous erythropoiesis, which could be done by blood transfusion or starvation. In this assay, it was achieved by inducing polycythaemia by exposing the animals to air at reduced pressure. This allowed appropriate numbers of animals in a similar state to be prepared. Each step in the assay was made as reproducible as possible and this explains its precision.

References

Cotes PM (1982). Immunoreactive erythropoietin in serum. I. Evidence for the validity of the assay method and the physiological relevance of estimates. *Br J Haematol* **50**, 427–438.

Cotes PM and Bangham DR (1966). The International Reference Preparation of Erythropoietin. *Bull World Health Organ* **35**, 751–760.

18.3 Purification of human erythropoietin

Authors

T Miyake, CKH Kung, E Goldwasser

Reference

Journal of Biological Chemistry 1977, **252**, 5558–5564.

Abstract

Human erythropoietin, derived from urine of patients with aplastic anemia, has been purified to apparent homogeneity. The seven-step procedure, which included ion exchange chromatography, ethanol precipitation, gel filtration, and adsorption chromatography, yielded a preparation with a potency of 70,400 units/mg of protein in 21% yield. This represents a purification factor of 930. The purified hormone has a single electrophoretic component in polyacrylamide gels at pH 9, in the presence of sodium dodecylsulfate at pH 7, and in the presence of Triton X-100 at pH 6. Two fractions of the same potency and molecular size, by sodium dodecyl sulfate gel electrophoresis, but differing slightly in mobility at pH 9, were obtained at the last step of fractionation. The nature of the difference between these two components is not yet understood.

Importance

This work was a tour de force requiring the collection of 2550 litres of urine from patients with aplastic anaemia. It was an essential prerequisite for the structural characterization of the hormone (Lai *et al.*, 1986); for the development of a radio-immunoassay for erythropoieitin, which allowed later study of the concentrations of erythropoieitin in diseases characterized by anaemia and polycythemia (Garcia *et al.*, 1979); and for the design of probes needed for cloning of the gene (see paper 18.4). The protein, which is highly conserved across species (mouse, monkey, and man), was shown to contain 193 amino acids, one of which is cleaved off. It was found to have a molecular weight of 32 kDa, 40% of which was accounted for by carbohydrate. When assembled, it was found to be a four-helix bundle structure interacting with its receptor, which was identified by D'Andrea *et al.* (1989). The effect of the binding of erythropoietin to its receptor is to rescue erythroid progenitors from apoptosis.

References

D'Andrea AD, Lodish HF, Wong GG (1989). Expression cloning of the murine erythropoietin receptor. *Cell* **57**, 277–285.

Garcia JF, Sherwood J, Goldwasser E (1979). Radioimmunoassay for erythropoietin. *Blood Cells* **5**, 405–19.

LaiPH, Everett R, Wang FF, Arakawa T, Goldwasser E (1986). Structural characterisation of human erythropoieitin. *J Biol Chem* **26**, 3116–3121.

18.4 Cloning and expression of the human erythropoietin gene

Authors

FK Lin, S Suggs, CH Lin, JK Browne, R Smalling, JC Egrie, KK Chen, GM Fox, F Martin, Z Stabinsky, SM Badrawi, PH Lai, E Goldwasser

Reference

Proceedings of the National Academy of Sciences USA 1985, **82**, 7580–7584.

Abstract

The human erythropoietin gene has been isolated from a genomic phage library by using mixed 20-mer and 17-mer oligonucleotide probes. The entire coding region of the gene is contained in a 5.4-kilobase *Hind*III-*Bam*HI fragment. The gene contains four intervening sequences (1562 base pairs) and five exons (582 base pairs). It encodes a 27-amino acid signal peptide and a 166-amino acid mature protein with a calculated M_r of 18,399. The erythropoietin gene, when introduced into Chinese hamster ovary cells, produces erythropoietin that is biologically active *in vitro* and *in vivo*.

Importance

This paper should be read in conjunction with that of Jacobs *et al.* (1986). They were published in the same year, but the Jacobs paper was in print earlier. The work by Lin and colleagues is chosen as the landmark paper only because it was the recombinant erythropoietin they produced that was first shown to be effective in uraemic man (see paper 18.5). Those without any expertise in molecular biology read these papers in awe. The cloning of this gene was a huge challenge. Firstly, there was relatively little pure erythropoietin protein to provide amino acid sequence information, and the design of oligonucleotide probes had to cover for the degeneracy of the DNA code. There was no enriched source of human erythropoietin mRNA to make a cDNA library. Both groups fished for the erythropoietin gene in a human fetal genomic library and used probes designed to find different parts of the gene simultaneously. Lin and colleagues used two probes screening 1.5 million phage clones and identified four that hybridized with both probe mixtures. They called this their 'two-site' confirmation approach. This worked, and they were fortunate in getting one clone that contained the complete erythropoietin gene. This was introduced into a cell line and active hormone was harvested. They had a cunning back-up strategy. They produced a cDNA library from the mRNA extracted from the kidney of a monkey that had been made anaemic with phenylhydrazine. They reasoned that there would be a substantial degree of sequence homology, which could have made the design of probes easier. As it happened, their 17-mer probe did not hybridise to the monkey erythropoietin gene because one of the amino acid differences was in this area (Lin *et al.*, 1986). Jacobs *et al.* (1986) had used three probes and obtained a portion of the erythropoietin gene from which they could produce a probe to find erythropoietin mRNA in fetal liver. They isolated cDNA clones from the cDNA library constructed from fetal liver mRNA and used this to transfect COS-1 cells, which produced the active hormone. These cloning achievements allowed accurate description of the protein's structure and identification of its glycosylation sites. They also resolved a few existing controversies—there was no precursor molecule 'erythropoietinogen' and it was not related to angiotensinogen. Both clones led to the production of therapeutic recombinant erythropoietin—'epoetin-α' from the Lin clone and 'epoetin-β' from the Jacobs clone.

References

Jacobs K, Shoemaker C, Rudersdorf R, *et al.* (1986). Isolation and characterization of genomic cDNA clones of human erythropoietin. *Nature* **313**, 806–810.

Lin FK, Lin CH, Lai PH, *et al.* (1986). Monkey erythropoietin gene: cloning expression and comparison with the human erythropoietin gene. *Gene* **44**, 201–209.

18.5 Effect of human erythropoietin derived from recombinant DNA on the anaemia of patients maintained by chronic hemodialysis

Authors

CG Winearls, DO Oliver, MJ Pippard, C Reid, MR Downing, PM Cotes

Reference

Lancet 1986, **ii**, 1175–1181.

Abstract

Ten patients with end-stage renal failure and anaemia (mean haemoglobin 6.1 g/dl, range 4.6–8.8 g/dl) on thrice-weekly haemodialysis were treated with human erythropoietin derived from recombinant DNA (rHuEPO). This was given as an intravenous bolus after each dialysis in rising doses within the range 3–192 IU/kg. All patients showed increases in reticulocyte numbers and haemoglobin concentration and after the first week of treatment none of the four previously transfusion-dependent patients needed further transfusions. In nine patients treated for 12 weeks haemoglobin rose to a mean of 10.3 g/dl, range 9.5 to 12.8 g/dl. Thereafter the dose of erythropoietin was adjusted to avoid a further rise in haemoglobin. During treatment one patient had an episode of hypertensive encephalopathy and two had clotting in their arteriovenous fistulas (complete in one). rHuEPO is an effective treatment for the anaemia of end-stage renal failure but longer-term observations are needed on the consequences of increasing the haematocrit.

Importance

This was a simple unequivocal report of one of the two pilot studies of the effect of recombinant human erythropoietin (rHuEPO) on the anaemia of uraemia. The other was conducted by Eschbach and colleagues (1987) in Seattle, the cradle of maintenance haemodialysis treatment for end-stage renal disease. It was an 'Everest' moment for the lead investigator, Dr P. Mary Cotes, who had been working on the biology and measurement of erythropoietin for over 20 years. Having predicted the effective dose, she had designed the protocol with the scientists from Amgen, who had synthesized the rHuEPO, and her nephrology colleagues. These ten responding patients underwent intense study of the handling of rHuEPO, their responses being judged by ferrokinetics and the behaviour of their red-cell progenitors (Reid *et al.*, 1988; Cotes *et al.*, 1989). The half-life of rHuEPO was 6–8 h and had not changed after the reversal of the anaemia, red-cell survival remained reduced, and the iron uptake of the erythron was supranormal, implying a need to compensate for the shorter red-cell lifespan. The Eschbach protocol compared a range of doses and showed that the rate of response was directly related to the dose. Both groups gave rHuEPO as an intravenous bolus at the time of dialysis for convenience and to ensure complete delivery. Neither knew whether the marrow needed exposure to high doses to imitate the concentrations found in non-renal anaemias or more sustained but smaller increases in the concentration. It was later shown that subcutaneous delivery was effective and more economical (Bommer *et al.*, 1988). Anyone reading this and Eschbach's paper now cannot fail to notice the danger flags that were raised—hypertensive encephalopathy and vascular access thrombosis were both reported. They also observed the high iron needs of the responders but found no antibodies to rHuEPO. These three issues—cardiovascular effects of rthe HuEPO, iron supplementation, and the development of pure red-cell aplasia caused by neutralizing antibodies—would later dominate research in the therapeutic use of rHuEPO.

References

Bommer J, Ritz E, Weinreich T, Bommer G, Ziegler T (1988). Subcutaneous erythropoietin. *Lancet* **ii**, 406.

Cotes PM, Pippard MJ, Reid CDL, Winearls CG, Oliver DO, Royston JP (1989). Characterisation of the anaemia of chronic renal failure and the mode of its correction by a preparation of erythropoietin (r-HuEpo). An investigation of the pharmacokinetics of intravenous r-HuEpo and it effect on erythrokinetics. *Quart J Med* **70**, 113–137.

Eschbach JW, Egrie JC, Downing MR Browne JK, Adamson JW (1987). Correction of the anemia of end-stage renal disease with recombinant human erythropoietin. Results of a Phase I and II clinical trial. *N Engl J Med* **316**, 73–78.

Reid CDL, Fidler J, Oliver DO, Cotes PM, Pippard MJ, Winearls CG (1988). Erythroid progenitor cell kinetics in chronic haemodialysis patients responding to treatment with recombinant human eythropoeitin. *Br J Haematol* **70**, 375–380.

18.6 The effects of normal as compared with low hematocrit values in patients with cardiac disease who are receiving hemodialysis and epoetin

Authors

A Besarab, WK Bolton, JK Browne, JC Egrie, AR Nissenson, DM Okamoto, SJ Schwab, DA Goodkin

Reference

New England Journal of Medicine 1998, **339**, 584–590.

Abstract

Background: In patients with end-stage renal disease, anemia develops as a result of erythropoietin deficiency, and recombinant human erythropoietin (epoetin) is prescribed to correct the anemia partially. We examined the risks and benefits of normalizing the hematocrit in patients with cardiac disease who were undergoing hemodialysis.

Methods: We studied 1233 patients with clinical evidence of congestive heart failure or ischemic heart disease who were undergoing hemodialysis: 618 patients were assigned to receive increasing doses of epoetin to achieve and maintain a hematocrit of 42 percent, and 615 were assigned to receive doses of epoetin sufficient to maintain a hematocrit of 30 percent throughout the study. The median duration of treatment was 14 months. The primary end point was the length of time to death or a first nonfatal myocardial infarction.

Results: After 29 months, there were 183 deaths and 19 first nonfatal myocardial infarctions among the patients in the normal-hematocrit group and 150 deaths and 14 nonfatal myocardial infarctions among those in the low-hematocrit group (risk ratio for the normal-hematocrit group as compared with the low-hematocrit group, 1.3; 95 percent confidence interval, 0.9 to 1.9). Although the difference in event-free survival between the two groups did not reach the prespecified statistical stopping boundary, the study was halted. The causes of death in the two groups were similar. The mortality rates decreased with increasing hematocrit values in both groups. The patients in the normal-hematocrit group had a decline in the adequacy of dialysis and received intravenous iron dextran more often than those in the low-hematocrit group.

Conclusions: In patients with clinically evident congestive heart failure or ischemic heart disease who are receiving hemodialysis, administration of epoetin to raise their hematocrit to 42 percent is not recommended.

Importance

This clinical trial was a bold enterprise that sought an answer to a perfectly reasonable question. Why not aim for complete anaemia correction in patients with end-stage renal disease? By analogy with other hormone-deficiency states the aim was to restore normality, be it euglycaemia, euthyroidism, or corticosteroid replacement. It was bold because there were underlying concerns that uraemic subjects might be put at risk of thrombotic events, a rise in blood pressure, and reduced dialysis efficiency (Anon., 1987). Before the advent of rHuEPO, a few dialysis patients—usually those with inherited polycystic kidney disease or acquired cystic disease—maintained a normal haematocrit without ill-effects. Indeed, they seemed to be healthier than their anaemic peers. There was no policy of venesecting them to target a lower haemoglobin. The choice of patients with cardiac disease to test the effect of a higher haematocrit was also reasonable. These were patients who had the most to gain from improved tissue oxygenation and would have a high enough event rate to make the trial yield a result with a manageable number of study subjects followed for a limited period. The result came as a complete surprise. Not only was the intervention not beneficial, it was close to being shown to be harmful. The paradox was made more difficult to explain by the finding that achieving a higher haematocrit was not associated with the adverse outcomes. The hormonal analogy was, of course, flawed. Anaemic chronic kidney disease (CKD) patients are not, in absolute terms, erythropoietin deficient. They are relatively deficient, and the hormone needs to be present in supranormal concentrations to restore the haematocrit to normal. Moreover, the anaemia is not a pure hormone-deficiency state. To achieve a normal haematocrit in the face of confounding factors such as inflammation, iron deficiency, and shortened red-cell survival, requires hyperstimulation of the erythron and high doses of iron. Many explanations for this unexpected result have been advanced but none are completely satisfying. What one could conclude was that attempting to achieve a normal haematocrit in haemodialysis patients with cardiac disease was neither justified nor prudent. What is not clear is whether the achievement of a normal haematocrit, either spontaneously or with modest erythropoietin supplements, is dangerous. Once again, the power of randomized trials was vindicated.

References

Anon. (1987). Erythropoietin. *Lancet* **329**, 392.

18.7 Pure red-cell aplasia and antierythropoietin antibodies in patients treated with recombinant erythropoietin

Authors

N Casadevall, J Nataf, B Viron, A Kolta, JJ Kiladjian, P Martin-Dupont, P Michaud, T Papo, V Ugo, I Teyssandier, B Varet, P Mayeux

Reference

New England Journal of Medicine, 2002, **346**, 469–467.

Abstract

Background: Within a period of three years, we identified 13 patients in whom pure red-cell aplasia developed during treatment with recombinant human erythropoietin (epoetin). We investigated whether there was an immunologic basis for the anemia in these patients.

Methods: Serum samples from the 13 patients with pure red-cell aplasia were tested for neutralizing antibodies that could inhibit erythroid-colony formation by normal bone marrow cells in vitro. The presence of antierythropoietin antibodies was identified by means of binding assays with the use of radiolabeled intact, deglycosylated, or denatured epoetin.

Results: Serum from all 13 patients blocked the formation of erythroid colonies by normal bone marrow cells. The inhibition was reversed by epoetin. Antibodies from 12 of the 13 patients bound only conformational epitopes in the protein moiety of epoetin; serum from the remaining patient bound to both conformational and linear epitopes in erythropoietin. In all the patients, the antibody titer slowly decreased after the discontinuation of treatment with epoetin.

Conclusions: Neutralizing antierythropoietin antibodies and pure red-cell aplasia can develop in patients with the anemia of chronic renal failure during treatment with epoetin.

Importance

This paper caused great consternation in the renal community but probably should not have done so. The problem of the development of neutralizing antibodies had not arisen, despite over a decade of use of rHuEPO. Something had changed to cause this devastating complication that rendered the patients resistant to their own native erythropoietin. It was suggested that this was a rare but not unexpected consequence of administration of any recombinant protein. Actually, most of these cases had received a particular formulation of epoetin-α. The working explanations were that the protein had been rendered immunogenic by aggregation in the absence of albumin as a stabilizer, which had been withdrawn from the formulation; breaks in the cold chain of storage and transport; and the effect of leachates derived from the syringe rubber, which acted as an adjuvant when rHuEpo was injected subcutaneously. When these concerns were attended to, the incidence reduced. The problem has, however, not gone away. There are now reported cases that have occurred with other formulations including epoetin-β, darbepoetin-α, and some biosimilars. The best guess is that the erythropoietin becomes immunogenic because of aggregation, and this is favoured by the lack of an effective stabilizer, mishandling, and the presence of tungsten in the syringes. Patients do recover after withdrawal of rHuEPO, and this may be hastened by immunosuppressive treatment and, if possible, renal transplantation. The effect of the neutralizing antibodies can be avoided by the administration of a peptide erythropoietin receptor agonist (see paper 18.9). This topic has recently been reviewed and updated (Macdougall *et al.*, 2012).

Reference

Macdougall IC, Roger S, de Francisco A, *et al.* (2012). Antibody-mediated pure red cell aplasia in patients receiving ESA therapy: new insights. *Kidney Int* **81**, 727–732.

18.8 Normalization of hemoglobin level in patients with chronic kidney disease and anemia

Authors

TB Drüeke, F Locatelli, N Clyne, KU Eckardt, IC Macdougall, D Tsakiris, HU Burger, A Scherhag, for the CREATE Investigators

Reference

New England Journal of Medicine 2006, **355**, 2071–2084.

Abstract

Background: Whether correction of anemia in patients with stage 3 or 4 chronic kidney disease improves cardiovascular outcomes is not established.

Methods: We randomly assigned 603 patients with an estimated glomerular filtration rate (GFR) of 15.0 to 35.0 ml per minute per 1.73 m^2 of body-surface area and mild-to-moderate anemia (hemoglobin level, 11.0 to 12.5 g per deciliter) to a target hemoglobin value in the normal range (13.0 to 15.0 g per deciliter, group 1) or the subnormal range (10.5 to 11.5 g per deciliter, group 2). Subcutaneous erythropoietin (epoetin beta) was initiated at randomization (group 1) or only after the hemoglobin level fell below 10.5 g per deciliter (group 2). The primary end point was a composite of eight cardiovascular events; secondary end points included left ventricular mass index, quality-of-life scores, and the progression of chronic kidney disease.

Results: During the 3-year study, complete correction of anemia did not affect the likelihood of a first cardiovascular event (58 events in group 1 vs. 47 events in group 2; hazard ratio, 0.78; 95% confidence interval, 0.53 to 1.14; P = 0.20). Left ventricular mass index remained stable in both groups. The mean estimated GFR was 24.9 ml per minute in group 1 and 24.2 ml per minute in group 2 at baseline and decreased by 3.6 and 3.1 ml per minute per year, respectively (P = 0.40). Dialysis was required in more patients in group 1 than in group 2 (127 vs. 111, P = 0.03). General health and physical function improved significantly (P = 0.003 and P < 0.001, respectively, in group 1, as compared with group 2). There was no significant difference in the combined incidence of adverse events between the two groups, but hypertensive episodes and headaches were more prevalent in group 1.

Conclusions: In patients with chronic kidney disease, early complete correction of anemia does not reduce the risk of cardiovascular events.

Importance

This paper should be read with that of Singh *et al.* (2006) describing the Correction of Hemoglobin in Outcomes and Renal Insufficiency (CHOIR) trial study published in the same issue of the *New England Journal of Medicine*. Nephrologists wanted to know what the objectives were of treating the renal anaemia of patients with CKD, given that it was milder than that of haemodialysis patients, many of whom were disabled by anaemia and were transfusion dependent. There was a subjective impression that well-being was improved and plausible reasons to believe that anaemia treatment could improve outcomes by a beneficial effect on the heart. Of course, there were fears that treatment might accelerate the progression of CKD and exacerbate hypertension. That erythropoiesis-stimulating agents (ESAs) are effective at reversing anaemia was not at issue, but the proportional benefit for the change in haemoglobin was. The trials therefore compared patients allocated to higher and lower haemoglobin targets. In the Drueke trial [Cardiovascular risk Reduction by Early Anemia Treatment with Epoetin Beta (CREATE) trial], the results were mixed: there was no beneficial effect on cardiovascular events, but health improved without accelerating a decline in function, despite some adverse effects on blood pressure. The Singh trial (CHOIR) found an excess of cardiovascular events in the higher haemoglobin group without any difference in quality of life. This led to widespread clinical policy changes: lowering the target haemoglobin and not allowing patients to achieve a normal haemoglobin concentration. These trials have been much discussed (Levin, 2007). CREATE was judged to be a good randomized controlled trial but unfortunate in that the event rate was lower than expected and so it was 'underpowered.' CHOIR was criticized because of some imbalance in the baseline characteristics between the groups, the high drop-out rate, protocol changes, and apparent erythropoietin resistance in the higher haemoglobin target group (this is a surrogate for co-morbidity). Most nephrologists took one message from these trials—that although higher haemoglobins are associated with better patient outcomes, there was no trial evidence to justify striving to achieve higher haemoglobin targets. The last words on this controversy have not been spoken (Roger and Levin, 2007).

References

Levin A (2007). Understanding recent trials in CKD: methods and lesson learned from CREATE and CHOIR. *Nephrol Dial Transplant* **22**, 309–312

Roger SD, Levin A (2007). Epoetin trials: randomised control trials don't always mimic observational data. *Nephrol Dial Transplant* **22**, 684–686.

Singh A, Szczech L, Tank KL, *et al.* (2006). Correction of anemia with epoetin alfa in chronic kidney disease. *New Engl J Med* **355**, 2085–2098.

18.9 A peptide-based erythropoietin-receptor agonist for pure red-cell aplasia

Authors

IC Macdougall, J Rossert, N Casadevall, RB Stead, AM Duliege, M Froissart, KU Eckardt

Reference

New England Journal of Medicine 2009, **361**, 1848–1855.

Abstract

Background: We investigated whether a novel, synthetic, peptide-based erythropoietin-receptor agonist (Hematide, Affymax) can stimulate erythropoiesis in patients with anemia that is caused by antierythropoietin antibodies.

Methods: In this open-label, single-group trial, we enrolled patients with chronic kidney disease who had pure red-cell aplasia or hypoplasia due to antierythropoietin antibodies and treated them with a synthetic peptide-based erythropoietin-receptor agonist. The agonist was administered by subcutaneous injection at an initial dose of 0.05 mg per kilogram of body weight every 4 weeks. The primary end point was a hemoglobin concentration above 11 g per deciliter without the need for transfusions.

Results: We treated 14 patients with the peptide agonist for a median of 28 months. The median hemoglobin concentration increased from 9.0 g per deciliter (with transfusion support in the case of 12 patients) before treatment to 11.4 g per deciliter at the time of the last administration of the agonist; transfusion requirements diminished within 12 weeks after the first dose, after which 13 of the 14 patients no longer required regular transfusions. Peak reticulocyte counts increased from a median of 10×10^9 per liter before treatment to peak counts of greater than 100×10^9 per liter. The level of antierythropoietin antibodies declined over the course of the study and became undetectable in six patients. One patient who initially responded to treatment had a diminished hematologic response a few months later despite increased doses of the agonist and required transfusions again; this patient was found to have antibodies against the agonist. One patient died 4 months after the last dose of the agonist, and a grade 3 or 4 adverse event occurred in seven other patients during the study period.

Conclusions: This novel agonist of the erythropoietin receptor can correct anemia in patients with pure red-cell aplasia caused by antierythropoietin antibodies.

Importance

There is a surfeit of ESAs, all competing for a limited but lucrative market. The agent described in this paper was novel and not a 'me too' recombinant protein or a modified formulation. One assumes that the idea behind designing a small molecule agonist was that it would be cheaper to manufacture. It arrived at a serendipitous time when the whole hormone was eliciting the production of function-neutralizing antibodies in a small but worrying number of subjects. It was therefore a possible rescue treatment for patients with ESA-induced pure red-cell aplasia, and so it proved. This suggested that the anti-erythropoietin antibodies in patients with pure red-cell aplasia were not directed at the actual binding motif but at a nearby epitope, thus preventing the locking of the hormone to its receptor. However, one patient developed antibodies to the peptide agonist. It was administered subcutaneously, which increases the risk of antibody development hugely. It may be safer to administer it intravenously to patients with pure red-cell aplasia (cumbersome though this may be). Since this description of its efficacy in this rather special circumstance, it has been tested in patients with CKD not on dialysis and found to be effective. It is called peginesatide, a synthetic PEGylated peptide-based ESA. Different doses, routes, and injection frequencies have been tested in 139 patients (Macdougall *et al.*, 2011). It was effective by both routes and predictably there were brisker responses with higher and more frequent dosing: once every 4 week subcutaneous administration would be satisfactory.

Reference

Macdougall IC, Wiecek A, Tucker B, *et al.* (2011). Dose-finding study of peginesatide for anaemia correction in chronic kidney disease patients. *Clin J Am Soc Nephrol* **6**, 2579–86

18.10 A trial of darbepoetin alfa in type 2 diabetes and chronic kidney disease

Authors

MA Pfeffer, EA Burdmann, CY Chen, ME Cooper, D de Zeeuw, KU Eckardt, JM Feyzi, P Ivanovich, R Kewalramani, AS Levey, EF Lewis, JB McGill, JJ McMurray, P Parfrey, HH Parving, G Remuzzi, AK Singh, SD Solomon, R Toto, for the TREAT Investigators

Reference

New England Journal of Medicine 2009, **361**, 2019–2032.

Abstract

Background: Anemia is associated with an increased risk of cardiovascular and renal events among patients with type 2 diabetes and chronic kidney disease. Although darbepoetin alfa can effectively increase hemoglobin levels, its effect on clinical outcomes in these patients has not been adequately tested.

Methods: In this study involving 4038 patients with diabetes, chronic kidney disease, and anemia, we randomly assigned 2012 patients to darbepoetin alfa to achieve a hemoglobin level of approximately 13 g per deciliter and 2026 patients to placebo, with rescue darbepoetin alfa when the hemoglobin level was less than 9.0 g per deciliter. The primary end points were the composite outcomes of death or a cardiovascular event (nonfatal myocardial infarction, congestive heart failure, stroke, or hospitalization for myocardial ischemia) and of death or end-stage renal disease.

Results: Death or a cardiovascular event occurred in 632 patients assigned to darbepoetin alfa and 602 patients assigned to placebo (hazard ratio for darbepoetin alfa vs. placebo, 1.05; 95% confidence interval [CI], 0.94 to 1.17; P = 0.41). Death or end-stage renal disease occurred in 652 patients assigned to darbepoetin alfa and 618 patients assigned to placebo (hazard ratio, 1.06; 95% CI, 0.95 to 1.19; P = 0.29). Fatal or nonfatal stroke occurred in 101 patients assigned to darbepoetin alfa and 53 patients assigned to placebo (hazard ratio, 1.92; 95% CI, 1.38 to 2.68; P < 0.001). Red-cell transfusions were administered to 297 patients assigned to darbepoetin alfa and 496 patients assigned to placebo (P < 0.001). There was only a modest improvement in patient-reported fatigue in the darbepoetin alfa group as compared with the placebo group.

Conclusions: The use of darbepoetin alfa in patients with diabetes, chronic kidney disease, and moderate anemia who were not undergoing dialysis did not reduce the risk of either of the two primary composite outcomes (either death or a cardiovascular event or death or a renal event) and was associated with an increased risk of stroke. For many persons involved in clinical decision making, this risk will outweigh the potential benefits.

Importance

The Trial to Reduce Cardiovascular Events with Aranesp Therapy (TREAT) changed clinical practice and so acquired landmark status. In light of the findings from the CHOIR and CREATE trials (see paper 18.8), there was a view that this TREAT trial was neither necessary nor prudent. However, its design was significantly different, and it had the potential to resolve the uncertainties that lingered. (Levin, 2007). The strengths were its size, that it was placebo controlled, that the endpoints were relevant, and that the recruited subjects were from a defined group with the commonest cause of CKD, diabetes mellitus, who because of co-morbidity would have the most to gain from an effective intervention. The results of the TREAT trial persuaded nephrologists to conclude that attempting to reverse (not ameliorate) anaemia with an ESA in CKD does not improve survival or reduce the incidence of cardiovascular events, does not delay progression of renal dysfunction, and gives symptomatic benefits that were at best modest, although blood transfusions and interventions for ischaemic heart disease were deployed less frequently. Patients with a history of stroke or at higher risk of cardiovascular events will default to ESA-sparing therapy for their anaemia. This trial settled the issue of whether nephrologists should be striving for 'eu-haemoglobinaemia'. As there were no benefits, the issue of justifying the cost of higher doses of ESA does not arise. Moreover, there was another reason not so to strive—strokes occurred more often in the intervention group and deaths from cancer in subjects with a history of cancer were more frequent. The increase in stroke was not a complete surprise, for there had long been a concern that treatment with ESAs might have effects on rheology and coagulation.

There are, however, still some doubts about how to treat anaemic patients with CKD. More than 60% of the trial subjects had a history of cardiovascular disease, so there remains doubt as to whether the results of TREAT can be extrapolated to non-diabetic patients who have a much lower vascular risk. Secondly, the trial showed that striving for eu-haemoglobinaemia was not justified but did not prove that there were no benefits to partial correction. A subsequent analysis of the trial has raised the conundrum of why striving for a higher haemoglobin achieves little and may be dangerous but achieving it is not (Solomon *et al.*, 2010).

CKD patients, especially those with diabetes mellitus, have a complex mix of factors that affect their health and survival, so perhaps it was naïve to attribute to anaemia so important a place in the pathophysiology of their cardiovascular disease (Muntner *et al.*, 2005).

Nephrologists have taken from this trial a simple message: ESAs should be used sparingly and with care in the sick co-morbid majority of patients with CKD (Goldsmith and Covic, 2010).

References

Goldsmith D, Covic A (2010). Time to reconsider evidence for anaemia treatment (TREAT) = Essential Safety Arguments (ESA). *Nephrol Dial Transplant* **25**, 1734–1737.

Levin A (2007). Understanding recent trials in CKD: methods and lesson learned from CREATE and CHOIR. *Nephrol Dial Transplant* **22**, 309–312.

Muntner P, He J, Astor BC, Folsom AR, Coresh J (2005). Traditional and nontraditional risk factors predict coronary heart disease in chronic kidney disease: results from the atherosclerosis risk in communities study. *J Am Soc Nephrol* **16**, 529–538.

Solomon SD, Uno H, Lewis EF, *et al.* (2010). Erythropoietic response and outcomes in kidney disease and type 2 diabetes. *N Engl J Med* **363**, 1146–1155.

Chapter 19

Clinical epidemiology

Robert N. Foley

Introduction

Nephrology has some important and well-described overlaps with common non-communicable disease, particularly hypertension and diabetes. Nevertheless, most 'pure' nephrological conditions are comparatively rare, and this rarity has made for difficulty in trying to establish informative observational studies. One aspect of nephrology, however, has proved almost ideal for observational studies, because of captive populations and reasonable numbers of affected individuals: renal replacement therapy.

As maintenance dialysis and kidney transplantation emerged as viable therapies in the 1970s, the need to collect reliable and comprehensive data soon followed, driven by a number of factors, not least the very high costs of these treatments, which justified thorough audits of efficacy. In some health economies, most notable the USA, the link of patient information to physician reimbursement quickly drove universal coverage and the comprehensive collection of data. High mortality rates and accelerated cardiovascular risk soon emerged as major concerns in these patients.

In the last decade, observational studies have focused increasingly on chronic kidney disease (CKD) in settings other than renal replacement therapy. In particular, a major public health advance has been the recognition that apparently small decrements in kidney function are important markers of adverse events including death, cardiovascular disease, and hospitalization.

The ten landmark papers selected here in chronological order reflect these developments, starting with detailed observations on only 39 patients—among the earliest in the world treated for substantial periods with maintenance haemodialysis—and moving on through studies of increasingly large patient populations. Eight of these landmark studies are based on dialysis populations, one on both dialysis and transplant populations, and one applies to CKD in the general population.

19.1 Accelerated atherosclerosis in prolonged maintenance hemodialysis

Authors

A Lindner, B Charra, DJ Sherrard, BH Scribner

Reference

New England Journal of Medicine 1974, **290**, 697–701.

Abstract

The survival experience of 39 patients receiving long-term regular hemodialysis in Seattle since 1960 was studied with particular reference to mortality and morbidity from arteriosclerotic cardiovascular complications. Mean age ($\pm$ 1 S.D.) was 37.0 ± 9.5 years for the group at the start of dialysis. Mean duration of treatment was 6.5 years (range, one to 13). Overall mortality was 56.4 per cent at the end of the 13-year follow-up period, and 14 of 23 deaths could be attributed to arteriosclerotic complications: myocardial infarction was responsible for eight, strokes for three, and refractory congestive heart failure for three deaths.

The incidence of these complications was many times higher than for normal and hypertensive groups of comparable age, and similar to rates found in Type 2 hyperlipoproteinemia. These results indicate that accelerated atherosclerosis is a major risk to long-term survivors on maintenance hemodialysis.

Importance

This was a retrospective study detailing the unexpectedly high mortality of 39 patients receiving long-term regular haemodialysis in Seattle from 1960. The introduction to the article is almost conversational, describing the sad demise of the first patient to be placed on chronic haemodialysis in the pioneering Seattle haemodialysis programme after 11 years of treatment. It was stated that the fact that the patient 'died in his sleep while on haemodialysis at home had, in retrospect, a prophetic meaning'. The comparatively young age of the patient, the unexpected death, and the autopsy findings of a severity of 'arteriosclerosis' beyond anything previously seen prompted the investigators to address the hypothesis that accelerated arteriosclerosis was the 'major factor limiting survival of patients on dialysis'.

It is noticeable that the paper has discordant pathological descriptions: with the terms 'accelerated atherosclerosis' (which is in the article title) and 'accelerated arteriosclerosis' often used interchangeably.

The methods used in this study are also worthy of a little scrutiny. This was a retrospective study of all 44 patients who started maintenance haemodialysis in Seattle between 1960 and 1966, at a time when a selection committee decided which patients with end-stage renal disease (ESRD) could be treated, and 'freedom from preexistent vascular or systemic disease was required for acceptance to the program'. Only five of the 44 patients were older than 50 years. A notable feature of the study, which almost certainly could never be replicated today, was the near-complete availability of autopsy data. Finally, the delivery of haemodialysis for this population was dramatically different from current norms. In general, the patients were dialysed twice weekly, for 12–16 h per treatment, before 1964 and three times weekly, for 8–10 h per treatment after 1964.

The mean age at inception of dialysis was 37 years, and 56.4% of the study population died during a mean follow-up of 6.5 years. The abstract reports that 14 of 23 deaths could be attributed to 'arteriosclerotic complications', which the authors interpreted as good evidence that 'accelerated atherosclerosis' was a major impediment to long-term survival in the maintenance haemodialysis population.

This study was instrumental in linking cardiovascular and renal disease, and accelerating the pace of research in this field. This study was one of the first to suggest that mortality rates in dialysis patients are many times higher than expected, even in populations without other co-morbid illnesses. In spite of the small numbers in this study, the finding that half of all deaths were attributed to cardiovascular causes has since been replicated in a remarkable variety of settings. The authors also commented that 'earlier analyses of life expectancy of patients on chronic hemodialysis suggest that most deaths occur during the first 1 to 2 years of regular dialysis treatment' and indicated current belief in 1974 that 'once a patient has survived for a few years, he may survive indefinitely, since no upper limit for the duration of survival on maintenance dialysis has been recognized' (Anon., 1970)—an optimism that has turned out to be unfounded.

With the benefit of hindsight, interpretation of the main findings was not entirely correct. The study was thought to implicate atheroma, and failed adequately to distinguish arterial stiffening from atheroma. Subsequently, it has also become evident that uraemia is a cardiomyopathic condition, and very little convincing evidence has emerged to support the concept of accelerated atheroma in uraemia. Nevertheless, the notion of accelerated atheroma has influenced research in this area: for example, the majority of large randomized controlled trials (RCTs) investigating cardiovascular disease in dialysis patients have used primary composite outcomes of death or myocardial infarction but have ignored more common events, notably congestive heart failure and major dysrhythmic events. In addition, the suggestion that uraemia accelerates atheroma was a negative selection factor for deciding the appropriateness of dialysis therapy for several decades: 'The high incidence of cardiovascular complications reported here suggests that it may not be wise to provide chronic hemodialysis patients who already have symptomatic cardiovascular disease as a result of a coexistent disorder such as diabetes or severe hyperlipemia.'

Reference

Anon. (1970). Editorial. Mortality during regular dialysis treatment. *Lancet* **2**, 968.

19.2 Predicting survival in adults with end-stage renal disease: an age equivalence index

Authors

TA Hutchinson, DC Thomas, B MacGibbon

Reference

Annals of Internal Medicine 1982, **96**, 417–423.

Abstract

To quantify prognosis in patients with end-stage renal disease, we evaluated pretreatment clinical state and ascertained the outcome of all 220 patients who began therapy at two hospitals from 1970 to 1975. Each of three pretreatment characteristics made a statistically significant independent contribution to the relative risk of death: age (relative risk for 10-year increments = 2.2, $p < 0.001$); duration of diabetes (relative risk for 10-year increments = 2.2, $p < 0.001$); and left-sided heart failure (relative risk = 2.0, $p < 0.001$). We combined the effects of these factors in an age-equivalence index that showed a strong gradient in survival rates from lower to higher values; the 5-year survival rate differed between 92% in patients with a score of 30 or less and 6% in patients with a score over 70. This index, which is simple to use, should prove helpful in patient care and can improve the scientific validity of therapeutic comparisons in patients with end-stage renal disease by identifying and adjusting for the selection biases that occur in the allocation of different treatments.

Importance

This was a retrospective, inception cohort study from Montreal examining associations between mortality and baseline characteristics at an institution of dialysis therapy. The cohort included 220 patients at two hospitals between 1970 and 1975. Although modest by current standards, the sample size of 220 was large for studies published at that time. The analytical approach used here was one of the first to take into account the growing reality in dialysis units that patients were starting dialysis with ever-increasing co-morbidity, which was very likely to co-segregate with other markers of poor survival. When imbalanced overlap patterns were taken into account, which conditions would remain important? Ultimately, this study showed that three characteristics showed statistically independent associations with death, each with a mortality risk ratio of approximately 2: age (relative risk for 10-year increments = 2.2), duration of diabetes (relative risk for 10-year increments = 2.2), and congestive heart failure (relative risk = 2.0). The authors then incorporated all three associations into a simple three-item index, which, not unexpectedly, showed potent survival discrimination.

This study arrived at conclusions that remain true today. Whilst associations between higher mortality rates and age and diabetes were to be expected, quantifying associations like these is always useful. Apart from age and diabetes, this study was the first to establish the primacy of congestive heart failure as a prognostic marker in dialysis patients, a finding that still resonates in contemporary dialysis populations.

To this day, this study reads like a 'modern' epidemiological study of contemporary dialysis patients. This was one of the first observational studies to recognize the complexity of dialysis patients, and a very rational attempt was made to disentangle this complexity. In particular, it was one of the very first to use multivariate statistics appropriately and to integrate the totality of evidence presented in the study into a tool to help patients and caregivers make difficult decisions. The methods used in this study represented a quantum leap in the haemodialysis literature. This remains a landmark study, not least as a teaching tool for budding observational researchers.

19.3 The urea reduction ratio and serum albumin concentration as predictors of mortality in patients undergoing hemodialysis

Authors

WF Owen Jr, NL Lew, Y Liu, EG Lowrie, JM Lazarus

Reference

New England Journal of Medicine 1993, **329**, 1001–1006.

Abstract

Background: Among patients with end-stage renal disease who are treated with hemodialysis, solute clearance during dialysis and nutritional adequacy are determinants of mortality. We determined the effects of reductions in blood urea nitrogen concentrations during dialysis and changes in serum albumin concentrations, as an indicator of nutritional status, on mortality in a large group of patients treated with hemodialysis.

Methods: We analyzed retrospectively the demographic characteristics, mortality rate, duration of hemodialysis, serum albumin concentration, and urea reduction ratio (defined as the percent reduction in blood urea nitrogen concentration during a single dialysis treatment) in 13,473 patients treated from October 1, 1990, through March 31, 1991. The risk of death was determined as a function of the urea reduction ratio and serum albumin concentration.

Results: As compared with patients with urea reduction ratios of 65 to 69 percent, patients with values below 60 percent had a higher risk of death during follow-up (odds ratio, 1.28 for urea reduction ratios of 55 to 59 percent and 1.39 for ratios below 55 percent). Fifty-five percent of the patients had urea reduction ratios below 60 percent. The duration of dialysis was not predictive of mortality. The serum albumin concentration was a more powerful (21 times greater) predictor of death than the urea reduction ratio, and 60 percent of the patients had serum albumin concentrations predictive of an increased risk of death (values below 4.0 g per deciliter). The odds ratio for death was 1.48 for serum albumin concentrations of 3.5 to 3.9 g per deciliter and 3.13 for concentrations of 3.0 to 3.4 g per deciliter. Diabetic patients had lower serum albumin concentrations and urea reduction ratios than nondiabetic patients.

Conclusions: Low urea reduction ratios during dialysis are associated with increased odds ratios for death. These risks are worsened by inadequate nutrition.

Importance

Among the quirks of maintenance dialysis in the USA is the willingness of the government to cover the costs of treatment. A by-product of the supporting registration system is that incidence rates and survival can be tracked accurately. In 1990, US dialysis care was under a cloud, as annual mortality rates were approximately 25%, far in excess of those reported in other countries. Although differences in co-morbidity, both measured and unmeasured, were frequently advanced as mitigating factors, there was concern that other factors might be at play.

Although the National Cooperative Dialysis Study RCT of 1981 had shown that neither the length of dialysis treatment nor greater dialytic urea removal had an effect on a primary outcome of survival (Lowrie *et al.*, 1981), a post hoc observational analysis of *Kt/V* (the product of dialyser urea clearance and treatment time divided by body urea volume) and urea-based protein catabolic rate suggested that 'clinical failure' suddenly worsened at specific values (Gotch and Sargent, 1985).

This notion was not accepted universally, not least because urea, with a molecular weight of 60 Da, was not considered a significant uraemic toxin. The role of malnutrition in dialysis outcomes was also being actively questioned.

The data for this retrospective observational study of 13,473 study subjects on three times weekly haemodialysis in the USA in 1990 came from a large provider of haemodialysis services. A very useful feature of this study was the availability of commonly used clinical laboratory values, including serum albumin and pre- and post-dialysis urea levels. A quarter of the study population received haemodialysis for 3 h or less per treatment, and another quarter for 4 h or more.

The average of age of the study population was 59 years and 52% were white. The length of dialysis treatment was not associated with death in this study, possibly, as the authors speculated, because the distribution of treatment times was narrow. Urea reduction values below 60% were associated with mortality and a dose–response relationship between falling serum albumin levels and death risk was easily discernible.

Estimates of co-morbidity in this study were limited. In addition, some of the major associations in the study had been seen in other studies. Nevertheless, this study is a landmark because of its very large sample size and wide availability of routinely used clinical measurements. With hindsight, it is notable that urea reduction values had a far weaker association with outcomes than did hypoalbuminaemia, perhaps anticipating the failure of the large Haemodialysis (HEMO) trial to show that aiming for high Kt/V values in haemodialysis patients had an effect on patient survival (Eknoyan *et al.*, 2002). At the time, it was the most definitive study linking hypoalbuminaemia to mortality. Whilst it has long been know that serum albumin is a negative acute-phase reactant, studies like this ushered in a new era of investigation that remains active to this day: investigating the inter-relationships of uraemia, dialysis, cardiovascular outcomes, and the inflammatory state.

References

Eknoyan G, Beck GJ, Cheung AK, *et al.* (2002). Effect of dialysis dose and membrane flux in maintenance hemodialysis. *N Engl J Med*, **347**, 2010–2019.

Gotch FA, Sargent JA (1985). A mechanistic analysis of the National Cooperative Dialysis Study (NCDS). *Kidney Int* **28**, 526–534.

Lowrie EG, Laird NM, Parker TF, Sargent JA (1981). Effect of the hemodialysis prescription of patient morbidity: report from the National Cooperative Dialysis Study. *N Engl J Med* **305**, 1176–1181.

19.4 Survival as an index of adequacy of dialysis

Authors

B Charra, E Calemard, M Ruffet, C Chazot, JC Terrat, T Vanel, G Laurent

Reference

Kidney International 1992, **41**, 1286–1291.

Abstract

To examine how patient survival substantiates dialysis adequacy, 20-year actuarial survival experience was calculated for 445 unselected hemodialysis (HD) patients (97 patients accepted on a temporary basis—and usually kept on their regular dialysis scheme—were left out). The dose of dialysis has been the same and unchanged for all patients since beginning: 24 square meter hours of Kiil dialysis (cuprophane) per week with acetate buffered dialysate. KT/V mean (SD) was 1.67 (0.41). Six months after starting dialysis, 98% of patients were normotensive and off all blood pressure (BP) medication. The mean population hematocrit, excluding the only 6 patients receiving erythropoietin supplementation, was 28%. Survival rate was 87% at 5 years, 75% at 10 years, 55% at 15 years, and 43% at 20 years of HD. The satisfactory control of BP without using potentially toxic BP drugs and the higher than usual dose of dialysis are two possible explanations for survival data better than usually reported. We suggest that patient survival should be considered as the best overall index of adequacy of dialysis.

Importance

This article began with a short editorial from the late Dr Belding Scribner, one of the pioneers of maintenance dialysis therapy:

> Shortly after our first patient, Mr. Clyde Shields, began long term hemodialysis in March of 1960, he developed malignant hypertension, and death seemed imminent…. Since we were unable to control his blood pressure with the few antihypertensive drugs then available, we decided that our only hope of saving him was to try aggressive removal of extracellular fluid by ultrafiltration during his once weekly 24-hour hemodialysis. During the subsequent weeks cramping was severe as we tried to maximize fluid removal during each dialysis. Gradually, however, his blood pressure came under control. Eventually he became normotensive off medication, and remained so until his death from a myocardial infarction in 1971. This dramatic episode made a lasting impression on our approach to the control of blood pressure in our hemodialysis patients. Even after effective antihypertensive medications became available, we continued to make control of the extracellular volume the cornerstone of treatment of hypertension.

Charra and colleagues reported their experience among 445 maintenance haemodialysis patients dialysed at Tassin, France, from the 1960s to 1990. The cause of ESRD was mixed, but it was notable that diabetes mellitus and systemic diseases were present in less than 10%. In addition, the mean age at inception of dialysis was younger than would be seen currently, varying from 36.2 years before 1970 to 52.9 years for 1986–1990. All patients received the same treatment: 24 h per week on 1 m² flat plate Kiil cuprophan dialysers, with blood flow at 200 ml/min and dialysis flow at 500 ml/min. Acetate was used as a buffer, and transfusion was almost never used in this study, which predated the use of erythropoiesis-stimulating agents. Controlled ultrafiltration was the method used to lower blood pressure (BP). In addition, salt restriction was advocated. The mean inter-dialytic weight gain was 1.9 kg. With this regimen, excellent BP controlled was achieved, usually within 6 months. Less than 2% of the patient population ultimately required anti-hypertensive medication. Half-time survival was a truly remarkable 17 years. Not unexpectedly, survival was related to older age. Regarding modifiable associations, mortality was clearly associated with higher mean arterial BP, but not with Kt/V.

No other centre has come close to equalling the survival rates in Tassin. BP control remains one of the more unfashionable elements in the day-to-day management of ESRD. Targeting dry weight remains very challenging for many patients and caregivers. This study, which was entirely observational, is often used for moral support when the right thing to do appears to be more ultrafiltration and longer treatment times. This study remains highly relevant today, and since its publication, interest in longer, slower, and more frequent dialysis treatments has mushroomed. RCTs with outcomes including left ventricular mass and quality of life suggest that this approach may yet prove fruitful (Culleton *et al.*, 2007; Chertow *et al.*, 2010).

References

Chertow GM, Levin NW, Beck GJ, *et al.* (2010). In-center hemodialysis six times per week versus three times per week. *N Engl J Med* **363**, 2287–300.

Culleton BF, Walsh M, Klarenbach SW, *et al.* (2007). Effect of frequent nocturnal hemodialysis vs conventional hemodialysis on left ventricular mass and quality of life: a randomized controlled trial. *JAMA* **298**, 1291–1299.

19.5 EPIBACDIAL: a multicenter prospective study of risk factors for bacteremia in chronic hemodialysis patients

Authors

B Hoen, A Paul-Dauphin, D Hestin, M Kessler

Reference

Journal of the American Society of Nephrology 1998, **9**, 869–876.

Abstract

Bacteremic infections are a major cause of mortality and morbidity in chronic hemodialysis patients. New developments in managing these patients (erythropoietin therapy, nasal mupirocin, long-term implanted catheters, and synthetic membranes) may have altered the epidemiologic patterns of bacteremia in dialysis patients. This multicenter prospective cross-sectional study was carried out to determine the current incidence of and risk factors for bacteremia in chronic hemodialysis patients in France. A total of 988 adults on chronic hemodialysis for 1 mo or longer was followed up prospectively for 6 mo in 19 French dialysis units. The factors associated with the development of at least one bacteremic episode over 6 mo were determined using the multivariate Cox proportional hazards model. *Staphylococcus aureus* ($n = 20$) and coagulase-negative staphylococci ($n = 15$) were responsible for most of the 51 bacteremic episodes recorded. The incidence of bacteremia was 0.93 episode per 100 patient-months. Four risk factors for bacteremia were identified: (*1*) vascular access (catheter *versus* fistula: RR = 7.6; 95% CI, 3.7 to 15.6); (*2*) history of bacteremia (≥ 2 *versus* no previous episode: RR = 7.3; 95% CI, 3.2 to 16.4); (*3*) immunosuppressive therapy (current *versus* no: RR = 3.0; 95% CI, 1.0 to 6.1); and (*4*) corpuscular hemoglobin (per 1 g/dl increment: RR = 0.7; 95% CI, 0.6 to 0.9). Catheters, especially long-term implanted catheters, were found to be the leading risk factor of bacteremia in chronic hemodialysis patients. There was a trend toward recurrence of bacteremia that was not associated with chronic staphylococcal nasal carriage. Synthetic membranes were not associated with a lower risk of bacteremia in this population of well dialyzed patients, but anemia linked to resistance to erythropoietin appeared to be a possible risk factor for bacteremia.

Importance

This was a prospective study of 988 adult patients undergoing haemodialysis in 19 French units. Patients on regular haemodialysis for at least 30 days were followed for 6 months. For case definition, only episodes with documented bacteraemia were considered. Single blood cultures positive for coagulase-negative staphylococci, *Corynebacteria* or *Bacillus* sp. were treated as contaminants not included in the formal analysis. Fifty-one bacteraemic episodes were noted in 50 patients, and the expected distribution of pathogens was seen: most common were *Staphylococcus aureus* in 20, and coagulase-negative staphylococci in 15. Six bacteraemic episodes resulted in death and the pathogens in these cases were *S. aureus* in two, *Pseudomonas* sp. in two, *Escherichia coli* in ine, and *Listeria monocytogenes* in one. Although not formally reported in the study, simple calculation indicates that case fatality rates were approximately 12%. The overall incidence of bacteraemic episodes was 0.93 per 100 patient-months.

When multivariate analysis was performed, modifiable risk factors for bacteraemia were present, including catheters for vascular access (relative risk compared to arteriovenous fistulas = 6.6); a previous history of bacteraemia (relative risk 7.3), and immunosuppressive therapy (relative risk of 3.0).

This was a well-designed and carefully performed study of an issue that has been scantily studied for years. Although infection is usually the second most commonly reported cause of death in dialysis patients, the potential for nosocomial infections is high, and the use of dialysis catheters remains stubbornly common. The issue of major infections in dialysis patients remains a Cinderella subject by comparison with cardiovascular disease. In the USA, infection rates continue to rise annually, and it is has become apparent that herein lies a major impediment to improving survival on dialysis. Many more studies like this one are sorely needed.

19.6 Poor long-term survival after acute myocardial infarction among patients on long-term dialysis

Authors

CA Herzog, JZ Ma, AJ Collins

Reference

New England Journal of Medicine 1998, **339**, 799–805.

Abstract

Background: Cardiovascular disease is common in patients on long-term dialysis, and it accounts for 44 percent of overall mortality in this group. We undertook a study to assess long-term survival after acute myocardial infarction among patients in the United States who were receiving long-term dialysis.

Methods: Patients on dialysis who were hospitalized during the period from 1977 to 1995 for a first myocardial infarction after the initiation of renal-replacement therapy were retrospectively identified from the U.S. Renal Data System data base. Overall mortality and mortality from cardiac causes (including all in-hospital deaths) were estimated by the life-table method. The effect of independent predictors on survival was examined in a Cox regression model with adjustment for existing illnesses.

Results: The overall mortality (±SE) after acute myocardial infarction among 34,189 patients on long-term dialysis was 59.3±0.3 percent at one year, 73.0±0.3 percent at two years, and 89.9±0.2 percent at five years. The mortality from cardiac causes was 40.8±0.3 percent at one year, 51.8±0.3 percent at two years, and 70.2±0.4 percent at five years. Patients who were older or had diabetes had higher mortality than patients without these characteristics. Adverse outcomes occurred even in patients who had acute myocardial infarction in 1990 through 1995. Also, the mortality rate after myocardial infarction was considerably higher for patients on long-term dialysis than for renal-transplant recipients.

Conclusions: Patients on dialysis who have acute myocardial infarction have high mortality from cardiac causes and poor long-term survival.

Importance

As paper 19.4 recalls, the first true maintenance haemodialysis patient died from a myocardial infarction after 11 years of therapy. The seminal paper on this issue (paper 19.1) included only 44 patients. The study of Herzog and colleagues revisited this issue, and asked a very simple but important question: what is the survival after myocardial infarction in patients on renal replacement therapy? At the time this study was developed, the mortality rate for US dialysis patients was beginning to reach its peak, and cardiac disease, as now, was believed to underlie about half of all deaths.

This study used data from 627,983 patients registered in the US Renal Data System database to examine the outcome of 34,189 patients after experiencing a first acute myocardial infarction between 1977 and 1995, as identified from Medicare reimbursement claims. There was a suggestion that there is an early risk of acute myocardial infarction associated with the initiation of dialysis, as 29% of infarctions occurred within 1 year and 52% within 2 years after the initiation of dialysis.

In-hospital mortality rates were 26% for all dialysis patients, 21% for patients under 65 years of age, and 30% for those of 65 years or more. In-hospital mortality rates were even higher in those with co-existing diabetes. Longer-term survival rates were dismal, with over 70% dead at 2 years. Strikingly, remembering the benefits of coronary reperfusion therapy in the general population, patients with acute myocardial infarctions between 1990 and 1995 had higher mortality rates than those who had had myocardial infarctions between 1977 and 1984 or between 1985 and 1989.

Although based on administrative reimbursement claims, and ignoring the issue of out-of-hospital cardiac events, this study had a very clear message, the catastrophic effect of cardiac events in dialysis patients. Whilst this was not an entirely new concept after 35 years of maintenance dialysis therapy, the large sample size allowed a precise estimate of prognostic associations. The findings were truly grim. In many ways, this was a call to arms and made the powerful case that the time had come for the nephrology community to re-evaluate how it approached cardiac disease in dialysis patients.

19.7 Sudden and cardiac death rates in hemodialysis patients

Authors

AJ Bleyer, GB Russell, SG Satko

Reference

Kidney International 1999, **55**, 1553–1559.

Abstract

Background: Sudden and cardiac death (including death from congestive heart failure, myocardial infarction, and sudden death) are common occurrences in hemodialysis patients. The intermittent nature of hemodialysis may lead to an uneven distribution of sudden and cardiac death throughout the week. The purpose of this study was to assess the septadian rhythm of sudden and cardiac death in hemodialysis patients.

Methods: Data from the United States Renal Data System (USRDS) were obtained to examine the day of death for United States hemodialysis and peritoneal dialysis patients from 1977 through 1997. The days of death were also determined for patients in the Case Mix Adequacy Study of the USRDS.

Results: There was an even distribution of sudden and cardiac deaths for patients on peritoneal dialysis, and hemodialysis patients dying of noncardiac deaths also had an even distribution. For all hemodialysis patients, Monday and Tuesday were the most common days of sudden and cardiac death. For patients in the Case Mix Adequacy Study designated as Monday, Wednesday, and Friday dialysis patients, 20.8% of sudden deaths occurred on Monday compared with the 14.3% expected ($P = 0.002$). Similarly, 20.2% of cardiac deaths occurred on Monday compared with the 14.3% expected ($P = 0.0005$). Similar trends were found on Tuesday for Tuesday, Thursday, and Saturday dialysis patients.

Conclusions: The intermittent nature of hemodialysis may contribute to an increased sudden and cardiac death rate on Monday and Tuesday for patients enrolled in the USRDS.

Importance

In the vast majority of cases, maintenance haemodialysis is performed three times per week, with two 1-day and one 2-day interval between dialysis sessions. This pragmatic configuration of dialysis delivery is not ideal given that those with ESRD have limited capacity to deal with excursions from normal fluid volumes and potassium loads, and most patients begin maintenance dialysis with cardiovascular disease.

In this simple study, the authors used data from the US Renal Data System to examine the day of the week of death for all haemodialysis and peritoneal dialysis patients from 1977 to 1997. As haemodialysis scheduling could not be determined in the overall population, the authors studied a subpopulation within US Renal Data System where data collection was more extensive and haemodialysis schedules were known (the Case Mix Adequacy Study).

There was an even distribution of sudden and cardiac deaths for patients on peritoneal dialysis, and for non-cardiac death in haemodialysis. For haemodialysis patients, however, sudden deaths and cardiac deaths were commonest on Monday and Tuesday. For patients dialysing on Monday, Wednesday, and Friday, 20.8% of sudden deaths occurred on Monday compared with the expected proportion of 14.3%; septadian trends, with Tuesdays being the outlier, were also seen in patients dialysing on Tuesday, Thursday, and Saturday.

This was a beautifully simple study, and an advanced degree in biostatistics is not required to fully appreciate its implications. Daily haemodialysis treatment, which has the potential to allay these concerns, has been the focus of considerable interest in recent years, and initial findings with daily haemodialysis have been encouraging.

It is rare these days to see observational studies that do not include multivariate analysis to adjust for the fact that dialysis patients typically have multiple co-morbid illnesses that could affect prognosis. For an issue like death on different days of the week, however, multivariate analysis has no use, as the same population is being examined for events on different days. That is not to say that all patients are the same, and appropriately selected subgroup analyses could still be enlightening. Only a direct effect of interdialytic interval on outcomes or different behaviour patterns on different days of the week could explain these findings. More than a decade on, this study still suggests that RCTs to assess different dialysis delivery schedules (such as alternate day) need to be performed.

19.8 Comparison of mortality in all patients on dialysis, patients on dialysis awaiting transplantation, and recipients of a first cadaveric transplant

Authors

RA Wolfe, VB Ashby, EL Milford, AO Ojo, RE Ettenger, LY Agodoa, PJ Held, FK Port

Reference

New England Journal of Medicine 1999, **341**, 1725–1730.

Abstract

Background: The extent to which renal allotransplantation—as compared with long-term dialysis—improves survival among patients with end-stage renal disease is controversial, because those selected for transplantation may have a lower base-line risk of death.

Methods: In an attempt to distinguish the effects of patient selection from those of transplantation itself, we conducted a longitudinal study of mortality in 228,552 patients who were receiving long-term dialysis for end-stage renal disease. Of these patients, 46,164 were placed on a waiting list for transplantation, 23,275 of whom received a first cadaveric transplant between 1991 and 1997. The relative risk of death and survival were assessed with time-dependent nonproportional-hazards analysis, with adjustment for age, race, sex, cause of end-stage renal disease, geographic region, time from first treatment for end-stage renal disease to placement on the waiting list, and year of initial placement on the list.

Results: Among the various subgroups, the standardized mortality ratio for the patients on dialysis who were awaiting transplantation (annual death rate, 6.3 per 100 patient-years) was 38 to 58 percent lower than that for all patients on dialysis (annual death rate, 16.1 per 100 patient-years). The relative risk of death during the first 2 weeks after transplantation was 2.8 times as high as that for patients on dialysis who had equal lengths of follow-up since placement on the waiting list, but at 18 months the risk was much lower (relative risk, 0.32; 95 percent confidence interval, 0.30 to 0.35; P < 0.001). The likelihood of survival became equal in the two groups within 5 to 673 days after transplantation in all the subgroups of patients we examined. The long-term mortality rate was 48 to 82 percent lower among transplant recipients (annual death rate, 3.8 per 100 patient-years) than patients on the waiting list, with relatively larger benefits among patients who were 20 to 39 years old, white patients, and younger patients with diabetes.

Conclusions: Among patients with end-stage renal disease, healthier patients are placed on the waiting list for transplantation, and long-term survival is better among those on the waiting list who eventually undergo transplantation.

Importance

The outcome of renal transplantation continues to evolve. By the mid 1990s, whilst there was little doubt that transplantation was a cheaper treatment option that offered better quality of life, it was still unclear whether it also afforded longer survival. Although direct survival comparisons strongly favoured transplantation over dialysis, even when adjustment was made for age, sex, race, and known co-morbidity, there was legitimate concern that none of the existing conclusions was fair, as potent selection factors had not been incorporated in survival comparisons. This study of Wolfe and colleagues took a novel approach to minimizing the impact of unmeasured co-morbidity on survival comparisons of dialysis and transplant by asking a simple question: among dialysis patients on the transplant waiting list, what was the impact on survival of actual transplantation?

As expected, transplant-censored mortality for dialysis patients on the transplant list was substantially lower than in the overall population of dialysis patients. Among patients on the transplant waiting list, deceased-donor renal transplantation was associated with an overall reduction in death risk; risk profiles, however, varied considerably in relation to the time elapsed following transplantation. The relative risk of death during the first 2 weeks after transplantation was 2.8 times as high as that for patients on dialysis who had equal lengths of follow-up since placement on the waiting list; at 18 months, the corresponding relative risk was 0.32. Thus, an initial early risk seemed to be more than compensated for by a later survival benefit, which appeared to come into play by approximately 3 months.

This was not a randomized trial of transplantation compared with remaining on dialysis. Even in the early 1990s, the quality-of-life differences were so apparent that such a trial could hardly be considered ethical. Whilst this study had the weaknesses of all retrospective, registry-based studies, it had the advantages of having a large sample size and being nationally representative. Although the statistics may be slightly difficult, this study used an intuitive approach towards minimizing the major niggling question of selective enrolment onto transplant waiting lists.

19.9 Association of comorbid conditions and mortality in hemodialysis patients in Europe, Japan, and the United States: the Dialysis Outcomes and Practice Patterns Study (DOPPS)

Authors

DA Goodkin, JL Bragg-Gresham, KG Koenig, RA Wolfe, T Akiba, VE Andreucci, A Saito, HC Rayner, K Kurokawa, FK Port, PJ Held, EW Young

Reference

Journal of the American Society of Nephrology 2003, **14**, 3270–3277.

Abstract

Mortality rates among hemodialysis patients vary greatly across regions. Representative databases containing extensive profiles of patient characteristics and outcomes are lacking. The Dialysis Outcomes and Practice Patterns Study (DOPPS) is a prospective, observational study of representative samples of hemodialysis patients in France, Germany, Italy, Japan, Spain, the United Kingdom, and the United States (US) that captures extensive data relating to patient characteristics, prescriptions, laboratory values, practice patterns, and outcomes. This report describes the case-mix features and mortality among 16,720 patients followed up to 5 yr. The crude 1-yr mortality rates were 6.6% in Japan, 15.6% in Europe, and 21.7% in the US. After adjusting for age, gender, race, and 25 comorbid conditions, the relative risk (RR) of mortality was 2.84 ($P < 0.0001$) for Europe compared with Japan (reference group) and was 3.78 ($P < 0.0001$) for the US compared with Japan. The adjusted RR of mortality for the US versus Europe was 1.33 ($P < 0.0001$). For most comorbid diseases, prevalence was highest in the US, where the mean age (60.5 ± 15.5 yr) was also highest. Older age and comorbidities were associated with increased risk of death (except for hypertension, which carried a multivariate RR of mortality of 0.74 [$P < 0.0001$]). Variability in demographic and comorbid conditions (as identified by dialysis facilities) explains only part of the differences in mortality between dialysis centers, both for comparisons made across continents and within the US. Adjustments for the observed variability will allow study of association between practice patterns and outcomes.

Importance

RCTs in dialysis populations have, to date, proved incapable of identifying practices that optimize survival expectations. This sad state of affairs may, perhaps, be explained by picking the 'wrong' intervention for testing. Non-experimental observational studies can help in this regard. For example, in populations not expected to change profoundly in small increments of time, sudden changes in mortality that are related temporally to a single change in treatment approach would immediately suggest an intervention for testing in trials.

For similar reasons, variability in outcomes within and between countries is also fertile ground for targeting interventions for large-scale trials. It has long been known that there are large, unexplained differences in mortality between different national registries, but it has been impossible to refute the suggestion that these differences reflect the inherent impossibility of true comparison between national registries, which differ with regard to critical data elements such as co-morbid illnesses, laboratory-based indicators of care, medications, dialysis prescription, and access to transplantation.

The Dialysis Outcomes and Practice Patterns Study (DOPPS) is a prospective, multicountry observational study of representative haemodialysis patients designed to collect comprehensively all these data elements with homogeneous data-capturing strategies. The current study was a comprehensive description of mortality experiences in DOPPS detailing survival experiences in 16,720 haemodialysis patients in France, Germany, Italy, Japan, Spain, the UK, and the USA. Unadjusted analysis revealed annual mortality rates of 6.6% in Japan, 15.6% in Europe, and 21.7% in the USA. Critically, mortality differences persisted when adjustment was made for age, sex, race, and a comprehensive array of prospectively defined co-morbid conditions. For example, relative death relative risk was 2.84 for Europe compared with Japan, 3.78 for the USA compared with Japan, and 1.33 for the USA compared with Europe. Thus, whilst burdens of co-morbidity increased with higher overall mortality rates, differences in co-morbidity came nowhere close to explaining differences in survival.

This was an extremely well-constructed study. It also showed that large-registry comparisons tend to show similar findings to studies with pristine prospective designs. Whilst unmeasured co-morbidity is, by definition, unknown, it is hard to see how much more could have been done to rule out this possibility. At some stage, alternative explanations should be explored. One potential explanatory hypothesis runs as follows: dialysis patients survive longer in some countries because age-adjusted survival rates in the underlying general populations are longer. Whilst this idea is not new, the study of Goodkin and colleagues suggested that comparisons of dialysis survival might not be complete without also seeing parallel comparisons in the general population.

19.10 Chronic kidney disease and the risks of death, cardiovascular events, and hospitalization

Authors

AS Go, GM Chertow, D Fan, CE McCulloch, CY Hsu

Reference

New England Journal of Medicine 2004, **351**, 1296–1305.

Abstract

Background: End-stage renal disease substantially increases the risks of death, cardiovascular disease, and use of specialized health care, but the effects of less severe kidney dysfunction on these outcomes are less well defined.

Methods: We estimated the longitudinal glomerular filtration rate (GFR) among 1,120,295 adults within a large, integrated system of health care delivery in whom serum creatinine had been measured between 1996 and 2000 and who had not undergone dialysis or kidney transplantation. We examined the multivariable association between the estimated GFR and the risks of death, cardiovascular events, and hospitalization.

Results: The median follow-up was 2.84 years, the mean age was 52 years, and 55 percent of the group were women. After adjustment, the risk of death increased as the GFR decreased below 60 ml per minute per 1.73 m^2 of body-surface area: the adjusted hazard ratio for death was 1.2 with an estimated GFR of 45 to 59 ml per minute per 1.73 m^2 (95 percent confidence interval, 1.1 to 1.2), 1.8 with an estimated GFR of 30 to 44 ml per minute per 1.73 m^2 (95 percent confidence interval, 1.7 to 1.9), 3.2 with an estimated GFR of 15 to 29 ml per minute per 1.73 m^2 (95 percent confidence interval, 3.1 to 3.4), and 5.9 with an estimated GFR of less than 15 ml per minute per 1.73 m^2 (95 percent confidence interval, 5.4 to 6.5). The adjusted hazard ratio for cardiovascular events also increased inversely with the estimated GFR: 1.4 (95 percent confidence interval, 1.4 to 1.5), 2.0 (95 percent confidence interval, 1.9 to 2.1), 2.8 (95 percent confidence interval, 2.6 to 2.9), and 3.4 (95 percent confidence interval, 3.1 to 3.8), respectively. The adjusted risk of hospitalization with a reduced estimated GFR followed a similar pattern.

Conclusions: An independent, graded association was observed between a reduced estimated GFR and the risk of death, cardiovascular events, and hospitalization in a large, community-based population. These findings highlight the clinical and public health importance of chronic renal insufficiency.

Importance

There are now literally hundreds of studies showing associations between low glomerular filtration rates (GRFs) estimated from serum creatinine and adverse health outcomes. This, however, was the first study to address this question, and it had the twin advantages of being broadly (if imperfectly) representative of the community and having a massive sample size.

Estimated GFR (eGFR) was calculated among 1,120,295 adults within a large, integrated system of healthcare delivery in whom serum creatinine had been measured between 1996 and 2000. Over a median follow-up of 2.84 years, the co-morbidity-adjusted risk of death increased as the eGFR decreased below 60 ml/min/1.73 m^2. For example, compared with an eGFR above 60, adjusted hazard ratios for death were 1.2, 1.8, 3.2, and 5.9 for GFR 45–59, 30–44, 15–29 and <15 ml/min/1.73 m², respectively. Corresponding adjusted hazards ratios for cardiovascular events were 1.4, 2.0, 2.8, and 3.4. Hospitalization risk showed similar associations with GFR.

Like all observational studies, this study has some elements that are imperfect. As it was a study of routine clinical care, estimates of the GFR were not available for the entire source population. In addition, an indicator of proteinuria would have been helpful. But this simple, elegant, and powerful study was a critical element in making the case for the public health importance of CKD.

Chapter 20

Health-related quality of life and the patient perspective

Fredric O. Finkelstein and Susan H. Finkelstein

Introduction

All nephrologists are aware of the compromised health-related quality of life (HRQOL) of patients with end-stage renal disease (ESRD). Early studies from the 1970s and 1980s, shortly after routine ESRD treatments became standard management, clearly document these impairments. The impact of the disease and its treatment was in many ways obvious—the patient lived a clearly compromised existence. A variety of well validated instruments were then developed to document the impaired HRQOL of patients with chronic kidney disease. The importance of the reduced HRQOL measurements was underscored by the association of these scores with mortality and hospitalization rates in CKD patients. These studies, recognized the importance of understanding how patients perceive their illness.

The impact of these impairments on individual patients needs systematic evaluation. It turns out that health care professionals have difficulties in recognizing and understanding patients' symptoms. Clinical staff, despite seeing haemodialysis patients three times per week, do not fully comprehend the symptoms which patient's experience and the severity of these symptoms as perceived by the patient. Nor do they appreciate the impact of the dialysis treatment regimen itself on the individual patient. The differential impact of peritoneal dialysis, conventional hemodialysis, and modifications of the conventional haemodialysis regimen on patient perceptions has only recently been recognized and studied systematically. This draws attention to the importance for clinicians to look not only at biological outcomes but also at the patients' perceptions of their quality of life to properly assess patient status. Attention should also be paid to understanding the variable impact of the dialysis treatment regimen itself on the patients' perception of their HRQOL. This becomes particularly important as the length of time of renal replacement therapy increases. In general, there is a deterioration over time of HRQOL scores reported by patients; it is necessary that these changes be acknowledged and monitored. This is particularly true now that studies have begun to explore treatment options to improve patient-related outcomes. For example, alterations in the dialysis treatment regimen can have positive impacts on various patient-related outcomes. Treatment of depression can not only improve depressive symptoms but other HRQOL measures as well.

Lastly, efforts are needed to educate patients about end of life care options and develop pathways for palliative care management. This will be particularly important as the number of older people receiving renal replacement therapy increases over the next decade. The limited work done thus far suggests that patients are not well informed about appropriate palliative care options. Health policy decisions will need to be made about levels of care provided to these patients—an informed, educated patient population is critical to rational shared decision making.

20.1 The quality of life of patients with end-stage renal disease

Authors

RW Evans, DL Manninen, LP Garrison Jr, LG Hart, CR Blagg, RA Gutman, AR Hull, EG Lowrie

Reference

New England Journal of Medicine 1985, **312**, 553–559.

Abstract

We assessed the quality of life of 859 patients undergoing dialysis or transplantation, with the goal of ascertaining whether objective and subjective measures of the quality of life were influenced by case mix or treatment. We found that 79.1 per cent of the transplant recipients were able to function at nearly normal levels, as compared with between 47.5 and 59.1 per cent of the patients treated with dialysis (depending on the type). Nearly 75 per cent of the transplant recipients were able to work, as compared with between 24.7 and 59.3 per cent of the patients undergoing dialysis. On three subjective measures (life satisfaction, well-being, and psychological affect) transplant recipients had a higher quality of life than patients on dialysis. Among the patients treated with dialysis, those undergoing treatment at home had the highest quality of life. All quality-of-life differences were found to persist even after the patient case mix had been controlled statistically. Finally, the quality of life of transplant recipients compared well with that of the general population, but despite favorable subjective assessments, patients undergoing dialysis did not work or function at the same level as people in the general population.

Importance

This is one of the first papers discussing the HRQOL of patients with ESRD. The differences noted between the dialysis patients and transplant patients are striking and these differences have remained one of the cardinal teachings in the world of nephrology (Tonelli *et al.*, 2011).

This study was cross-sectional in design, examining patients maintained on in-centre haemodialysis, home haemodialysis, and continuous ambulatory peritoneal dialysis and after transplantation. 'Objective measures' of quality of life that were used included an assessment of functional impairment (using the Karnofsky Index) and the ability to work for pay. 'Subjective measures' assessed included the Index of Well-Being, the Index of Overall Life Satisfaction, and the Index of Psychological Affect. After correction for case-mix variables, the transplant patients clearly had the best scores—particularly on the 'objective measures'. In fact, their scores on both 'objective' and 'subjective' measures were not different from those of the general population. The dialysis patients all had worse scores—particularly on the 'objective' measures, with the home haemodialysis patients clearly having the best scores on these measures compared with other dialysis patients.

However, what puzzled the authors in this study was the observation that, although the dialysis patients had significant functional impairments, their scores on the 'subjective' measures were not as low as might have been expected. Thus, the authors commented that '…patients on dialysis are clearly not functioning like people who are well, despite the fact that they are enjoying life…Whereas documentation of the objective aspects may be relatively straightforward, most of the subjective aspects of the quality of life…are highly problematic.' It remained for future studies to better define how these 'subjective' assessments could be done. Importantly, these future studies would then address the relationships of these 'subjective' assessments to patient outcomes, the impact of the dialysis regimen itself on these assessments, and how the reduced quality of life measures could in fact be improved (see papers 20.2–20.8 and 20.10).

Reference

Tonelli M, Wiebe N, Knoll G, *et al.* (2011). Systematic review: kidney transplantation compared with dialysis in clinically relevant outcomes. *Am J Transplant* **11**, 2093–2109

20.2 Multiple measurements of depression predict mortality in a longitudinal study of chronic hemodialysis outpatients

Authors

P Kimmel, RA Peterson, KL Weihs, SJ Simmens, S Alleyne, I Cruz, JH Veis

Reference

Kidney International 2000, **57**, 93–98.

Abstract

Background: The medical risk factors associated with increased mortality in hemodialysis (HD) patients are well known, but the psychosocial factors that may affect outcome have not been clearly defined. One key psychosocial factor, depression, has been considered a predictor of mortality, but previous studies have provided equivocal results regarding the association. We sought to determine whether depressive affect is associated with mortality in a longitudinal study of end-stage renal disease (ESRD) patients treated with HD, using multiple assessments over time.

Methods: Two hundred ninety-five outpatients with ESRD treated with HD were recruited from three outpatient dialysis units in Washington D.C. to participate in a prospective cohort study with longitudinal follow-up. Patients were assessed every six months for up to two years using the Beck Depression Inventory (BDI), age, serum albumin concentration, Kt/V, and protein catabolic rate (PCR). A severity index, previously demonstrated to be a mortality marker, was used to grade medical comorbidity. The type of dialyzer with which the patient was treated was noted. Patient mortality status was tracked for a minimum of 20 and a maximum of 60 months after the first interview. Cox proportional hazards models, treating depression scores as time-varying covariates in a univariable analysis, and controlling for age, medical comorbidity, albumin concentration, and dialyzer type and site in multivariable models, were used to assess the relative mortality risk.

Results: The mean (± SD) age of our population at initial interview was 54.6 ± 14.1 years. The mean PCR was 1.06 ± 0.27 g/kg/day, and the mean Kt/V was 1.2 ± 0.4 at baseline, suggesting that the patients were well nourished and dialyzed comparably to contemporary U.S. patients. The patients' mean BDI at enrollment was 11.4 ± 8.1, in the range of mild depression. Patients' baseline level of depression was not a significant predictor of mortality at 38.6 months of follow-up. In contrast, when depression was treated as a time-varying covariate based on periodic follow-up assessments, the level of depressive affect was significantly associated with mortality in both single variable and multivariable analyses.

Conclusions: Higher levels of depressive affect in ESRD patients treated with HD are associated with increased mortality. The effects of depression on patient survival are of the same order of magnitude as medical risk factors. Our findings using both controls for factors possibly confounded with depressive affect in patients with ESRD and time-varying covariate analyses may explain the inconsistent results of previous studies of depression and mortality in ESRD patients. Time-varying analyses in longitudinal studies may add power to defining and sensitivity to establishing the association of psychosocial factors and survival in ESRD patients. The mechanism underlying the relationship of depression and survival and the effect of interventions to improve depression in HD outpatients and general medical inpatients should be studied.

Importance

The impaired HRQOL reported by ESRD patients had been confirmed in various studies subsequent to the 1985 paper of Evans and colleagues (see paper 20.1). Few studies, however, had examined the relationship between these factors and hospitalization and mortality rates of ESRD patients. One of the challenges in these analyses is that patient perceptions change over time, shifting as a result of various medical, social, and psychological issues. This paper introduced the concept of time-varying analysis as a way of dealing with this issue. The paper focused attention on depressive symptoms of haemodialysis patients using a standardized scoring instrument, the Beck Depression Inventory (BDI). Depression scores were reanalysed every 6 months in a cohort of 295 ESRD patients maintained on conventional thrice weekly in-centre haemodialysis, and mortality rates were examined in the 6 months following completion of the BDI. The mean BDI scores at baseline for these patients was 11.4 ± 8.1, providing a standard measure of depressive symptoms in ESRD patients (this mean score has been confirmed in subsequent studies and set a standard against which other investigations could be judged) (Watnick *et al.*, 2005; Wuerth *et al.*, 2005; Hedayati and Finkelstein, 2009). Importantly, the association of BDI scores with mortality was not demonstrated if just the baseline BDI scores were used in the analysis. However, with the time-varying analysis, a significant association with mortality emerged. The reasons for this association were not examined in this study and the causes of death were not analysed. The authors pointed out the association between depression and mortality in patients hospitalized with a myocardial infarction or other general medical illnesses. Subsequent studies have discussed the possible contribution of depression to mortality by pointing out the association with cardiovascular events, withdrawal from dialysis, and poor compliance (Hedayati and Finkelstein, 2009).

References

Hedayati S, Finkelstein FO (2009). Epidemiology, diagnosis and management of depression in patients with chronic kidney disease. *Am J Kidney Dis* **54**,741–752.

Watnick S, Wang PL, Demadura T, *et al.* (2005). Validation of two depression screening tools in dialysis patients. *Am J Kidney Dis* **46**, 919–924.

Wuerth D, Finkelstein SH, Finkelstein FO (2005). The identification and treatment of depression in patients maintained on chronic peritoneal dialysis: results of an eight year experience. *Semin Dialysis* **18**, 123–127.

20.3 Health-related quality of life as a predictor of mortality and hospitalization: the Dialysis Outcomes and Practice Patterns Study (DOPPS)

Authors

D Mapes, AA Lopes, S Satayathum, KP McCullough, DA Goodkin, F Locatelli, S Fukuhara, EW Young, K Kurokawa, A Saito, J Bommer, FA Wolfe, PJ Held, FK Port

Reference

Kidney International 2003, **64**, 339–349.

Abstract

Background: We investigated whether indicators of health-related quality of life (HRQOL) may predict the risk of death and hospitalization among hemodialysis patients treated in seven countries, taking into account serum albumin concentration and several other risk factors for death and hospitalization. We also compared HRQOL measures with serum albumin regarding their power to predict outcomes.

Methods: We analyzed data from the Dialysis Outcomes and Practice Patterns Study (DOPPS), an international, prospective, observational study of randomly selected hemodialysis patients in the United States (148 facilities), five European countries (101 facilities), and Japan (65 facilities). The total sample size was composed of 17,236 patients. Using the Kidney Disease Quality of Life Short Form (KDQOL-SF™), we determined scores for three components of HRQOL: (*1*) physical component summary (PCS), (*2*) mental component summary (MCS), and (*3*) kidney disease component summary (KDCS). Complete responses on HRQOL measures were obtained from 10,030 patients. Cox models were used to assess associations between HRQOL and the risk of death and hospitalization, adjusted for multiple sociodemographic variables, comorbidities, and laboratory factors.

Results: For patients in the lowest quintile of PCS, the adjusted risk (RR) of death was 93% higher (RR = 1.93, $P < 0.001$) and the risk of hospitalization was 56% higher (RR = 1.56, $P < 0.001$) than it was for patients in the highest quintile level. The adjusted relative risk values of mortality per 10-point lower HRQOL score were 1.13 for MCS, 1.25 for PCS, and 1.11 for KDCS. The corresponding adjusted values for RR for first hospitalization were 1.06 for MCS, 1.15 for PCS, and 1.07 for KDCS. Each RR differed significantly from 1 ($P < 0.001$). For 1 g/dL lower serum albumin concentration, the RR of death adjusted for PCS, MCS, and KDCS and the other covariates was 1.17 ($P < 0.01$). Albumin was not significantly associated with hospitalization (RR = 1.03, $P > 0.5$).

Conclusion: Lower scores for the three major components of HRQOL were strongly associated with higher risk of death and hospitalization in hemodialysis patients, independent of a series of demographic and comorbid factors. A 10-point lower PCS score was associated with higher elevation in the adjusted mortality risk, as was a 1 g/dL lower serum albumin level. More research is needed to assess whether interventions to improve quality of life lower these risks among hemodialysis patients.

Importance

The Dialysis Outcomes and Practice Patterns Study (DOPPS) database has provided some of the most significant information concerning the association between various HRQOL measures and mortality and hospitalization rates of haemodialysis patients. The strengths of the DOPPS studies include the large number of patients, the international data base, and the detailed adjustments for various confounding variables.

This study clearly documented the strong association between patient-reported outcomes and mortality and hospitalization rates of haemodialysis patients, after adjustments had been made for various and appropriate co-morbidities. This study employed a widely used and standard HRQOL instrument—the physical component and mental component scores (PCS and MCS) of the SF-36 Health Survey. A time-varying analysis (see paper 20.2) was not used in this study; nevertheless, a robust association between HRQOL scores and outcomes was still clearly demonstrated—probably reflecting the large sample size. There was a stepwise increment in mortality and hospitalization rates as PCS and MCS scores decreased (reduced HRQOL). Patients with scores on the PCS of <25 had a nearly twofold increase in mortality compared with patients with scores of >46 and patients with MCS scores of <34 had a nearly 1.5-fold increase in mortality compared with patients with scores of >50. These relationships and strong associations have been confirmed in other studies in single countries. For example, data from the large Fresenius Medical Care database in the USA involving over 44,000 haemodialysis patients noted virtually identical findings with the PCS and MCS scores, without using a time-varying analysis (Lacson *et al.*, 2010).

The DOPPS database, in a subsequent analysis, examined the relationship between depressive symptoms, as assessed by the Center for Epidemiologic Studies Depression (CES-D) questionnaire, and mortality and hospitalizations (Lopes *et al.*, 2002). The findings in this study were equally robust. There was a stepwise increase in mortality rates as CES-D scores increased, with patients with scores of 15–30 having a greater than 1.8-fold higher mortality rate compared with patients with scores of 0–4. Importantly, this study also noted a strong association between withdrawal from dialysis and CES-D scores; patients with scores of 15–40 had a greater than twofold likelihood of withdrawing from dialysis compared with patients with scores of 0–4. However, withdrawal from dialysis was not the only reason that patients with high CES-D scores died. Thus, the association between CES-D scores and death persisted even after excluding death due to dialysis withdrawal. This relationship between depressive symptoms and mortality has been confirmed in several other studies, such as paper 20.4.

What remains uncertain from the information provided in these studies is whether there is a causal relationship between the depressive symptoms or reduced PCS or MCS scores and worse outcomes. The question remains as to whether the association can be explained by the fact that not all confounding variables can be accounted for in these databases, or whether the data suggest that understanding and treating the underlying problem (depression, reduced perception of mental or physical health) can directly result in reduced mortality and hospitalization rates. These important questions are now being addressed in prospective studies. In addition, a variety of differing treatment approaches are now being implemented and investigated to improve the depressive symptoms and impaired HRQOL of ESRD patients (see papers 20.8 and 20.10).

References

Lacson E Jr, Xu J, Lin SF, Dean SG, Lazarus JM, Hakim RM (2010). A comparison of SF-36 and SF-12 composite scores and subsequent hospitalization and mortality risks in long-term dialysis patients. *Clin J Am Soc Nephrol* **5**, 252–260.

Lopes AA, Bragg J, Young E, *et al.* (2002). Depression as a predictor of mortality and hospitalization among hemodialysis patients in the United States and Europe. *Kidney Int* **62**, 199–207.

20.4 Death or hospitalization of patients on chronic hemodialysis is associated with a physician-based diagnosis of depression

Authors

SS Hedayati, H Bosworth, L Briley, RJ Sloane, CF Pieper, PL Kimmel, LA Szczech

Reference

Kidney International 2008, **74**, 930–936.

Abstract

Depressive symptoms, assessed using a self-report type of questionnaire, have been associated with poor outcomes in dialysis patients. Here we determined if depressive disorders diagnosed by physicians are also associated with such outcomes. Ninety-eight consecutive patients on chronic hemodialysis underwent the Structured Clinical Interview for Diagnostic and Statistical Manual of Mental Disorders administered by a physician. Depression was diagnosed in about a quarter of the patients. Associations adjusted for age, gender, race, time on dialysis and co-morbidity were determined using survival analysis. Using time to event (death or hospitalization) models of analysis the hazard ratios were 2.11 and 2.07 in unadjusted and adjusted models respectively. The finding of poor outcome using a formal structured physician interview suggests that a prospective study is needed to determine whether treatment of depression affects clinical outcomes.

Importance

This paper is one of the most important dealing with the problem of interpreting patient-reported outcomes and incorporating them into an appropriate clinical context. The frequent occurrence of depressive symptoms and the association of these symptoms with mortality and hospitalizations in ESRD patients had been well documented at the time of the publication of this study (see paper 20.2 and studies reviewed by Hedayati and Finkelstein, 2009). However, this paper underscored the need to examine the results of patient symptoms in a systematic clinical context. It is important to remember that questionnaires (such as the BDI or CES-D) inform and alert healthcare professionals about the presence of symptoms experienced by a patient (see papers 20.1 and 20.2). However, to establish a diagnosis of a mental health condition, such as depression, a direct patient interview by an appropriately trained healthcare professional is required.

That is what was done in this study: 98 consecutive haemodialysis patients were interviewed with one of the accepted instruments to diagnosis clinical depression [the Structured Clinical Interview for Depression (SCID)]. Depression was diagnosed using the standard Diagnostic and Statistical Manual of Mental Disorders, 4th edition (DSM-IV) criteria;, and 25% of haemodialysis patients were diagnosed with clinical depression, findings confirmed in other studies. The association of increased hospitalizations and mortality with depression was confirmed in this study, supporting the findings in papers 20.2 and 20.3. However, in this study, standard DSM-IV criteria to diagnose clinical depression were used, whereas previous studies relied on patient-reported symptoms.

This study then raises two important issues. Firstly, why do patients diagnosed with clinical depression have higher mortality and hospitalization rates? Among factors that have been considered are withdrawal from dialysis, poor compliance with complex medical regimens, and increases in cardiovascular complications (Hedayati and Finkelstein, 2009). Secondly, this work underscores the need to test the hypothesis (in a prospective study) that treating depression could result in an improvement in patient outcomes. But importantly, this study emphasizes that the design of such a prospective study should include a structured interview by a trained clinician to make the diagnosis of clinical depression.

Reference

Hedayati SS, Finkelstein FO (2009). Epidemiology, diagnosis, and management of depression in patients with CKD. *Am J Kidney Dis* **54**, 741–752.

20.5 Renal provider recognition of symptoms in patients on maintenance hemodialysis

Authors

SD Weisbord, LF Fried, MK Mor, AL Resnick, ML Unruh, PM Palevsky, DJ Levenson, SH Cooksey, MJ Fine, PL Kimmel, RM Arnold

Reference

Clinical Journal of the American Society of Nephrology 2007, **2**, 960–967.

Abstract

Background and objectives: Although several studies have found that the burden of symptoms in patients who are on maintenance hemodialysis is substantial, little is known about renal providers' awareness of these symptoms. The aim of this study was to assess renal provider recognition of symptoms and their severity in hemodialysis patients.

Design, setting, participants, & measurements: The Dialysis Symptom Index, a 30-item measure of symptoms and their severity, was administered to patients during a routine hemodialysis session. Immediately after surveying patients, the renal provider who evaluated the patient completed the Dialysis Symptom Index to report the symptoms that he or she believed were present in that patient. Sensitivity, specificity, and positive and negative predictive values of provider reports of symptoms were calculated using patient reports as the reference standard. Patient-provider agreement on the presence and severity of symptoms was assessed using the κ statistic.

Results: Surveys were completed by 75 patients and 18 providers. For 27 of 30 symptoms, the sensitivity of provider responses was <50%, and provider responses for 25 symptoms were characterized by positive predictive values of <75%. κ scores for 25 symptoms including those pertaining to pain, sexual dysfunction, sleep disturbance, and psychologic distress were <0.20, indicating poor provider recognition of these symptoms. Providers underestimated the severity of 19 of 30 symptoms.

Conclusions: Renal providers are largely unaware of the presence and severity of symptoms in patients who are on maintenance hemodialysis. Implementation of a standardized symptom assessment process may improve provider recognition of symptoms and promote use of symptom-alleviating treatments.

Importance

This is a landmark paper in the field; it underscored the value of patient-reported outcomes and the need to routinely measure such outcomes. It also emphasized the uncomfortable notion that healthcare professionals, despite meeting patients three times a week during haemodialysis treatment sessions, do not really understand the symptoms of which dialysis patients complain, and do not appreciate the significance of these symptoms for the patients. The paper was therefore critical in emphasizing why patient-reported outcomes need to be incorporated into the routine care of dialysis patients.

Seventy-five in-centre haemodialysis patients, who were receiving haemodialysis treatments three times per week, were studied. The authors surveyed patients and the healthcare professionals caring for these patients in terms of patients' symptoms and the severity of the symptoms experienced by patients. The results indicated the marked discrepancy in what the patients reported their experience to be and what the providers understood the patients' experiences to be, despite the high frequency of visits and encounters. The findings suggested that, during these patient encounters, healthcare professionals do not fully appreciate the patients' experiences, supporting the notion that there needs to be a more formal, systematic means for healthcare professionals to obtain this information. This study concluded with the very reasonable suggestion that use of an appropriate clinical tool (such as a patient-outcome scale) could be incorporated into routine clinical care. Studies to evaluate the impact of such routine assessments of patient experiences would be of much interest. Attention needs to be focused not only on patients' HRQOL but also on the impact of the dialysis treatment itself (see paper 20.6).

The study also emphasized the remarkably high prevalence of symptoms reported by the dialysis patients. A similar high symptom burden has also been reported in patients with stage 4–5 CKD not on dialysis using a patient-outcome scale assessing 17 frequently reported symptoms (Murphy *et al.*, 2009).

Reference

Murphy EL, Murtagh FE, Carey I, Sheerin NS (2009). Understanding symptoms in patients with advanced chronic kidney disease managed without dialysis: use of a short patient-completed assessment tool. *Nephron Clin Prac* **111**, c74–c80.

20.6 Hemodialysis and peritoneal dialysis: patients' assessment of their satisfaction with therapy and the impact of the therapy on their lives

Authors

E Juergensen, D Wuerth, SH Finkelstein, PJ Juergensen, A Bekui, FO Finkelstein

Reference

Clinical Journal of the American Society of Nephrology 2006, **1**, 1191–1196.

Abstract

This study was undertaken to examine patient satisfaction with peritoneal dialysis (PD) and hemodialysis (HD) therapies, focusing attention on the positive and negative impact of the therapies on patients' lives. Patients were recruited from a free-standing PD unit and two free-standing HD units. A total of 94% ($n = 62$) of eligible PD and 84% ($n = 84$) of eligible HD patients participated. HD patients were significantly older and had higher Charlson Comorbidity Index scores than the PD patients, but there were no differences in duration of dialysis treatment, prevalence of diabetes, educational backgrounds, or home situations. Patients were asked to rate their overall satisfaction with and the overall impact of their dialysis therapy on their lives, using a 1 to 10 Likert scale. In addition, patients were asked to rate the impact of their therapy on 15 domains that had been cited previously as being important for patients' quality of life. The mean satisfaction score for PD patients (8.02 ± 1.41) was higher than for HD patients (7.4 ± 1.4; $P = 0.15$). PD patients indicated that there was less impact of the dialysis treatment on their lives globally (7.25 ± 2.12 versus 6.19 ± 2.83; $P = 0.019$). In addition, PD patients noted less impact of the therapy in 14 of the 15 domains examined. With the use of a proportional odds model analysis, the only significant predictor of overall satisfaction and impact of therapy was dialysis modality ($P = 0.037$ and $P = 0.021$, respectively). Patients also were asked to comment freely on the positive and negative effects of the dialysis treatments on their lives, and a taxonomy of patient perceptions and concerns was developed. This study suggests that PD patients in general are more satisfied with their overall care and believe that their treatment has less impact on their lives than HD patients.

Importance

'Patient-centred care' has become the new 'buzz word' in healthcare delivery. This, in many ways, represents a paradigm shift in physicians' approach to healthcare delivery. Patient preferences for and patient satisfaction with fundamental aspects of healthcare delivery are now recognized as important variables for healthcare providers to integrate into practice patterns.

This paper focused our attention on patient satisfaction with care by comparing the perceptions of patients maintained on peritoneal dialysis and haemodialysis. In addition, it examined the impact of the treatment regimen itself on patients' life experiences. Juergensen and colleagues looked at approximately 150 prevalent ESRD patients who had been maintained on dialysis for about 3 years. Importantly, peritoneal dialysis patients appeared to be more satisfied with their care and perceived that the therapy had less of a negative impact on their lives. These findings supported those of Rubin *et al.* (2004) in the Choices for Healthy Outcomes in Caring for End-stage Renal Disease (CHOICE) study, which prospectively examined a cohort of incident ESRD patients starting haemodialysis or peritoneal dialysis who completed questionnaires at an average of 7 weeks after the start of therapy. They also found that patients receiving peritoneal dialysis rated their care higher than those receiving haemodialysis.

The significance of these findings involves the recognition that the impact of the treatment modality for ESRD patients needs to be explored and understood in more detail. This is particularly important as treatment options for ESRD patients continue to expand. The impact on the patient needs to be compared in a standardized and systematic fashion. The potential positive and negative effects experienced by the individual patient of more frequent and nocturnal haemodialysis sessions (in-centre or at home) as compared with the more traditional conventional three times per week in-centre haemodialysis needs to be examined. In addition, these effects need to be compared with the impact of manual and automated peritoneal dialysis treatment regimens.

Reference

Rubin HR, Fink NE, Plantinga LC, Sadler JH, Kliger AS, Powe NR (2004). Patient ratings of dialysis care with peritoneal dialysis vs hemodialysis. *JAMA* **291**, 697–703.

20.7 Health-related quality of life predicts outcomes but is not affected by peritoneal clearance: the ADEMEX trial

Authors

R Paniagua, D Amato, E Vonesh, A Guo, S Mujais, for the Mexican Nephrology Collaborative Study Group

Reference

Kidney International 2005, **67**, 1093–1104.

Abstract

Background: We hypothesized that increasing small solute clearance in peritoneal dialysis (PD) would lead to improvements in patient health-related quality of life (HRQOL).

Methods: Patients were randomized to a control group [standard 4×2L continuous ambulatory peritoneal dialysis (CAPD)] and an intervention group (CAPD with a target creatinine clearance $\geq 60L/$ week/1.73 m²). The Kidney Disease Quality of Life Short Form was obtained at baseline and at 6, 12, and 24 months. Physical (PCS), mental (MCS), and kidney disease component summary (KDCS) scores were computed.

Results: The two groups were comparable at baseline with respect to HRQOL. Baseline variables highly predictive of better QOL included absence of diabetes, younger age, higher starting GFR, and serum albumin. Baseline values of QOL were highly predictive of survival and hospitalizations. An unadjusted comparison revealed that patients in the intervention group had significantly higher PCS and KDCS scores at six months. However, there were no significant differences between the intervention and control patients at 12 or 24 months. When similar analyses were carried out adjusting for different patterns of patient dropout, there were no significant differences between the two groups at any time point in terms of PCS, MCS, and KDCS scores.

Conclusion: We found no evidence of a long-term benefit in HRQOL of CAPD patients by increasing peritoneal small-solute clearances when HRQOL parameters were adjusted for patient dropout. Measures of HRQOL have a significant predictive value for patient survival and hospitalizations.

Importance

This paper was a randomized controlled trial (RCT) examining the impact of increasing small-molecule clearances in a large cohort ($n = 965$) of ESRD patients maintained on peritoneal dialysis in Mexico. The description of impaired HRQOL in people with ESRD raised the question whether improving the delivery of dialysis would improve HRQOL. This study gave the opportunity to investigate this possibility, as patients were randomized to a control group receiving a standard continuous ambulatory peritoneal dialysis regimen of four 2 l exchanges per day and an intervention group receiving a modified peritoneal dialysis prescription aimed at achieving a creatinine clearance of 60 l per week per 1.73 m². The Kidney Disease Quality of Life Short Form (KDQOL-SF) was used to assess the impact of the different regimens on patient-reported quality of life.

After appropriate adjustments, no significant differences were noted in patient-reported quality of life in the two groups at 12 and 24 months after the start of the study. These findings echoed the results of the Haemodialysis (HEMO) trial in which increasing the 'dose' of haemodialysis did not result in a significant improvement in HRQOL (Unruh *et al.*, 2004).

This study also reported the change in HRQOL over time and the predictive value of baseline HRQOL measurements on patient outcomes. In both the control and intervention group, there was a progressive decline in both the physical and mental component scores of the SF-36 Health Survey, suggesting that, despite a standard and 'acceptable' treatment regimen, the HRQOL of patients declined over time. In addition, this study confirmed the DOPPS findings in haemodialysis patients (see paper 20.3) in a cohort of PD patients. The PCS and MCS were strong predictors of mortality; 5-point decrements in the PCS and MCS were associated with an increased risk of death of 1.13 and 1.07, respectively. In addition, a 5-point decrease in the Kidney Disease Composite Score from the KDQOL-SF was associated with increased risk of death of 1.14. Thus, what had been clearly shown in haemodialysis patients also applies to peritoneal dialysis patients.

Reference

Unruh M, Benz R, Greene T, *et al.* (2004). Effects of hemodialysis dose and membrane flux on health-related quality of life in the HEMO Study. *Kidney Int* **66**, 355–366.

20.8 Effect of daily hemodialysis on depressive symptoms and postdialysis recovery time: interim report from the FREEDOM study

Authors

BL Jaber, Y Lee, AJ Collins, AR Hull, MA Kraus, J McCarthy, BW Miller, L Spry, FO Finkelstein, FREEDOM Study Group

Reference

American Journal of Kidney Diseases 2010, **56**, 531–539.

Abstract

Background: Clinical depression and postdialysis fatigue are important concerns for patients with kidney failure and can have a negative impact on quality of life and survival.

Study design: The FREEDOM (Following Rehabilitation, Economics and Everyday-Dialysis Outcome Measurements) Study is an ongoing prospective cohort study investigating the clinical and economic benefits of daily (6 times per week) hemodialysis (HD). In this interim report, as part of an a priori planned analysis, we examine the long-term impact of daily HD on depressive symptoms, measured using the Beck Depression Inventory (BDI) survey, and postdialysis recovery time, measured using a previously validated questionnaire.

Setting and participants: Adult patients initiating daily HD with a planned 12-month follow-up.

Outcomes and measurements: The BDI survey and postdialysis recovery time question were administered at baseline, and changes were assessed at months 4 and 12.

Results: 239 participants were enrolled (intention-to-treat cohort) and 128 completed the study (per-protocol cohort). Mean age was 52 years, 64% were men, 55% had an arteriovenous fistula, and 90% transitioned from in-center HD therapy. In the per-protocol cohort, there was a significant decrease in mean BDI score over 12 months (11.2 [95% CI, 9.6–12.9] vs 7.8 [95% CI, 6.5–9.1]; $P < 0.001$). For robustness, the intention-to-treat analysis was performed, yielding similar results. The percentage of patients with depressive symptoms (BDI score >10) significantly decreased during 12 months (41% vs 27%; $P = 0.03$). Similarly, in the per-protocol cohort, there was a significant decrease in postdialysis recovery time over 12 months (476 [95% CI, 359–594] vs 63 minutes [95% CI, 32–95]; $P < 0.001$). The intention-to-treat analysis yielded similar results. The percentage of patients experiencing prolonged postdialysis recovery time (≥60 minutes) also significantly decreased (81% vs 35%; $P = 0.001$).

Limitations: Observational study with lack of control arm.

Conclusions: Daily HD is associated with long-term improvement in depressive symptoms and postdialysis recovery time.

Importance

The previous landmark papers in this chapter have documented unequivocally the marked impairment in HRQOL of ESRD patients, but few studies have examined interventions that could result in improvements in these HRQOL measures. The impact of the dialysis treatment regimen itself on patient-reported outcomes is an area that is attracting much interest now that an increasing variety of ESRD treatment options are available. The assumption that increasing the 'dose' of dialysis would improve outcomes has, perhaps surprisingly, not been substantiated: trials that increased the 'dose' of dialysis [as measured by Kt/V_{urea} (the product of dialyser urea clearance and treatment time divided by body urea volume) or creatinine clearance] did not result in an improvement in HRQOL measures (see paper 20.7). However, there is more to dialysis than simply the 'dose'; for example, the relative impact of the dialysis treatment regimen on patients needs to be considered (see paper 20.6). For peritoneal dialysis patients, there may be a difference between automated peritoneal dialysis with night-time cycling with or without daytime exchanges and continuous ambulatory peritoneal dialysis with two to five manually done exchanges spaced out during the day with a long night-time dwell. In addition, the various options for haemodialysis treatment regimens have been expanding with the use of more frequent in-centre and home haemodialysis, longer haemodialysis treatments, and nocturnal in-centre and home haemodialysis.

Recently, studies have begun to examine the impact of these varying haemodialysis treatment regimens on patient outcomes. For example, studies have suggested that longer treatment times, lower ultrafiltration rates, and more frequent haemodialysis may have a positive effect on various outcomes, including HRQOL measures. The study selected here is important in that the investigators utilized various HRQOL indicators as primary and secondary outcomes in a randomized prospective cohort design. Changing ESRD patients from conventional three times a week in-centre haemodialysis to six times a week home haemodialysis resulted in a significant improvement in BDI scores and the time to recovery after a haemodialysis session. This latter finding was particularly impressive, as the average time it took patients to resume their usual activities after completion of dialysis was reduced from 473 to 63 min. These findings support the observations made in the Frequent Hemodialysis Network RCT (see paper 12.10), in which patients randomized to more frequent in-centre haemodialysis compared with conventional three times a week haemodialysis had a significant improvement in the physical-health composite score of the RAND 36-item health survey and a non-significant improvement in the BDI score.

These two studies are of major importance for two reasons. Firstly, they represent the beginning of an effort to explore strategies to improve the HRQOL of patients. Secondly, they address the contribution of the dialysis treatment regimen itself to the impaired HRQOL of ESRD patients—an issue that has received far too little attention.

20.9 End-of-life care preferences and needs: perceptions of patients with chronic kidney disease

Authors

SN Davison

Reference

Clinical Journal of the American Society of Nephrology 2010, **5**, 195–204.

Abstract

Background and objectives: Despite high mortality rates, surprisingly little research has been done to study chronic kidney disease (CKD) patients' preferences for end-of-life care. The objective of this study was to evaluate end-of-life care preferences of CKD patients to help identify gaps between current end-of-life care practice and patients' preferences and to help prioritize and guide future innovation in end-of-life care policy.

Design, setting, participants, and measurements: A total of 584 stage 4 and stage 5 CKD patients were surveyed as they presented to dialysis, transplantation, or predialysis clinics in a Canadian, university-based renal program between January and April 2008.

Results: Participants reported relying on the nephrology staff for extensive end-of-life care needs not currently systematically integrated into their renal care, such as pain and symptom management, advance care planning, and psychosocial and spiritual support. Participants also had poor self-reported knowledge of palliative care options and of their illness trajectory. A total of 61% of patients regretted their decision to start dialysis. More patients wanted to die at home (36.1%) or in an inpatient hospice (28.8%) compared with in a hospital (27.4%). Less than 10% of patients reported having had a discussion about end-of-life care issues with their nephrologist in the past 12 months.

Conclusions: Current end-of-life clinical practices do not meet the needs of patients with advanced CKD.

Importance

The understanding of patient preferences concerning end-of-life care is becoming a more important subject as nephrologists are faced with an aging population, which has a markedly higher incidence of CKD. Understanding how patients make decisions concerning treatment options for ESRD is a major element to be considered. A recent systematic review of qualitative studies concerning decision-making and choices of ESRD options (Morton *et al.*, 2010) confirmed that few studies have addressed this issue in a meaningful way. What was perhaps most striking in this review was the observation that the desires and requirements of patients and their carers were not being met, and the authors presented a series of recommendations for healthcare professionals, including: (i) the formal incorporation of peers (other patients) as mentors and educators, (ii) providing education to patients who are at stage 4 CKD, (iii) the development of formal care pathways for pre-emptive transplantation, home dialysis (peritoneal and home haemodialysis), and (iv) the development of palliative care pathways for those patients who choose not to receive renal replacement therapy.

In this context, this paper by Davison is a noteworthy landmark; the importance of palliative care pathways for CKD patients is discussed in depth. The author developed a survey instrument to examine patients' (and their families') preferences and expectations for quality end-of-life care. Importantly, patients had poor knowledge of palliative care options and few patients reported having had end-of-life discussions with their nephrologists in the past 12 months. Surprisingly, 61% of dialysis patients reported regretting their decision to start dialysis. This percentage seems remarkably high, and may perhaps suggest that the patients recruited to a study whose known purpose was to examine end-of-life preferences were not representative of all ESRD patients. Nevertheless, the findings of this paper, especially in the context of the systematic review by Morton *et al.* (2010) challenge us to rethink and expand our approach to informing patients with ESRD about palliative care options and sharing decision-making with them.

Reference

Morton RL, Tong A, Howard K, Snelling P, Webster AC (2010). The views of patients and carers in treatment decision making for chronic kidney disease: systematic review and thematic synthesis of qualitative studies. *Brit Med J* **340**, c112.

20.10 Cognitive-behavioral group therapy is an effective treatment for major depression in hemodialysis patients

Authors

PS Duarte, MC Miyasaki, SL Blay, R Sesso

Reference

Kidney International 2009, **76**, 414–421.

Abstract

Depression is an important target of psychological assessment in patients with end-stage renal disease because it predicts their morbidity, mortality, and quality of life. We assessed the effectiveness of cognitive-behavioral therapy in chronic hemodialysis patients diagnosed with major depression by the Mini International Neuropsychiatric Interview (MINI). In a randomized trial conducted in Brazil, an intervention group of 41 patients was given 12 weekly sessions of cognitive-behavioral group therapy led by a trained psychologist over 3 months while a control group of 44 patients received the usual treatment offered in the dialysis unit. In both groups, the Beck Depression Inventory, the MINI, and the Kidney Disease and Quality of Life-Short Form questionnaires were administered at baseline, after 3 months of intervention or usual treatment, and after 9 months of follow-up. The intervention group had significant improvements, compared to the control group, in the average scores of the Beck Depression Inventory overall scale, MINI scores, and in quality-of-life dimensions that included the burden of renal disease, sleep, quality of social interaction, overall health, and the mental component summary. We conclude that cognitive-behavioral group therapy is an effective treatment of depression in chronic hemodialysis patients.

Importance

Papers 20.7 and 20.8 showed how strategies to optimize dialysis regimens have so far been disappointing in their ineffectiveness in improving the quality of life and patient-reported outcomes for patients with ESRD. What about other interventions not directly related to treatment of kidney failure? Few other studies have used RCT methodology to explore such options to improve patient-reported outcomes of ESRD patients. This landmark paper was one of the first to utilize a randomized control design, and examined the impact of cognitive behavioural therapy (CBT) on depressive symptoms of patient maintained on haemodialysis in Brazil.

CBT is a well-documented treatment option for patients with a range of psychiatric disorders. It is based on the premise that poor decisions, ineffective problem-solving, and distorted or emotional thinking can result from 'automatic thoughts' in response to strong negative feelings and/or emotions. CBT uses well-structured techniques to support logical thinking and reorganize negative thoughts. This allows improved problem-solving and decision-making and consequently improved mood.

This study reported a 9-month trial of CBT involving 85 haemodialysis patients who met the criteria for a major depressive disorder on standardized interviewing. These depressed patients were randomized to receive standard care or CBT therapy with a trained psychologist. Group sessions (average of four patients per group) were held weekly for 12 weeks and monthly maintenance sessions were then continued. BDI scores decreased from about 25 in both groups to 10.8 ± 8.8 in the treatment group compared with 17.6 ± 11.2 in the control group ($P < 0.002$). These significant improvements in depressive symptoms in the treatment group were confirmed with standardized patient interviews. Several domains on the KDQOL-SF also improved. However, the relationships between the improvement in depressive symptoms and other HRQOL measures were not examined.

There is increased interest in treating depressive symptoms in ESRD patients, and this is long overdue (Hedayati *et al.*, 2011). Whether the treatment of depression will result in improvement in hospitalization and mortality rates remains to be determined. Nevertheless, improvement in patients' depressive symptomatology is of itself a valid goal (Hedayati *et al.*, 2011). This study is particularly noteworthy, as it used a randomized trial design and demonstrated that a well-validated intervention, CBT, can improve patient-reported outcomes. Hopefully, this signifies a new era for HRQOL research for CKD patients with a shift from simply documenting the problem to investigating the impact of interventions with randomized study designs. In addition to CBT and changes in the dialysis treatment regimen (see paper 20.8), exercise therapy and anti-depressant medications are also reported to be useful for treatment of depression in CKD patients (Hedayati *et al.*, 2011), but these now need to be tested properly in RCTs.

Reference

Hedayati SS, Yalamanchili V, Finkelstein FO (2011). A practical approach to the treatment of depression in patients with chronic kidney disease and end-stage renal disease. *Kidney Int* **81**, 247–255.

Index